Exercise Metabolism

Mark Hargreaves, PhD
The University of Melbourne

Editor

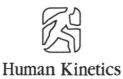

Human Kinetics

Library of Congress Cataloging-in-Publication Data

Exercise metabolism / Mark Hargreaves, editor.
    p.   cm.
    Includes bibliographical references and index.
    ISBN 0-87322-453-1 (hardcover)
    1. Exercise--Physiological aspects. 2. Energy metabolism.
  3. Metabolism. I. Hargreaves, Mark, 1961-
    [DNLM: 1. Energy Metabolism. 2. Exertion. 3. Muscle, Skeletal-
  -metabolism. QU 125 E955 1995]
  QP301.E967   1995
  612'.044--dc20
  DNLM/DLC
  for Library of Congress   95-3325
                                          CIP

ISBN: 0-87322-453-1

Acquisitions Editor: Rik Washburn; **Developmental Editors:** Lori Garrett, Glennda Kouts, and Elaine Mustain; **Assistant Editors:** Anna Curry and Ed Giles; **Copyeditor:** Nedra Lambert; **Proofreader:** Karin Leszczynski; **Indexer:** Barbara Cohen; **Typesetting and Layout:** Julie Overholt; **Text Designer:** Robert Reuther; **Cover Designer:** Hunter Design Associates; **Printer:** Edwards Brothers

Printed in the United States of America
10 9 8 7 6 5 4 3 2 1

Human Kinetics
P.O. Box 5076, Champaign, IL 61825-5076
1-800-747-4457

Canada: Human Kinetics, Box 24040, Windsor, ON N8Y 4Y9
1-800-465-7301 (in Canada only)

Europe: Human Kinetics, P.O. Box IW14, Leeds LS16 6TR, England
(44) 532 781708

Australia: Human Kinetics, 2 Ingrid Street, Clapham 5062, South Australia
(08) 371 3755

New Zealand: Human Kinetics, P.O. Box 105-231, Auckland 1
(09) 309 2259

Contents

List of Contributors   iv

Preface   v

About the Editor   vi

Credits   vii

Chapter 1   **Anaerobic Metabolism During High-Intensity Exercise**   **1**
Lawrence L. Spriet

Chapter 2   **Skeletal Muscle Carbohydrate Metabolism During Exercise**   **41**
Mark Hargreaves

Chapter 3   **Hepatic Fuel Metabolism During Exercise**   **73**
Michael Kjær

Chapter 4   **Lipid Metabolism During Exercise**   **99**
Lorraine P. Turcotte, Erik A. Richter, and Bente Kiens

Chapter 5   **Skeletal Muscle Amino Acid Metabolism and Ammonia Production During Exercise**   **131**
Terry E. Graham, James W.E. Rush, and Dave A. MacLean

Chapter 6   **Metabolic Adaptations to Endurance Training: Substrate Metabolism During Exercise**   **177**
Andrew R. Coggan and Bradley D. Williams

Chapter 7   **Metabolic Determinants of Activity Induced Muscular Fatigue**   **211**
Howard J. Green

Index   257

List of Contributors

Lawrence L. Spriet, PhD
University of Guelph, Ontario, Canada

Mark Hargreaves, PhD
The University of Melbourne, Australia

Michael Kjær, MD, DMSc
University of Copenhagen, Denmark

Lorraine P. Turcotte, PhD
University of Southern California, Los Angeles, United States

Erik A. Richter, MD, DMSc
University of Copenhagen, Denmark

Bente Kiens, PhD
University of Copenhagen, Denmark

Terry E. Graham, PhD
University of Guelph, Ontario, Canada

James W.E. Rush, MSc
State University of New York at Syracuse, United States

Dave A. MacLean, PhD
Copenhagen Muscle Research Centre, Denmark

Andrew R. Coggan, PhD
Shriners Burns Institute, Galveston, Texas, United States

Bradley D. Williams, BS
Shriners Burns Institute, Galveston, Texas, United States

Howard J. Green, PhD
University of Waterloo, Ontario, Canada

Preface

The general aim of this book is to provide, at a reasonably advanced level, an overview of the metabolic processes that occur during exercise. During exercise, the continual supply of ATP to the myofilaments within active skeletal muscle is critical for the maintenance of ongoing contractile activity. The increase in ATP resynthesis that occurs during exercise is the result of activation of a number of metabolic pathways within contracting muscle. This involves, and requires, the mobilization and utilization of both intra- and extramuscular fuel reserves. Although most attention is focused on contracting skeletal muscle, the important role of the liver and adipose tissue is also discussed. We hope that this book will be a useful resource for those biochemists, dietitians, and physiologists with a particular interest in the metabolic response to exercise.

The first five chapters summarize the metabolic responses to exercise. Metabolism during high-intensity exercise is covered in chapter 1, which details the regulation of the so-called anaerobic energy pathways. Chapter 2 discusses the effects of exercise on muscle glycogenolysis and glucose uptake and summarizes the potential regulatory mechanisms. Because the liver has a critical role in maintaining glucose homeostasis during exercise, this is discussed in chapter 3, which also includes a brief summary of some of the other metabolic functions of the liver during exercise. Together with carbohydrates, lipids provide the vast majority of energy during prolonged exercise. The sources, role, and regulation of lipid metabolism during exercise are discussed in detail in chapter 4. Chapter 5 describes the emerging role of protein metabolism in the metabolic response to exercise and the potential interactions between amino acid, purine nucleotide, and ammonia metabolism. Whereas the first five chapters provide an overview of exercise metabolism, the final two chapters of the book describe the metabolic adaptations to endurance training (chapter 6) and the potential metabolic bases of fatigue (chapter 7). Wherever possible, authors have reviewed the most recent literature, and although an attempt has been made to avoid significant overlap, there are instances where a particular topic has been covered by more than one author.

This book would not have been possible without the support and encouragement of Rainer Martens and all the staff at Human Kinetics, and for that I thank them. I would particularly like to thank all the authors for their efforts in preparing and writing their chapters and for making my job as an editor an extremely easy one.

Mark Hargreaves
Melbourne, 1995

About the Editor

Mark Hargreaves, PhD, brings a wealth of experience to his role as editor of *Exercise Metabolism*, as evidenced by his research on the subject since 1983. He is a senior lecturer in the Department of Physiology at the University of Melbourne in Australia, where he earned his PhD in physiology in 1989. His master's degree, in exercise physiology, is from Ball state University.

Dr. Hargreaves was honored by the American College of Sports Medicine with a 1994 New Investigator Award. Also in 1994, he was awarded the McIntyre Prize by the Australian Physiological and Pharmacological Society. Hargreaves lives in Hawthorn, a suburb of Melbourne, with his wife, Sue, and their son, Christopher.

Credits

Figure 4.5 is from "Skeletal Muscle Substrate Utilization During Submaximal Exercise in Man: Effect of Endurance Training" by B. Kiens, B. Essen-Gustavsson, N.J. Christensen, and B. Saltin, 1993, *J. Physiol. Lond.*, **469**, 459-478. Copyright 1993 by the Physiological Society. Adapted by permission.

Figure 4.6 is from "Saturation Kinetics of Palmitate Uptake in Perfused Skeletal Muscle" by L.P. Turcotte, B. Kiens, and E.A. Richter, 1991, *FEBS Lett.*, **279**(2), 327-329. Copyright 1991 by the Federation of European Biochemical Societies. Reprinted by permission.

Figure 4.7 is from "Muscle Malonyl-CoA Decreases During Exercise" by W.W. Winder, J. Arogyasami, R.J. Barton, I.M. Elayan, and P.R. Vehrs, 1989, *J. Appl. Physiol.*, **67**, 2230-2233. Copyright 1989 by the American Physiological Society. Adapted by permission.

Figure 6.5 is from "Plasma Glucose Kinetics During Exercise in Subjects With High and Low Lactate Thresholds" by A.R. Coggan, R.J. Spina, W.M. Kohrt, J.P. Kirwan, D.M. Bier, and J.O. Holloszy, 1992, *J. Appl. Physiol.*, **73**, 1873-1880. Copyright 1992 by the American Physiological Society. Adapted by permission.

Chapter 1

Anaerobic Metabolism During High-Intensity Exercise

LAWRENCE L. SPRIET

This chapter examines the metabolism of 5'-adenosine triphosphate (ATP), phosphocreatine (PCr), glycogen, and lactate in skeletal muscle during both a single bout and repeated bouts of high-intensity, short-duration exercise. The pathways of anaerobic metabolism are examined in terms of how quickly they are activated, the rates at which ATP can be provided, and their capacity to provide ATP. This chapter also examines the regulation of the pathways and factors that influence anaerobic metabolism during high-intensity exercise, including diet, acid-base status, and sprint training. Adult human data are emphasized and supplemented with data from animal models where necessary. Readers should also consult previous reviews on the topic of anaerobic metabolism (29, 42, 81).

Anaerobic energy production is essential for the maintenance of high-intensity exercise when the demand for ATP is greater than can be provided aerobically. At the onset of high-intensity exercise, anaerobically derived ATP provides up to 80 to 90% of the total ATP required because oxygen (O_2) is in short supply, and the cardiovascular system increases O_2 delivery to the working muscles in an attempt to meet the metabolic demand. A significant anaerobic ATP production remains important when the working muscles reach maximal rates of O_2 uptake, because the ATP demand in sustained high-intensity exercise is much greater than the maximal aerobic ATP provision rate. For example, the approximate contributions of anaerobic and aerobic sources to total ATP production during high-intensity exercise lasting ~3 min are

1

- 80%/20% in the initial 30 s,
- 45%/55% from 60 to 90 s, and
- 30%/70% from 120 to 180 s.

Sources of Anaerobic ATP

The sources of anaerobic ATP are shown schematically in Figure 1.1. Significant amounts of anaerobically derived ATP can be provided from PCr degradation and the glycolytic pathway. The endogenous ATP store can also contribute a small amount of energy, as the [ATP] in muscle may fall by ~50% when the demand for ATP is extreme.

High-intensity exercise leading to exhaustion in 3 min or less increases the activity of the myosin, Ca^{2+}, and Na^+-K^+ ATPases that hydrolyze ATP to extreme levels;

$$ATP \xleftrightarrow{\text{ATPases}} ADP + P_i + H^+$$

where ADP is adenosine 5'-diphosphate and P_i is inorganic phosphate. Consequently, the extreme demand for energy requires that ATP is resynthesized anaerobically as described in the following pathways:

$$PCr + ADP + H^+ \xleftrightarrow{\text{CPK}} ATP + Cr$$

$$Glycogen + 3ADP + 3P_i \longrightarrow 3ATP + 2Lactate^- + 2H^+$$

$$2ADP \xleftrightarrow{\text{AK}} ATP + AMP$$

$$AMP + H^+ \xleftrightarrow{\text{AMP deaminase}} IMP + NH_4^+$$

where Cr is creatine, CPK is creatine phosphate kinase, AK is adenylate kinase, AMP is adenosine 5'-monophosphate, and IMP is inosine monophosphate. The equations demonstrate the potential for estimating anaerobic ATP provision in skeletal muscle. To assess the importance of

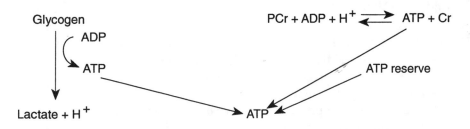

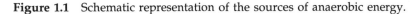

Figure 1.1   Schematic representation of the sources of anaerobic energy.

anaerobic ATP provision during high-intensity exercise, repeated measurements of the key substrates and metabolites in the preceding equations must be made. This is accomplished through biopsy sampling of contracting muscle at frequent intervals during high-intensity exercise. From these measurements the importance of the individual pathways of anaerobic ATP provision can be examined, and a total ATP provision during a high-intensity task can be calculated in units of mmol ATP/kg dry muscle (dm);

$$\text{Total ATP provision} = \Delta PCr + 1.5\ \Delta lactate + 2(\Delta ATP - \Delta ADP)$$

For every millimole of PCr degradation measured in muscle, an equal amount of ATP is liberated. The glycolytic ATP provision can be estimated by multiplying the muscle lactate accumulation and the lactate efflux from muscle by 1.5, because 3 mmol of ATP and 2 mmol of lactate are produced for each mmol of glucose moiety (derived from glycogen) metabolized. If the exercise is severe, a decrease in the muscle ATP store will also make a minor contribution to the provision of anaerobic ATP. This can be estimated by multiplying the decrease in [ATP] minus the increase in [ADP] by 2 (or simply [ATP] decrease × 2), because most of the depleted ATP ends up as IMP, thereby releasing 2 ATP. By metabolizing AMP to IMP, the regeneration of ATP from ADP in the adenylate kinase reaction is maintained.

In many situations, no decrease in muscle [ATP] will occur, and measurements of PCr and lactate will provide reasonable estimates of total anaerobic ATP provision. Estimates of glycolytic ATP provision from muscle lactate accumulation will in most situations of dynamic exercise be underestimations, unless the lactate that escaped the working muscle is also accounted for. In high-intensity exercise of very short duration, the amount of lactate efflux is not great, but the amount becomes substantial as the exercise is prolonged. Estimating the glycolytic ATP contribution in the aforementioned manner during high-intensity exercise also assumes a minimal uptake of glucose from outside the cell, minimal oxidation of lactate in the cell, and no significant accumulation of glycolytic intermediates that would alter the ratio between ATP yield and lactate accumulation. Fortunately, several studies have demonstrated that these assumptions are reasonable (19, 51, 54, 93).

How Quickly Are Anaerobic Pathways Activated?

Margaria et al. (59, 60) proposed that PCr degradation was the immediate and only substrate for ATP resynthesis during the early stages (<10 s) of intense exercise. Upon depletion of this substrate, glycogenolysis was activated to provide a continued ATP supply via glycolysis. For many years this "serial mobilization" theory of anaerobic ATP provision was used to explain how human skeletal muscle responded to the large demand for ATP during high-intensity exercise.

The experimental evidence that has accumulated since this time indicates that PCr degradation is instantaneous at the onset of exercise (Table 1.1). Muscle biopsies taken following as little as 1.28 to 10 s of electrical stimulation and sprint cycling confirmed the immediate and rapid breakdown of PCr (9, 44, 45, 51). These results are also consistent with the extremely high maximal activities of CPK measured *in vitro* and the near-equilibrium nature of the enzyme (71). Therefore, the PCr store is a powerful energy buffer, as small changes in ATP and ADP concentrations ensure rapid ATP resynthesis. In fact, several investigations have demonstrated that muscle [ATP] is maintained in the face of intense contractile activity until PCr is largely depleted (9, 79, 92).

The suggestion that anaerobic glycolysis was activated only when the PCr store became depleted in maximally contracting skeletal muscle is clearly not supported by experimental evidence. Saltin et al. (82) measured muscle [lactate] that was higher than normal resting values following 10 s of cycling at 110% $\dot{V}O_2$ max in two subjects, although resting contents were not reported (Table 1.1). Consequently, they proposed that anaerobic

Table 1.1 Experimental Evidence for the Rapid Onset of Anaerobic Glycolysis During Intense, Short-Term Muscular Activity

Reference	Activity	Time (s)	n	Lactate (mmol/kg dm) Rest	Exercise
Saltin et al. (82)	cycling (110% $\dot{V}O_2$ max)	10	2	—	~15.0
Boobis et al. (9)	cycling	6	4	9.3	28.4
Jacobs et al. (49)	cycling				
	(747 W)	10	15M	—	46.1
	(539 W)	10	7F	—	25.2
Jones et al. (51)	isok. cycling				
	(750 W, 60 rpm)	10	2	7.7	61.5
	(900 W, 140 rpm)	10	2	8.6	69.7
Hultman & Sjoholm	elect. stim.	5	4M,5F	~2	~9
(44)	(20 Hz)	10	4M,5F	~2	~17
Hultman & Sjoholm	elect. stim.	1.28	?	~2.5	~6
(45)	(50 Hz)	2.56	?	~2.5	~11
	(20 Hz)	3.0	?	~2	~9

References are listed chronologically. Abbreviations: W, watts; M, male; F, female; rpm, revolutions/min.

glycolysis commenced with the onset of muscular contraction (82). The findings of Jacobs et al. (49) supported this contention, as lactate accumulated to 46.1 and 25.2 mmol/kg dry muscle (dm) following 10 s of maximal cycling in males and females, respectively. Unfortunately, resting lactate and resting and 10 s PCr measurements were not reported. Two additional studies reported large accumulations in muscle lactate content (19-61 mmol/kg dm) following only 6 and 10 s of cycling at high power outputs (9, 51). These studies also measured PCr degradation and demonstrated that the PCr store was not depleted following 6 to 10 s of high-intensity exercise, but had decreased to ~25 to 33% of the resting content. The data suggested that PCr degradation and anaerobic glycolysis were activated simultaneously at the onset of high-intensity activity.

Compelling evidence that anaerobic glycolysis is activated at the onset of intense muscular contraction was provided by the electrical stimulation work of Hultman and Sjoholm (44, 45). They stimulated vastus lateralis (VL) muscle for 1.28-5 s at 20-50 Hz and consistently measured increases in muscle [lactate] (Table 1.1). Even a single contraction lasting 1.28 s increased muscle lactate from ~2 to ~6 mmol/kg dm (44; estimated values). In these experiments, the circulation to the muscle was occluded during stimulation and following the short stimulation periods to prevent metabolic recovery prior to biopsy sampling. One should remember that these were electrical stimulation experiments and not maximal dynamic exercise; but one would expect activation of all motor units during contraction in both situations.

Rates of Anaerobic ATP Provision

The rates that anaerobic pathways provide ATP are critical to the development and maintenance of high power outputs. Consistent with this is the ability to provide anaerobic ATP at a rate that is much greater than aerobic metabolism. However, as discussed in the next section, the capacity for anaerobic ATP provision is extremely limited. This is consistent with the ability of humans to attain power outputs that are 2 to 4 times that required to elicit maximal O_2 uptake ($\dot{V}O_2$ max), but only maintain them for short periods of time.

Estimates of anaerobic ATP provision rates have been calculated from the studies reporting intramuscular substrate and metabolite changes following intense exercise lasting from 1.28 to 200 s (Table 1.2). When examining these values, one must remember that as muscular activity extends beyond 10 s, power output will decline, and rates of glycolytic and PCr derived ATP provision will not be maximal. In addition, most of the glycolytic estimates involving dynamic exercise do not account for lactate that has escaped into the blood and are, therefore, underestimations.

Table 1.2   Rates of Anaerobic ATP Provision From Phosphocreatine Degradation and Glycolysis During High-Intensity Exercise

Reference	Type of exercise	Duration (s)	ATP provision (mmol/kg dm/s) PCr	Glycolysis
Hultman & Sjoholm	el stim	0-1.28	~9.0	~2.0
(45)	(50 Hz)	0-2.56	~5.0	~5.3
	(20 Hz)	0-3	~5.0	~2.8
Hultman & Sjoholm	el stim	0-5	~3.1	~2.1
(44)	(20 Hz)	0-10	~3.3	~2.3
		10-20	~2.0	~3.0
		20-30	~0.9	~3.8
		30-40	~0.7	~3.8
		40-50	~0.4	~4.1
		0-30	~2.1	~3.0
		0-50	~1.5	~3.4
Boobis et al. (9)	cycling	0-6	6.0	4.8
		0-30	1.9	4.0
Jacobs et al. (49)	(M) cycling	0-10	—	6.0
	(F) cycling	0-10	—	2.9
	(M) cycling	0-30	—	3.4
	(F) cycling	0-30	—	2.1
Jones et al. (51)	isok. cycling	0-10	5.1	8.0
	(60 rpm)	0-30	1.4	5.8
	(140 rpm)	0-10	4.4	9.3
		0-30	0.7	6.5
Boobis et al. (10)	cycling	0-30	2.0	4.4
McCartney et al. (62)	isok. cycling (100 rpm)	0-30	1.4	5.9
Cheetham et al. (19)	running	0-30	1.9	3.8
Jacobs et al. (48)	cycling	0-30	1.3	2.6
Nevill et al. (70)	running	0-30	1.9	4.1
Withers et al. (104)	cycling	0-30	1.3	3.7
		0-60	0.9	2.5
		0-90	0.5	1.7
Spriet et al. (92)	el stim	0-50	1.3	1.8
		50-150	0.1	1.1
		150-200	0.0	0.3
Costill et al. (23)	running, 125% $\dot{V}O_2$ max (G)	0-60	—	1.2
		0-60	—	1.3
	running 400m	0-60	—	2.1

Table 1.2   *(continued)*

Reference	Type of exercise	Duration (s)	ATP provision (mmol/kg dm/s)	
			PCr	Glycolysis
Hultman et al. (46)	cycling	0-77	0.8	—
Karlsson et al. (53)	isometric (50% MVC)	0-90	0.8	1.1
Karlsson & Saltin (52)	cycling	0-143	0.4	0.7
Bangsbo et al. (3)	isok. knee extensions	0-192	0.3	1.6

References are arranged with the shortest contraction periods listed first. Abbreviations: PCr, phosphocreatine; el stim, electrical stimulation; M, male; F, female; rpm, revolutions/minute; G, gastrocnemius; MVC, maximal voluntary contraction. All muscle biopsies were from the vastus lateralis unless noted otherwise.

The highest measured rates for PCr and glycolytic ATP provision during various contraction modes lasting from 1.28 to 10 s were ~6.0-9.0 and 6.0-9.3 mmol ATP/kg dm/s, respectively (Table 1.2). The two sources of anaerobic ATP combined to provide 10.3-11.0 mmol ATP/kg dm/s during electrical stimulation at 50 Hz lasting 1.28 to 2.56 s (45) and 10.8-13.7 mmol ATP/kg dm/s during sprint cycling for 6 to 10 s (9, 51).

The anaerobic ATP provision rates decrease when examined over longer periods of time. In the investigations (10 studies) that examined intense exercise for 30 s, the average ATP provision rates (mean ± SD) from PCr and glycolysis were 1.59 ± 0.44 and 4.38 ± 1.30 mmol ATP/kg dm/s. If it is assumed that ~25% of the produced lactate escaped the working muscle during 30 s of exercise, then the glycolytic estimate would increase to 5.84 mmol ATP/kg dm/s. The variation within these studies was large: 0.7-2.1 for PCr derived ATP and 2.6-6.5 mmol ATP/kg dm/s for glycolytic ATP. This may be due to differences in exercise mode (cycling, running, electrical stimulation), actual power output of high-intensity exercise (e.g., 125% vs. 200% $\dot{V}O_2$ max, 50% maximal voluntary contraction [MVC], 50 Hz electrical stimulation), depletion of the PCr store between 10 and 30 s, and varying amounts of escaped lactate.

When high-intensity exercise was maintained for ~50 to 90 s (5-7 studies), the average anaerobic ATP provision rates from PCr and glycolysis decreased further to 0.86 ± 0.29 and 1.67 ± 0.50 mmol ATP/kg dm/s. This indicated that no further PCr breakdown occurred from 30 to 60 s, as the PCr store was already depleted, and that the glycolytic average was actually less than one-half of the 0 to 30 s average. Because a glycolytic rate of less than zero from 30 to 60 s is not possible, the results suggest that the average power output that is sustained for 60 s is much lower than that sustained for 30 s, and that the escape of lactate during 60 s of exercise is considerable, leading to a larger underestimation of glycolytic ATP production than during 30 s of exercise.

In summary, the data in Table 1.2 demonstrate that the highest rates of anaerobic ATP provision from PCr and glycolysis during maximal or near maximal high-intensity exercise will be attained in the initial 10 s of exercise. If exercise is extended for 30 s, the PCr store will be depleted between 10 and 30 s, and the glycolytic ATP rate will be ~50% of the rate during the initial 10 s. The average glycolytic ATP provision rate during 30 s of high-intensity exercise will be ~3 to 4 times greater than the rate of ATP provided by PCr. With high-intensity exercise extended to ~60 to 90 s, estimations of glycolytic ATP provision are greatly underestimated due to the large amount of lactate that has escaped the muscle. It is interesting to note that when muscular contraction is intense but not maximal, anaerobic ATP provision from glycolysis will not reach maximal rates in the initial 10 s. For example, electrical stimulation at 20 Hz (rather than 50-100 Hz) produced glycolytic ATP provision rates of 2.3, 3.0, 3.8, 3.8, and 4.1 mmol/kg dm/s in 5 successive 10-s intervals (44; Table 1.2).

Capacity of Skeletal Muscle to Provide Anaerobic ATP

To accurately assess the anaerobic capacity of a given muscle or muscle group, measurements of ATP, PCr, and lactate contents are required from muscle biopsies obtained before and after an exhausting task. The total amount of lactate that has escaped the working muscles must also be estimated using arterial and venous catheters and blood flow measurements and then normalized to the mass of working muscle. While measurements of escaped lactate were not always made, estimates of total anaerobic ATP provision/kg dm were made using data from representative studies where the exercise task was exhaustive or intense and prolonged.

The data of Karlsson and Saltin (52) indicate a total anaerobic ATP provision of ~160 mmol/kg dm during intense cycling (Table 1.3). Glycolysis provided 60% of the ATP, PCr breakdown provided 33%, and depletion of the ATP store provided only 7%. During an isometric contraction to exhaustion at 50% MVC, the estimated anaerobic ATP was considerably greater at ~225 mmol/kg dm (53). The increase was due to a greater glycolytic contribution, which presumably resulted from lower leg blood flow and less lactate escape during the isometric contraction. Jones et al. (51) reported that 245 mmol ATP/kg dm were generated anaerobically

Table 1.3 Direct Measurements of the Capacity of Human Vastus Lateralis Muscle to Provide Anaerobic ATP From PCr Degradation, Glycolysis, and the ATP Store

Reference	Activity	Time (s)	Duty cycle	Anaerobic ATP provision (mmol/kg dm)			
				PCr	Glycolysis	ATP	Total
Karlsson & Saltin (52)	cycling (385 W)	143	~1/1	55	95+	10	160+
Karlsson et al. (53)	isometric (50% MVC)	~90	—	70	153+	3	226
Jones et al. (51)	isokinetic cycling (750 W)	30	~1/1	45	190+	10	245+
Spriet et al. (92)	electrical stimulation (20 Hz)	205	1/1	75	210	20	305
Bangsbo et al. (3)	knee extension (65 W)	192	~1/1	60	300 (193+95+12)	10	370

Abbreviations: W, watts; MVC, maximal voluntary contraction; +, indicates no attempt to include the lactate that escaped from muscle. Numbers in parentheses under glycolysis, from Bangsbo et al. (3), indicate ATP contributions from accumulated muscle lactate, escaped lactate, and accumulated glycolytic intermediates, respectively. Exercise was continued to fatigue in all studies except Jones et al. (51).

during 30 s of isokinetic cycling at extreme power outputs. The estimated ATP contribution from glycolysis based only on muscle measurements was high, suggesting that only a small amount of lactate escaped during the short exercise period, even though the muscle blood flow was undoubtedly high.

In a different approach, Spriet et al. (92) occluded the circulation to one leg and electrically stimulated the quadriceps muscles to fatigue. With a closed circulation, no significant amounts of glucose or O_2 could be taken up, and lactate could not escape the muscles. The electrical stimulation protocol was 1.6 s on, 1.6 s off at 20 Hz for ~200 s (1/1 duty cycle). During the final 50 s of continuing stimulation, peak tetanic tension decreased to less than 15% of initial tension, and no appreciable PCr degradation, glycolytic activity, or further reductions in [ATP] were measured, indicating that the muscles were fatigued. Energy contributions from PCr, ATP, and glycolysis were ~75, 20, and 210 mmol ATP/kg dm, respectively, for a total of ~305 mmol/kg dm (Table 1.3).

Bangsbo et al. (3) quantified the anaerobic ATP provision of quadriceps muscles during intense dynamic exercise to exhaustion with an open circulation. The task required subjects to extend the lower leg once per second against a resistance corresponding to a power output of ~130% of the knee extensors' peak aerobic power output. Recovery of the leg to the starting point was passive, and the work/rest duty cycle was 1/1. The mean time to exhaustion was 192 s. The criterion used to determine exhaustion was a decrease in the force magnitude or a drop in the rate of extensions. The anaerobic ATP contribution from glycolysis was estimated from knee extensor muscle lactate and glycolytic accumulations, and the lactate released from a known amount of extensor muscle (~2-3 kg), and from knowledge of knee flexor lactate involvement using leg arterial-venous difference and blood flow. The anaerobic ATP provision from PCr, ATP, and glycolysis was ~60, 10, and 300 mmol/kg dm, respectively, for a total of ~370 mmol/kg dm (Table 1.3). The data demonstrated that ~67% of the produced lactate remained in the muscle at exhaustion, and ~33% escaped into the circulation.

The total anaerobic ATP contribution from glycolysis during exhausting contractions with an open circulation was ~30% higher when compared with exhausting contractions with a closed circulation (300 vs. 210 mmol ATP/kg dm, Table 1.3). The escape of lactate and associated changes in ion movements increased the capacity to provide anaerobic ATP from glycolysis when the circulation was open. In other words, to attain the true anaerobic capacity of a muscle or muscle group, the circulation must be open during the high-intensity exercise.

Estimating Anaerobic Capacity: Direct and Indirect Approaches

It is of great practical importance to be able to measure anaerobic capacity or the maximum amount of ATP that can be supplied by the anaerobic energy pathways. As outlined earlier, direct measurements of the substrates, intermediates, and products of these pathways are required to establish an accurate determination of anaerobic capacity. Due to the invasiveness of this approach, however, a less invasive and more practical technique for indirectly estimating anaerobic capacity is required. The most commonly used indirect technique is to measure the maximal accumulated O_2 deficit during short-term intense exercise (42, 65, 67, 83). Ideally, the indirect approach should be validated against the direct approach, but this is very difficult to accomplish during whole-body exercise. To determine whole-body anaerobic capacity from direct measurements in one muscle group, one must assume that accurate estimates of total working muscle mass and the total amount of escaped lactate can be made, and that the sampled muscle represents all muscles involved in the exercise (104). Unfortunately, the difficulty with these assumptions and estimates does not allow for accurate indirect and direct comparisons of anaerobic capacity during whole-body exercise.

Bangsbo et al. (3), realizing the difficulties of whole-body comparisons, compared direct and indirect estimates of the anaerobic capacity in a workable experimental situation using an isolated human muscle preparation. In the knee extensor model, the working muscle mass is isolated and can be quantified, the muscle biopsies permit direct measurements of anaerobic energy release, and the O_2 deficit can be estimated. Arterial and femoral venous catheterization and blood flow measurements were used to measure leg O_2 uptake. A graded exercise test for the knee extensor muscles provided the relationship between O_2 uptake and power outputs below leg peak $\dot{V}O_2$, which was used to predict the energy demand of power outputs above leg peak $\dot{V}O_2$. The O_2 deficit during intense work was estimated as the difference between the energy demand and the aerobic energy provision.

The comparison of direct and indirect (O_2 deficit) methods for quantifying the anaerobic ATP capacity of the knee extensor muscles gave estimates of 91.2 and 91.6 mmol/kg wet muscle, respectively. In addition, the calculated O_2 deficits across the thigh and the lung were 0.46 and 0.44 L/kg active muscle, respectively, indicating that the O_2 deficit determined at the lung represented the anaerobic ATP capacity of the knee extensor muscle group. With the excellent match between direct and indirect estimations of anaerobic ATP capacity, frequent determinations of O_2 uptake and deficit during the exhausting exercise permitted an accurate partitioning of the proportions of energy arising from anaerobic and aerobic sources. As seen in Figure 1.2, the contributions from anaerobic and aerobic sources were

- 80%/20% in the initial 30 s,
- 45%/55% from 60-90 s, and
- 30%/70% from 120-192 s.

The average over the ~3 min of exercise was 45% anaerobic and 55% aerobic. The study also measured thigh and pulmonary O_2 debts (0.55 and 1.65 L/kg active muscle, respectively). It is obvious that O_2 debt values do not accurately estimate the anaerobic ATP capacity of the working muscle.

It remains to be determined if the aforementioned O_2 deficit findings are directly applicable to whole-body exercise situations. However, the results are encouraging and do suggest that an accurately obtained maximal O_2 deficit at the lung may well be a valid indirect method for quantifying a person's anaerobic capacity in other exercise situations. There have been concerns raised regarding the methodology and assumptions used to estimate the maximal O_2 deficit in certain situations (2, 64), but further study with this technique is certainly warranted (67, 83, 104).

Some investigations have estimated the contributions of the aerobic and anaerobic (PCr and glycolytic) energy systems during high-intensity exercise using measurements of O_2 uptake, total work output, and assumptions regarding the fuels oxidized, the mechanical efficiency of the exercise, and the time course and capacity of energy derived from PCr degradation. The anaerobic contribution is that which cannot be accounted for by aerobic metabolism after estimating mechanical efficiency. The partitioning of the anaerobic component into PCr and glycolytic contributions is entirely dependent on these assumptions regarding the use of PCr:

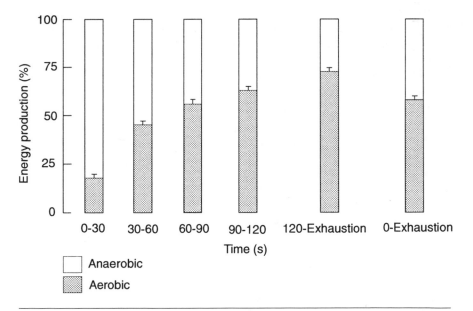

Figure 1.2   The relative contribution of aerobic and anaerobic energy production during 30 s intervals while performing exhausting exercise (~3 min) consisting of knee extensions. Reprinted with permission from Bangsbo et al. (1990).

1. All ATP was derived from the PCr/ATP system in the initial seconds until maximal power output was reached (2-3 s).
2. The PCr contribution lasted only 10 s at these high power outputs.
3. The decrement in the PCr derived energy was linear from the point of maximal power output to 10 s.

The remaining anaerobic contribution is then attributed to the glycolytic system. During the initial 10 s of cycling during a 30-s Wingate test, the respective contributions from PCr, glycolysis, and aerobic metabolism were 53%, 44%, and 3% (84). The direct measurements of ATP resynthesis from PCr and glycolysis in the initial 10 s of high-intensity exercise suggest that the assumptions used in the indirect estimations overestimate the importance of the PCr system and, therefore, underestimate the glycolytic contribution. These measurements suggest that by 10 s of high-intensity exercise, the glycolytic system has already contributed more anaerobic energy than the PCr system.

During a Wingate cycling test lasting 30 s, indirect estimates of energy provision were 23-28% from PCr, 49-56% from glycolysis (72-84% anaerobic), and 16-28% from oxidative metabolism (84, 87). In other studies, the energy contribution was 72-82% anaerobic and 18-28% aerobic (56, 104). The large variation in the aerobic component was the result of differences in estimating mechanical efficiency. However, the mean of the anaerobic/aerobic partitioning was similar to the 80%/20% reported during the initial 30 s of the direct study by Bangsbo et al. (3). When high-intensity cycling was extended to 90 s, anaerobic metabolism contributed 36-54% of the required energy, and the aerobic contribution was 46-64% (84, 104). Direct estimates of the anaerobic/aerobic contributions during 90 s of intense exercise were 60%/40% (3). Therefore, the indirect studies appear to underestimate the anaerobic contribution and overestimate the aerobic contribution when the intense exercise is prolonged.

Anaerobic Metabolism in Human Skeletal Muscle Fiber Types

Most investigations have examined the metabolic response of human skeletal muscle to high-intensity exercise by analyzing samples of whole muscle comprised of roughly equal proportions of type I and type II fibers. Naturally, conclusions from these studies represent only average responses and do not provide information regarding the responses of individual fiber types. A series of recent investigations has separated single fibers and measured glycogen, PCr, and ATP contents either in pools of one fiber type or in individual fibers of one fiber type at rest, during muscle contraction, and during recovery. This information is particularly valuable for the understanding of anaerobic metabolism during high-intensity exercise. A summary of the fiber type data at rest appears in Table 1.4. All of the subjects in these studies were engaging in some form of regular physical activity but could not be considered trained.

The content of ATP in type I and type II fibers is similar, with a tendency for a slightly higher content in type II fibers, although this difference is rarely significant (Table 1.4). Resting PCr contents in human type I fibers are 5-15% lower than contents in type II fibers, and in many cases this difference is significant. Resting glycogen content in type I fibers is consistently 10-25% lower than resting glycogen content in type II fibers.

During high-intensity exercise or electrical stimulation lasting ~10-30 s, there was a consistent trend toward a greater PCr degradation in type II vs. type I fibers (34, 91, 97). In addition, the rate of PCr degradation decreased by ~50% from 10-20 s of electrical stimulation compared with the 0-10 s rate in the type II fibers, whereas the corresponding rates in type I fibers were similar. There was also a tendency toward a greater decrease in type II fiber [ATP] during intense exercise (34, 91). The type I fibers resynthesized PCr (90, 97) and ATP (90) at a slightly greater rate than type II fibers in the first minute of recovery following exercise (Figure 1.3). It should be noted, however, that the magnitudes of the greater PCr and ATP degradation in type II fibers during high-intensity exercise and the greater PCr and ATP resynthesis in type I fibers during recovery were not large. It is also interesting that, after 15 min of recovery from ATP-lowering and PCr-depleting electrical stimulation, the ATP content in type II fibers was not fully recovered, but the PCr content was actually higher than before stimulation (Figure 1.3).

Measurements of glycogen in pools of single fibers following electrical stimulation have demonstrated a much higher glycogenolytic rate in type II fibers. When the circulation is intact, type II fiber glycogenolytic rates averaged 3.5-6.3 mmol glucosyl units/kg dm/s during 20-60 s of electrical stimulation at 20-50 Hz (33). In type I fibers, the rates were only 0.18-0.60 mmol/kg dm/s. When the circulation was occluded, the rates in type I and II fibers were 2.05 and 4.32 mmol/kg dm/s, respectively (35). The findings demonstrate a larger than expected difference in the glycogenolytic rates between the fiber types and suggest that the presence of oxygen (open circulation) plays a major role in modulating the low rate in type I fibers. However, the type I fiber glycogenolytic rate increased from 0.18 to 1.08 mmol/kg dm/s when epinephrine (~5 nM) was added to the circulation, while the rate in type II fibers was unaffected (33).

The same authors also examined fiber glycogenolytic rates during volitional high-intensity exercise (34). Subjects performed a 30-s maximal sprint on a frictionless treadmill. During the exercise the glycogenolytic rates in type I and II fibers were 2.57 and 4.21 mmol/kg dm/s, respectively. Therefore, during volitional exercise, glycogenolysis in type I fibers was 60% of the rate in type II fibers, a rate that was much higher than the rates reported for all experimental conditions using electrical stimulation.

Table 1.4 Resting Glycogen, Phosphocreatine, and ATP Contents in Type I and II Fibers in Human Skeletal Muscle

Reference	Glycogen		PCr		ATP	
	I	II	I	II	I	II
Tesch et al. (97)	—	—	73.1 ± 9.5	82.7 ± 11.2*	—	—
Soderlund & Hultman (89)	—	—	—	—	25.2 ± 4.0	25.9 ± 3.6
Soderlund & Hultman (90)	—	—	72.3 ± 4.5	83.3 ± 9.8*	23.9 ± 1.4	25.0 ± 1.2
Soderlund et al. (91)	399 ± 28	480 ± 33*	79.4 ± 2.4	89.6 ± 5.2*	23.7 ± 0.6	25.2 ± 0.6*
Greenhaff et al. (33)	399 ± 47	445 ± 47*	67.7	71.2	24.1	25.5
Greenhaff et al. (35)	364 ± 23	480 ± 24*	85.4 ± 2.8	88.5 ± 4.9	25.5 ± 0.5	25.7 ± 0.5

Data are means ± SE. Numbers in parentheses are references. Fiber types are designated type I or slow twitch and type II or fast twitch. Units for glycogen, phosphocreatine (PCr), and ATP are mmol/kg dry muscle. *, significantly different from type I fibers.

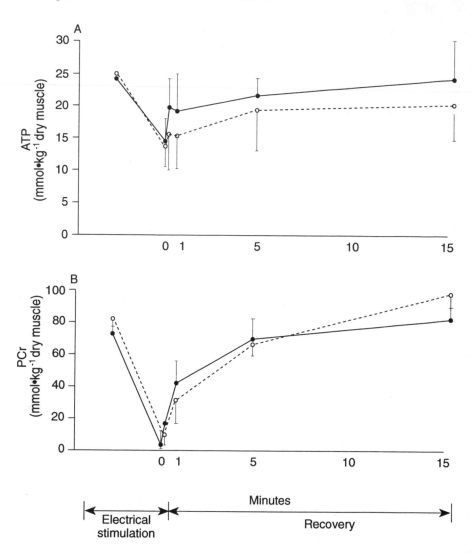

Figure 1.3 ATP (A) and phosphocreatine (PCr, B) contents in type I (O) and type II (●) fibers before and after electrical stimulation and during recovery. Reprinted with permission from Soderlund and Hultman (1991).

These exciting fiber type measurements hold much promise for future work examining the fiber type PCr and glycogenolytic responses to volitional high-intensity exercise and recovery from exercise and how these responses are affected by intermittent high-intensity exercise, sprint training, diet, active versus passive recovery, and other perturbations. For example, the ability to recover from exercise and maximally reactivate PCr degradation and glycogenolysis is essential for success in sports requiring intermittent bursts of high-intensity exercise. Future work may also be able to examine differences in anaerobic metabolism between type IIa and type IIb fibers.

Anaerobic Metabolism During Intermittent High-Intensity Exercise

Many sports require the athlete to repeatedly engage in high-intensity exercise with varying amounts of recovery time between bouts. Most of the energy for short bouts of high-intensity exercise is derived from anaerobic sources, and therefore the ability to recover during rest periods is essential for success. Many studies have examined the performance effects of intermittent high-intensity exercise, but few have examined the anaerobic metabolism associated with this type of metabolic stress. While several models of intermittent high-intensity exercise exist, two will be examined here to demonstrate that anaerobic metabolism is altered during this type of task.

In one model, an isokinetic cycle ergometer was used to examine muscle metabolism during three to four successive 30-s bouts of maximal cycling (100 rpm) with 4 min of rest between each bout (62, 94). The maximal average power during one pedal stroke (average power) was ~800-900 W in the initial seconds (~4-8 s) of cycling, decreasing to ~500 W at the end of the first bout (Figure 1.4). The generated power in the initial seconds was 2.5-3 times greater than the power required to elicit $\dot{V}O_2$ max (~300 W)! The average power over the entire 30-s bout was ~700 W, or ~2.5 times the power required to elicit $\dot{V}O_2$ max. However, as one can see in Figure 1.4, $\dot{V}O_2$ max is not reached in 30 s, and the total energy

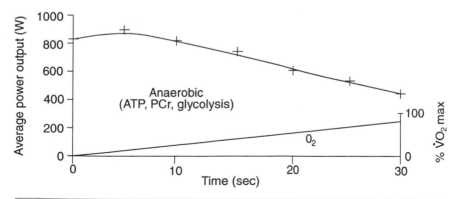

Figure 1.4   Average pedal stroke power output during 30 s of maximal isokinetic cycling at 100 rpm. Approximate O_2 uptake during the 30 s of cycling is also indicated on the right axis. Data from Spriet et al. (94).

contribution from aerobic metabolism is ~20% of the total (area under the $\dot{V}O_2$ curve), leaving anaerobic metabolism to provide the remainder. When three to four successive bouts were performed, the average power during the last bout decreased from ~550 to 300 W. The average over 30 s was ~425 W, or ~1.5 that of $\dot{V}O_2$ max power. Total work for the first and last bouts were ~21 and 12 kJ, respectively. The message from these data is that the power generated during maximal isokinetic cycle sprinting is extreme and decreases both within a bout and with successive bouts.

Muscle biopsy measurements demonstrated that PCr was decreased by ~75% (to < 15-20 mmol/kg dm), and ATP was decreased by 20-40% after all bouts (62, 94). Other reports have demonstrated that PCr and ATP are almost completely restored following 4 min of recovery, indicating that the energy contribution to successive bouts from PCr is unchanged (39, 80, 90). Muscle glycogenolysis was ~80 mmol/kg dm and 50-60 mmol/ kg dm during bouts 1 and 2, respectively. The decrease in bout 2 matched the ~20-25% decrease in total work that occurred (Figure 1.5). However, during the final 2 bouts, glycogenolysis decreased almost to zero (0-15 mmol/kg dm), while total work production was maintained at ~60% of that in bout 1 (Figure 1.5). Because anaerobic glycolysis is a major energy source for exercise of this type, it was surprising that the power output was so well maintained in the final 2 bouts.

Bangsbo et al. (4, 5) used a different model to examine repeated bouts of high-intensity exercise and reported similar findings. They used an

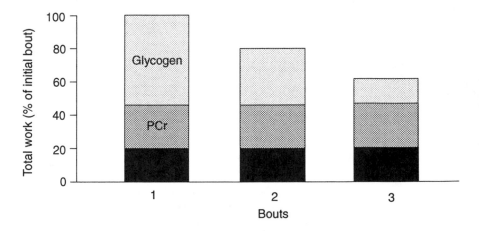

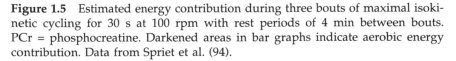

Figure 1.5 Estimated energy contribution during three bouts of maximal isokinetic cycling for 30 s at 100 rpm with rest periods of 4 min between bouts. PCr = phosphocreatine. Darkened areas in bar graphs indicate aerobic energy contribution. Data from Spriet et al. (94).

isolated knee extensor model where subjects exercised to exhaustion in ~3 min while working at a constant power output of ~130% of leg $\dot{V}O_2$ max. Their studies measured both muscle lactate accumulation and lactate efflux, enabling the calculation of total lactate production by the muscle. The first study involved 1 bout of exhausting exercise (~3 min), 10 min of rest, 3.5 min of intermittent high-intensity exercise, 2.5 min of rest, and a second bout of exhaustive exercise (5). Anaerobic ATP provision from PCr was similar in the 2 bouts, as PCr was nearly replenished at the start of the second bout. However, glycogenolysis was reduced by ~50%, lactate production by 60%, and NH_4^+ production by 30-40% during bout 2, whereas the total work done was reduced by only 20% (5, 30). A subsequent study demonstrated that glycogenolysis and lactate production during a second high-intensity exercise bout remained lower than during the initial exercise bout, even though there was a 1-hour recovery period between bouts (4).

The findings of these studies raise several questions regarding the metabolic and performance responses to intermittent, high-intensity exercise. One question to be answered is how are the muscles capable of maintaining high power outputs in repeated high-intensity bouts when anaerobic ATP from glycolysis is severely reduced. It has been proposed that a greater $\dot{V}O_2$ during later exercise bouts may be responsible, because small increases in O_2 uptake will translate into large amounts of extra ATP if carbohydrate (CHO) is oxidized instead of being metabolized to lactate. This will also reduce the need for CHO, although it is possible that intramuscular fat provides some of the extra substrate for oxidation. Only Bangsbo et al. (5) measured leg O_2 uptake, and they reported a 13% increase in the second bout when corrected for exhaustion time (1.32 vs. 1.17 L/min). Pulmonary $\dot{V}O_2$ data revealed the same tendency (5, 62). Other possibilities include greater free energy release for ATP hydrolysis due to higher muscle temperature and recruitment of a different fiber type profile and/or other muscles that normally play a secondary role in power generation. The former is a possibility because the indirectly determined O_2 deficit was not reduced during the second exhausting bout in the Bangsbo et al. study (5), whereas the directly measured ATP provision was lower.

It also remains to be explained why muscle glycogenolysis cannot be reactivated to the same degree with repeated bouts, and what causes fatigue during exercise when power output decreases during the bout, or when subjects exercise to exhaustion. The first question will be covered in the section examining the regulation of muscle glycogenolysis, and the second question will be examined here. Fatigue in the isokinetic cycling experiments was manifested as a decrease in power output during all bouts, occurring as early as 5-10 s into the bout. Much work has focused on the accumulation of metabolic by-products initiating the fatigue process at a site upstream from metabolism. However, it seems possible in this type of maximal exercise that an inability to maintain ATP provision is also a strong candidate. In a previous section, it was demonstrated that the highest rates of ATP provision occurred within 10 s of the onset of exercise when PCr degradation and glycolytic activity were maximum, and both contributed to the rephosphorylation of ADP. These findings coincide with the fact that peak average power for one pedal stroke also occurred within 10 s. With repeated bouts, the peak power for one pedal stroke was lower, and the pedal stroke where it occurred was delayed until ~10-12 s, which is consistent with decreased glycolytic ATP provision. In the later bouts, the initial anaerobic ATP provision relies more on PCr degradation, as the glycolytic contribution is no longer maximal, and therefore the ATP provision rate that can be attained is also lower.

In the Bangsbo et al. studies (4, 5), a constant power was generated and failure to maintain this power was the measure of fatigue. They demonstrated that the accumulation of metabolic intermediates could not be the sole reason for fatigue, as muscle H^+, lactate, and K^+ contents had recovered to resting levels prior to a second bout of exercise, but exhaustion time was reduced. Muscle and blood lactate accumulations were also lower at exhaustion in the second bout. The authors suggest that some long-term effect of prior high-intensity, exhaustive exercise may affect the Ca^{2+} kinetics of the sarcoplasmic reticulum system and/or produce a more rapid reduction in neural drive in the second exercise bout.

Effects of Sprint Training on the Anaerobic Capacity

Very few studies have determined whether the anaerobic capacity can be increased through sprint training. This is surprising, considering the impact that training-induced increases could have on the performance of high-intensity activities when anaerobic ATP provision is paramount. MacDougall et al. (58) subjected nine males with no previous experience to a 5-month weight-training program. Biopsies of the triceps brachii muscle before and after the training program demonstrated significant increases in PCr, ATP, and glycogen contents following training (Table 1.5). Although there is no relationship between resting substrate content and anaerobic ATP provision for anaerobic glycolysis, a higher [PCr] content translates into a greater anaerobic ATP potential during intense activity.

Boobis et al. (10) sprint trained subjects on a cycle ergometer and reported unchanged resting [ATP], whereas [PCr] decreased and glycogen increased (Table 1.5). The amount of anaerobic ATP provided per unit muscle mass from glycolysis, PCr degradation, and the ATP store during 30 s of maximal dynamic cycling was not significantly changed by training, although the glycolytic contribution and average power output increased

Table 1.5 Effects of Sprint Training on Resting PCr, ATP, and Glycogen Contents and Anaerobic ATP Provision During Intense Short-Term Exercise

Reference	Training	[Resting]			Anaerobic ATP provision		
		PCr	ATP	Glycogen	ATP	PCr	Glycolysis
MacDougall et al. (58)	4-5 months weight training	~5%	~18%	~32%			
Boobis et al. (10)	8wk, 5/wk cycling						
	30 s cycling	9%	—	36%	—	—	8%*
Nevill et al. (70)	8wk, 4/wk running						
	30 s running	—	11%*	10%*	—	—	20%
	2 min run (110% V̇O₂ max)	—	6%*	10%*	—	—	—

Resting PCr and ATP, mmol/kg dm; glycogen, mmol glucosyl units/kg dm; anaerobic ATP provision, mmol/kg dm. Blanks indicate no determination; —, indicates no changes from pretraining condition. *, *no* significant difference from pretraining value.

by 8%. It was suggested that the greater power output following training was due to the recruitment of a larger muscle mass. In a second study, recreational runners sprint trained for 8 weeks, and no significant training-induced changes in resting muscle fuels and metabolites were reported (70). The average power output during a 30-s maximal run increased by 6% following training. Anaerobic ATP provision from glycolysis increased significantly (20%) during the sprint following training, whereas the contributions from PCr and ATP did not change. Consequently, the total anaerobic ATP provision during the 30-s sprint increased by 14%. There were no training-associated changes in anaerobic ATP provision during a 2-min run at 110% of the pretraining $\dot{V}O_2$ max (70).

Medbø and Burgers (66) examined the effects of sprint training on the anaerobic capacity of men and women during a 2-3 min treadmill run to exhaustion. Anaerobic capacity was estimated indirectly by measuring the accumulated O_2 deficit. An initial cross-sectional analysis revealed no differences in the anaerobic capacity of untrained subjects and endurance trained athletes, whereas track sprinters had a 30% higher anaerobic capacity. A group of recreationally active subjects who were not engaging in any form of anaerobic training were then sprint trained (3 sessions/week) for 6 weeks and increased their anaerobic capacity by 10%.

Other studies have examined the effects of short-term, high-intensity training on muscle fiber type composition, and most have reported no effect of sprint training (23, 99). Only Jansson et al. (50) reported a decrease in type I (57 to 48%) and an increase in type II (32 to 38%) fibers following 4-6 weeks of sprint cycle training.

Regulation of Anaerobic Energy From Phosphocreatine

This section examines issues related to PCr degradation that are relevant to both the rate of ATP provision and the capacity of ATP derived from this source.

Resting Phosphocreatine Content

Several human investigations using ^{31}P nuclear magnetic resonance (NMR) have suggested that the resting muscle [PCr] is considerably higher than it is when measured chemically in biopsy samples (14, 26, 63, 96). The lower measurement from the biopsy samples could be caused by disruption of muscle membranes during the biopsy procedure, release of Ca^{2+}, activation of actomyosin ATPase, and subsequent PCr degradation to maintain the ATP concentration prior to freezing the sample. The freezing procedure itself may also cause some PCr degradation. If the resting [PCr] was truly greater than that reported with traditional bio-chemical analyses, estimates of anaerobic ATP provision from PCr degra-dation would be low.

However, the validity of the NMR measurements has been questioned, because chemical compounds in skeletal muscle have not been quantita-tively calibrated with this technique. Calibration is attempted by assuming that the area under the ATP peaks in the NMR spectra is equal to the chemically determined ATP content and by using this relationship to quantitate the area under the PCr peak. If the NMR technique does not see all of the intracellular ATP, the estimated [PCr] will be too high. Another problem contributing to the difficulty in attaching absolute num-bers to the NMR spectra is the difficulty in determining the true baselines of the ATP and PCr peaks for subsequent integration of the peak areas. The seriousness of these problems is demonstrated by the fact that several investigators have reported NMR-derived resting human PCr contents that are much higher (~170 mmol/kg dry muscle; 13, 14, 96, 98) than muscle *total* Cr content determined biochemically in a number of labora-tories (~115-140 mmol/kg dry muscle; 38, 70, 76, 94, 97). As a result of these problems, several investigators report NMR data only as a percentage of resting levels (68, 86, 103).

Hultman and Sjoholm (44) also have argued that the degradation rate of PCr during the 3-5 s it takes to obtain and freeze a biopsy sample would need to be as great or greater than the rates measured during maximal contractile activity (~10 mmol/kg dm/s) for the NMR estimates of [PCr] to be correct. This seems highly unlikely.

Essen (28) examined the effects of delayed freezing on the PCr content of human muscle biopsy samples and reported that delays of up to 60 s had no effect on [PCr] of resting or exercised samples. Soderlund and Hultman (88) also examined the effects of delayed freezing and the freez-ing procedure itself on resting [PCr] in biopsy samples. If freezing was delayed by 1 min following the biopsy, PCr content increased from 72 to 85 mmol/kg dm (16%). Further delays for up to 6 min had no additional effect, and the freezing also had no effect on resting [PCr]. The authors concluded that the biopsy procedure results in only a small degradation of PCr, which was much less than suggested by NMR studies. One may assume that this effect would be even smaller in exercised muscle where the [PCr] was lower at the time of sampling.

Creatine Supplementation

It is obvious from the discussions in this chapter that the energy stored as PCr is extremely important for the maintenance of ATP provision during high-intensity exercise. During repeated bouts of intense exercise, it is also important to quickly replenish the PCr store during recovery periods. This is especially true given the difficulty in reactivating the glycolytic pathway with intermittent high-intensity exercise. Therefore, the maintenance of optimal muscle creatine content is necessary to maintain high PCr stores. Total Cr (TCr) content in skeletal muscle is usually 115-140 mmol/kg dm (38) with ~60-65% of the Cr bound to phosphate (70-90 mmol/kg dm). The body absorbs creatine from dietary sources and synthesizes creatine in the liver to provide for the tissue needs. The fact that dietary creatine can enter the bloodstream directly suggests that muscle TCr and possibly PCr contents may be elevated through dietary means. If PCr stores could be elevated, it would immediately increase the capacity of this anaerobic energy source and may increase the rate of ATP provision during high-intensity exercise. There have been examinations of the effects of Cr supplementation in humans (24, 85), but until very recently no measurements of skeletal muscle TCr content had been reported.

Harris et al. (40) examined this issue and found that large oral doses of creatine could increase muscle TCr and PCr contents in recreationally active subjects. TCr increased from 126.8 ± 11.7 (mean ± SE) to 148.6 ± 5.0 mmol/kg dm in 17 subjects (5 females, 12 males) following 2-7 days of consuming 20-30 g of Cr/day. PCr was also increased from 84.2 ± 7.3 to 90.6 ± 4.8 mmol/kg dm following Cr supplementation, whereas muscle [ATP] was unaffected. Supplementation beyond 2-3 days produced no further increases, and the TCr increases were related to the starting content. For example, all but 2 of the 17 subjects demonstrated an increase in TCr, and the 2 nonresponders already had [TCr] above 145 mmol/kg dm prior to supplementation. Because TCr contents are higher in females, the success of this procedure was greater in males, as all subjects appeared to reach an upper TCr level of ~155 mmol/kg dm following supplementation.

Harris et al. (40) reported that creatine doses of 5 g, given 4-6 times/ day, were necessary to produce these results, presumably by increasing plasma creatine levels to 0.5-1.0 mM. Even with these large increases, creatine must be transported from plasma against a large concentration gradient into skeletal muscle. Consuming 20-30 g of creatine a day is a large dose, as the total body creatine store is ~120 g, and 5 g of creatine is the equivalent of 1.1 kg of fresh, uncooked steak. However, no side effects to the creatine supplementation were reported (40).

In an additional experiment, Harris et al. (40) examined the effects of previous intense exercise on the response to Cr supplementation. Five males exercised one leg as hard as possible for 1 hour/day for 4-7 days while ingesting 20-30 g of Cr/day. TCr increased from 118.1 ± 3.0 mmol/ kg in both legs before supplementation to 148.5 ± 5.2 in the nonexercised leg and 162.2 ± 12.5 mmol/kg in the exercised leg. Control PCr increased from 81.9 ± 5.6 mmol/kg to 93.8 ± 4.0 and 103.1 ± 6.2 mmol/kg in the nonexercised leg and exercised leg, respectively, whereas muscle ATP was again unchanged. These studies demonstrated that high doses of oral

Cr for 2-3 days can augment muscle TCr and PCr stores and that the response is greatest when coupled with intense exercise on a daily basis.

The same authors then examined whether the enhanced PCr and TCr contents following Cr supplementation were associated with improved muscle performance (or delayed fatigue) in high-intensity exercise. Greenhaff et al. (36) had subjects perform 5 bouts of 30 maximal voluntary isokinetic knee extensions at 180°/s, with recovery periods of 1 min between bouts, following placebo and Cr supplementation. After creatine ingestion, muscle peak torque was greater during the final 10 contractions of bout 1; during all contractions of bouts 2, 3, and 4; and during the middle 10 contractions of bout 5. The improvement in performance was attributed to greater muscle PCr contents prior to exercise, due to an increased ability to resynthesize PCr during the recovery periods. The increased availability of PCr may better maintain the required rate of ATP demand during exercise. This postulation was supported by lower accumulations of plasma NH_4^+ during exercise after creatine ingestion. Greenhaff et al. (37) then directly examined the effect of Cr ingestion on PCr resynthesis with muscle measurements. They electrically stimulated human VL and tibialis anterior muscles with leg blood flow occluded to deplete the PCr store before and after Cr supplementation (20 g/day for 5 days). Blood flow was then restored, and PCr resynthesis during 120 s of recovery was measured with needle biopsies or NMR. Following Cr supplementation, PCr was 20% higher in the VL ($p < 0.05$) and 11% higher in the tibialis anterior (not sig.) after 120 s of recovery.

The same group of investigators also carried out a field study examining the effects of Cr supplementation on performance during near-maximal short-term running (41). Ten trained middle distance runners were divided randomly into placebo and Cr groups in a double-blind fashion. All subjects performed 4 × 300 m and 4 × 1000 m runs with 3-4 min rest periods between repetitions before and after placebo or Cr supplementation. Improvements were noted in the Cr group during the final 300 m and 1000 m runs of each set of 4 runs as compared with the placebo group. The best 300 m and 1000 m times were also 0.3 s and 2.1 s faster, respectively, following Cr supplementation, but were unchanged in the placebo group.

Anaerobic Energy From Glycogenolysis/Glycolysis

The most significant source of anaerobic ATP during intense activities is from glycolysis. In exhausting exercise lasting ~3 min, glycolysis provides ~80% of the total anaerobic ATP. Although the energy yield of 3 mmol ATP/mmol glucosyl unit is low when compared with the aerobic energy yield, anaerobic glycolysis activates quickly during intense activity, provides ATP at high rates, and has a much larger capacity than PCr degradation. The predominant source of glucose moieties is from muscle glycogen, as the rate of exogenous glucose uptake by muscle is several fold lower than the flux through the pathway during maximal exercise (54). In addition, the accumulation of glucose-6-phosphate (G-6-P) is believed to inhibit glucose phosphorylation in the cell (20). Glycolysis is also associated with the accumulation of lactate and H^+ ions. It is interesting that the anaerobic glycolytic capacity during maximal contractile activity is reached well before the muscle glycogen store is depleted in well-fed and previously rested subjects.

Glycogenolytic/glycolytic regulation has received considerable attention in an attempt to account for the several hundredfold increase in net flux, which occurs at the onset of maximal activity. The key regulatory or rate-limiting enzymes in this pathway are glycogen phosphorylase (PHOS) and phosphofructokinase (PFK). Both are nonequilibrium enzymes, and PHOS is also flux-generating as the K_m of the enzyme for glycogen is ~1-2 mM (72).

It is not possible in this chapter to present a complete review of the regulation of these enzymes during maximal or near-maximal muscular contractions. Instead, this section will briefly highlight areas of existing controversy and exciting new ideas regarding the regulation of these enzymes.

Phosphorylase Regulation

There are several potential mechanisms that may be responsible for the regulation of PHOS: substrate regulation, interconversion between less active and more active forms, allosteric regulation, bound and free forms of the enzyme, and glycogen-glucose 1-phosphate (G-1-P) cycling.

Substrate Regulation.   For many years the two substrates of PHOS were not considered important in the regulation of the enzyme. In most situations glycogen is abundant in the muscle, and it was thought that an adequate amount of P_i, or the dianion form (HPO_4^{2-}), which is believed to be the active form, was always present in the cell.

In vitro experiments have demonstrated that the K_m of PHOS for glycogen is extremely low (~1-2 mM; 12). If these results are applicable to the *in vivo* muscle cell, glycogen should never limit the activity of PHOS. However, it has been reported that phosphorylase is bound to a glycogen-protein-sarcoplasmic reticulum complex in muscle (27). It has been suggested that the glycogen utilization accompanying exercise may cause the release of phosphorylase from the complex, thereby inactivating the enzyme. Although most evidence suggests that other exercise factors inhibit phosphorylase activation, the relationship between the preexercise muscle [glycogen] and the exercise glycogenolytic rate has drawn much attention.

There is a clear consensus on this topic in the human literature; glycogenolysis during short-term, high-intensity exercise or electrical stimulation is unaltered following increases or decreases in the resting or starting [glycogen] (4, 10, 47, 77, 95). It is equally apparent that previous exercise (especially high-intensity exercise, as discussed previously) does alter this relationship and makes it appear that a lower starting [glycogen] is associated with reduced glycogenolysis, when the previous exercise is the actual cause. The conclusions are based upon the studies that measured muscle glycogen directly and controlled for the effect of previous exercise when manipulating starting glycogen content through dietary and exercise means. In these studies, both exhaustive or near exhaustive exercise and high CHO diets are used to manipulate the starting [glycogen]. Other studies have suggested that muscle glycogenolysis increases following glycogen supercompensation (31, 32, 61). However, these conclusions were reached on the basis of performance and blood lactate measurements only and/or did not control for previous exercise. It should be noted that if the starting [glycogen] is reduced below the amount required to complete the high-intensity task, net glycogenolysis will be reduced (45). Therefore, supercompensating muscle glycogen content prior to high-intensity exercise will not result in greater glycogenolysis during the exercise. During the course of training on a given day, however, there could be some advantage to having high glycogen contents.

A series of studies by Hultman and coworkers confirmed the importance of P_i in the regulation of PHOS in human skeletal muscle, as suggested by Cori (21) in nonhuman muscle. Chasiotis et al. (15) demonstrated that the fraction of PHOS in the more active a form was ~20% at rest, although measured in $vivo$ PHOS activity was low. In addition, infusion of epinephrine greatly increased the fraction of PHOS a, yet the rate of glycogenolysis remained low (16). These results were explained by the low concentration of P_i in resting muscle and demonstrated that transformation of PHOS from the less active b form to the a form is not synonymous with enhanced glycogenolysis. During intense contractile activity, P_i rapidly accumulates in muscle at a rate that is approximately proportional to the rate of PCr degradation and permits rapid glycogenolysis to occur.

However, a recent study from the same laboratory questioned the high resting levels of PHOS a and reported that 5-10% may be more realistic (76). Additional work demonstrated that elevated [P_i] was not the only factor required for glycogenolysis to proceed during intense activity. Ren and Hultman (74) stimulated human muscle for 10 s to increase the [P_i], then occluded the circulation for 1 min while the muscle was at rest to prevent the recovery of metabolites. Epinephrine was also infused and present in the blood trapped in the leg to ensure a high proportion of PHOS *a*. Despite high levels of P_i and a high PHOS *a* fraction, glycogenolysis did not occur. In a subsequent study, epinephrine was infused during 10 s of stimulation at 15 Hz and 10 s at 50 Hz, with the circulation occluded (75). The fraction of PHOS *a* was constant at 86-92% in both stimulation conditions, yet the glycogenolytic rate, the force generation, and the total anaerobic ATP provision were twofold higher during stimulation at 50 Hz. These experiments demonstrate that rapid glycogenolysis during intense muscular contractions is not due only to increases in $[P_i]$ and transformation of PHOS *b* to *a*. Clearly, modulators associated with the rate of ATP utilization are also required to match the rate of glycogenolysis to the demand for ATP.

Interconvertible Forms.   It is generally believed that the transformation of PHOS *b* to *a* during high-intensity exercise occurs through activation of PHOS *b* kinase via Ca^{2+} liberated by contraction. It is known that epinephrine can also activate the transformation via an enzyme cascade initiated by increasing the concentration of cyclic AMP. However, this mechanism does not appear to be important during intense contractions. The muscle cyclic AMP content did not increase during an isometric contraction at 66% MVC to fatigue in humans (18), and perfusion with 15-35 nM epinephrine did not augment muscle glycogenolysis during 45 s of tetanic contractions in rat skeletal muscle (19a). However, the role of epinephrine in the activation of glycogenolysis during a single bout or repeated bouts of high-intensity exercise has not been systematically studied in the human.

There are suggestions that H^+ may play a role in interfering with activation of PHOS in human skeletal muscle. Chasiotis et al. (17) demonstrated that the transformation of PHOS *b* to *a* and the accumulation of cyclic AMP were depressed when muscles were acidotic. Spriet et al. (94) maximally exercised subjects for 30 s on an isokinetic cycle ergometer three times, with 4 min of rest between bouts. Estimations of muscle acidity and glycogenolysis during each bout demonstrated a relationship between increasing acidity and an inability to reactivate glycogenolysis with successive bouts. In this study, it was not possible to conclude whether the H^+ or some other contraction-mediated event interfered with the conversion of PHOS *b* to *a*. However, the study of Bangsbo et al. (4) demonstrated that the inability to reactivate glycogenolysis was not only a function of H^+. Muscle glycogenolysis during a second bout of high-intensity exercise remained lower than it was in the first bout, even though there was a 1 hour rest period between bouts and $[H^+]$ had recovered to resting levels before the second bout. Measurements of PHOS *a* and *b* fractions during repeated bouts of high-intensity exercise would help determine if the reduced glycogenolytic activity in later bouts was related to transformation from *b* to *a*, posttransformation regulation (allosteric regulation of PHOS *a*, see next section), or unrelated to PHOS and metabolism (e.g., neural activation).

The initial conversion of PHOS from *b* to *a* during high-intensity exercise is reversed with sustained activity (< 20-60 s), and PHOS is rapidly converted back to the *b* form (15, 16, 77). It is not known what causes the reconversion of PHOS to the *b* form. It is also not known whether the glycogenolysis that persists beyond ~30 s of high-intensity activity can be accounted for by the PHOS remaining in the *a* form, by an increased activity of the *b* form, or both.

Allosteric Regulation.   Most of the work examining allosteric regulation of this enzyme is associated with the *b* form. The *a* form appears to be active in the absence of allosteric regulators, although AMP decreases the K_m of the enzyme for P_i. The *b* form requires allosteric regulators to achieve significant activity; ATP, G-6-P, and H^+ are believed to be negative modulators, and free ADP and AMP, IMP and P_i have been reported to modulate the enzyme in a positive manner (1, 15, 72). A considerable amount of work is required where the actual activity of PHOS *b* and its putative modulators are measured during bouts of intense exercise in order to determine the *in vivo* significance of this form of the enzyme. If it can be demonstrated that there is post-transformation regulation of PHOS (allosteric regulation of the *a* form, by free AMP for example), similar measurements are required for PHOS *a*.

Other Regulatory Mechanisms.   As mentioned earlier, there have been suggestions that PHOS is bound to a glycogen-protein-sarcoplasmic reticulum complex *in vivo* (27). With sustained intense activity, PHOS may become unbound from this complex, reducing the ability of Ca^{2+} to catalyze PHOS *b* to *a* transformation. The potential significance of enzyme binding in glycogenolytic/glycolytic control has received much attention, and interested readers are advised to consult a recent review on this topic (73). Newsholme and Leech (72) also have proposed that a cycling between glycogen and G-1-P could increase the sensitivity of the system to the energy demands of the cell.

Phosphofructokinase Regulation

This section examines some recent advances regarding the allosteric regulation of PFK in human skeletal muscle during high-intensity exercise or contractions. Other mechanisms that may regulate PFK, such as enzyme binding, phosphorylation of the enzyme, binding to calmodulin, and fructose 6-phosphate (F-6-P)/fructose 1,6-diphosphate (F-1,6-DP) cycling will not be examined.

Allosteric Regulation.   It has been suggested that the most important mechanism for allosteric control of PFK is through an ATP-induced inhibition. The current theory suggests that ATP binds to the PFK molecule at two distinct sites, one catalytic and one allosteric. The ATP binds the catalytic site with high affinity, as it is one of the substrates of the enzyme. At resting concentrations in the cell (5-7 mM), ATP also binds a low-affinity allosteric site, which is responsible for inhibition of the enzyme (7, 8). ATP binding at the allosteric site also makes it more difficult for F-6-P to bind at its catalytic site. Most modulators of PFK appear to function by altering the affinity of ATP binding at the allosteric site. For example, accumulation of H^+, an inhibitor of PFK, enhances ATP binding at the allosteric site by increasing the ratio of protonated to unprotonated ionization groups at the binding site. Other inhibitors include citrate, 2- and 3-phosphoglycerate, phosphoenolpyruvate, and Mg^{2+} (102). Putative positive modulators include free AMP and ADP, P_i, NH_4^+, F-1,6-DP, fructose 2,6-diphosphate (F-2,6-DP), and glucose 1,6-diphosphate (G-1,6-DP) (102).

Most of the early work that identified the putative modulators of PFK involved *in vitro* experiments with PFK extracts from skeletal muscle of various species. The difficulty for physiologists has been to determine if the *in vitro* modulators are important *in vivo* modulators during high-intensity exercise in human skeletal muscle (11, 25, 93). The following discussion will examine the potential of these modulators in activating PFK and maintaining its activity during intense muscular contractions.

It is unlikely that muscle citrate is involved in regulating PFK activity during short-term, intense activity. The consensus regarding citrate seems to be that if it has a role in regulating PFK, it would occur during much less intense exercise, when oxidative metabolism dominates the provision of ATP. However, it is not known how quickly muscle [citrate] increases during high-intensity exercise, as O_2 uptake reaches ~70% and ~100% of maximal following 30 and 60 s, respectively. The concentrations of 2- and 3-phosphoglycerate and phosphoenolpyruvate do not accumulate to any large extent during high-intensity exercise and, therefore, do not appear to be important *in vivo* modulators. This leaves only the cytoplasmic ATP and H^+ contents as the major *in vivo* inhibitors of PFK. Conversely, the positive modulators free AMP and ADP, F-1,6-DP, P_i, and NH_4^+ are all present in the cell and can be measured or estimated.

At the onset of high-intensity exercise, increases in free AMP and ADP, P_i, and F-1,6-DP have been measured or estimated, and F-6-P content, the second substrate of the enzyme, also increases several fold (9, 19, 93). These accumulations appear to be responsible for activating PFK. It is likely that the true *in vivo* importance of the increases in free AMP and ADP is often overlooked in these discussions, as they are intimately related to the energy status of the cell, and the free concentrations can only be estimated. As much as 95% of these compounds may be bound at rest and, therefore, if the measured increases in total ADP and AMP with high-intensity exercise are actually increases in free contents, the relative increases would be several fold. No significant decreases in [ATP] or increases in [NH_4^+] occur within the initial few seconds of contraction, making it unlikely that they are involved in the initial activation of PFK (9, 19, 93). It is also possible that the cytoplasmic [H^+] may initially decrease, as the H^+ consumed during PCr degradation outbalance those liberated during lactate production. An initial decrease in [H^+] would assist in removing the ATP-induced inhibition of PFK. It is not known if this occurs in human skeletal muscle type II or type I fibers as glycolysis is activated at the onset of intense activity. This would be difficult to resolve in human muscle due to the finite time constraints with biopsy and NMR techniques, but it could be resolved with biopsy sampling before and after short periods of electrical stimulation with an occluded circulation, as described by Hultman and Sjoholm (44, 45).

The previous discussion has not considered the role of two modulators that have been shown to be potent activators of PFK *in vitro*: F-2,6-DP and G-1,6-DP. There appear to have been no attempts to evaluate F-2,6-DP in human skeletal muscle. *In vivo* animal studies have measured very low [F-2,6-DP] in skeletal muscle, with either no change, a small accumulation, or a decrease in [F-2,6-DP] during intense contractions (6, 69). Hue and Rider (43) concluded in their review paper that F-2,6-DP does not contribute significantly to the regulation of glycolysis during intense muscular contractions, when PFK activity is high.

The role of G-1,6-DP in PFK regulation during intense activity has been examined in human skeletal muscle, but the results are equivocal. The concentration of G-1,6-DP is higher than F-2,6-DP at ~70-100 µmol/kg dm. Isometric contraction of the knee extensor muscles to exhaustion in 67 s increased [G-1,6-DP] from 100 ± 12 µmol/kg dm at rest to 135 ± 17 and 150 ± 12 µmol/kg dm following 20 and 67 s, respectively (57). Katz et al. (55) also reported no increase in muscle [G-1,6-DP] following intense dynamic cycling to exhaustion in 4.8 min. It remains to be established if a small early increase in [G-1,6-DP] occurs during dynamic exercise and whether these small increases play a role in the activation of PFK during intense muscular contractions.

The conclusion from the existing literature regarding the potent *in vitro* PFK activators F-2,6-DP and G-1,6-DP is that they are unlikely to be potent *in vivo* activators in human skeletal muscle at the onset of high-intensity exercise. However, a large amount of work remains before this conclusion can be firmly established. Therefore, increases in the substrate [F-6-P] and increases in the allosteric activators free ADP and AMP, P_i, and F-1,6-DP appear to be related to the release of the ATP-induced inhibition of PFK at the onset of high-intensity exercise.

With sustained intense exercise, the contents of F-6-P, free ADP and AMP, P_i, and F-1,6-DP remain high (9, 93). The content of ATP in the cell begins to decrease with stoichiometric increases in IMP and NH_4^+ (78, 92). The accumulation of H^+ also becomes significant (78, 93) and should strengthen the ATP-induced inhibition as suggested by *in vitro* experiments (100, 101). Despite these changes, significant glycolytic activity persists, regardless of whether the tension production (ATP demand) is constant or decreases (44, 78, 93). The combination of decreasing [ATP], increased [F-6-P], and maintained or increasing accumulations of free ADP and AMP, P_i, NH_4^+, and F-1,6-DP is clearly associated with significant PFK activity that persists as intramuscular [H^+] increases. It has been proposed that these cellular changes decrease the pH-dependent ATP inhibition of PFK and extend the physiological or *in vivo* pH range of the enzyme to that normally encountered during high-intensity exercise (25, 93).

Other Regulatory Mechanisms.   Many additional mechanisms may contribute to the control of *in vivo* PFK activity. Binding of PFK to protein is again a potential mechanism (73). Newsholme and coworkers Start and Leech (71, 72) proposed a role for a F-6-P/F-1,6-DP substrate cycle that maintains PFK in a state of partial readiness facilitating full activation of the enzyme when high-intensity exercise begins. Preexercise plasma epinephrine concentrations and muscle cyclic AMP contents are essential components of the PFK substrate cycle mechanism. There is, however, little human study data to either refute or support this theory. Other mechanisms that may also be involved in PFK regulation are phosphorylation of the enzyme and interaction of the enzyme with calmodulin, but again little or no human data exist to evaluate their roles.

Summary

This chapter has examined directly obtained information regarding the ability of human skeletal muscle to provide ATP anaerobically during short-term, high-intensity exercise. Evidence suggests that both PCr and glycolysis are activated instantaneously with the onset of maximal activity. Maximal rates of directly measured anaerobic ATP provision from PCr degradation and glycolysis during intense muscular activity are each ~9-10 mmol ATP/kg dm/s. During high-intensity exercise the two sources combine to provide 10-14 mmol ATP/kg dm/s. The capacity of muscle to provide anaerobic ATP is ~370 mmol/kg dm during dynamic exercise lasting ~3 min. Anaerobic glycolysis provided ~80%, and PCr degradation contributed ~16% of the total. When the blood flow to the contracting muscle is occluded, the anaerobic ATP capacity decreases to ~310 mmol/kg dm. This reduction is due to a lower glycolytic capacity associated with an inability to remove lactate from the muscles.

The only study that compared direct and indirect estimates of the anaerobic capacity suggests that O_2 deficit measured at the mouth is a good predictor of the anaerobic capacity of a *single* muscle group of man, and that O_2 debt is a poor predictor. Therefore, estimating anaerobic capacity from the maximally accumulated O_2 deficit during *whole-body* exercise deserves further study.

Measurements in skeletal human muscle fiber types indicate that [ATP] is similar in type I and II fibers, whereas type II fibers have [PCr] that are 5-15% higher and [glycogen] that are 10-25% higher than type I fibers. Muscle PCr degradation and glycogenolysis are higher in type II fibers during high-intensity exercise, and PCr resynthesis is faster in type I fibers following exercise. Repeated bouts of exhaustive high-intensity exercise decrease the ability to reactivate the glycogenolytic pathways, thereby reducing the glycolytic anaerobic ATP provision while anaerobic PCr and aerobic energy contributions are maintained. The inability to reactivate glycogenolysis is maintained after muscle H^+, lactate, and K^+ are returned to resting levels. It is surprising that sprint training does little to increase the resting PCr content and only produces 10-20% increases in glycolytic ATP provision and 6-16% increases in total anaerobic ATP provision.

Several issues related to the capacity of the PCr, glycogenolytic, and glycolytic systems to provide ATP during intense activity are unresolved and require more investigation. Muscle total Cr and PCr contents can be elevated through dietary ingestion of Cr. Performance during one bout or repeated bouts of high-intensity exercise appears to be improved via the increased [PCr] and/or increased PCr resynthesis between exercise bouts. Recent work is directed toward understanding the *in vivo* regulation of the regulatory and flux-generating enzymes, PHOS and PFK, in human skeletal muscle. Evidence suggests that regulators associated with the energy status of the cell are critical in maintaining the activity of PHOS and PFK during sustained high-intensity exercise, despite significant increases in intramuscular [H^+].

Acknowledgments

I wish to thank the Natural Sciences and Engineering Research Council of Canada for supporting the work in my laboratory.

References

1. Aragon, J.J.; Tornheim, J.K.; Lowenstein, J.M. On a possible role of IMP in the regulation of phosphorylase activity in skeletal muscle. FEBS Lett. 117 (Suppl.):K56-K64; 1980.

2. Bangsbo, J. Is the O_2 deficit an accurate quantitative measure of the anaerobic energy production during intense exercise? J. Appl. Physiol. 73:1207-1208; 1992 (Letter to the editor).

3. Bangsbo, J.; Gollnick, P.D.; Graham, T.E.; Juel, C.; Kiens, B.; Mizuno, M.; Saltin, B. Anaerobic energy production and O_2 deficit-debt relationship during exhaustive exercise in humans. J. Physiol. Lond. 42:539-559; 1990.

4. Bangsbo, J.; Graham, T.E.; Kiens, B.; Saltin, B. Elevated muscle glycogen and anaerobic energy production during exhaustive exercise in man. J. Physiol. 451:205-227; 1992.

5. Bangsbo, J.; Graham, T.; Johansen, L.; Strange, S.; Christensen, C.; Saltin, B. Elevated muscle acidity and energy production during exhaustive exercise in humans. Am. J. Physiol. 263:R891-R899; 1992.

6. Bassols, A.M.; Carreras, J.; Cusso, R. Changes in glucose 1,6-bisphosphate content in rat skeletal muscle during contraction. Biochem. J. 240:747-751; 1986.

7. Bock, P.E.; Frieden, C. Phosphofructokinase I. Mechanism of the pH-dependent inactivation and reactivation of the rabbit muscle enzyme. J. Biol. Chem. 151:5630-5636; 1976.

8. Bock, P.E.; Frieden, C. Phosphofructokinase II. Role of ligands in pH-dependent structural changes of the rabbit muscle enzyme. J. Biol. Chem. 251:5637-5643; 1976.

9. Boobis, L.H.; Williams, C.; Wooton, S.A. Human muscle metabolism during brief maximal exercise. J. Physiol. Lond. 338:21P-22P; 1982 (Abstract).

10. Boobis, L.H.; Williams, C.; Wooton, S.A. Influence of sprint training on muscle metabolism during brief maximal exercise in man. J. Physiol. Lond. 342:36P-37P; 1983 (Abstract).

11. Bosca, L.; Aragon, J.J.; Sols, A. Modulation of muscle phosphofructokinase at physiological concentration of enzyme. J. Biol. Chem. 260:2100-2107; 1985.

12. Brown, D.H.; Cori, C.F. Animal plant polysaccharide phosphorylase. In: Boyer, P.D.; Lardy, H.; Myrback, K., eds. The enzymes. New York: Academic Press; 1961. (Vol. 5).

13. Burt, C.T.; Glonek, T.; Barany, M. Analysis of phosphate metabolites, the intracellular pH, and the state of adenosine triphosphate in intact muscle by phosphorous nuclear magnetic resonance. J. Biol. Chem. 251:2584-2591; 1976.

14. Chance, B.; Eleff, S.; Bank, W.; Leigh, J.S.; Warnell, R. ^{31}P NMR studies of control of mitochondrial function in phosphofructokinase-deficient human skeletal muscle. Proc. Nat. Acad. Sci. 79:7714-7718; 1982.

15. Chasiotis, D.; Sahlin, K.; Hultman, E. Regulation of glycogenolysis in human muscle at rest and during exercise. J. Appl. Physiol. 53:708-715; 1982.

16. Chasiotis, D.; Sahlin, K.; Hultman, E. Regulation of glycogenolysis in human muscle in response to epinephrine infusion. J. Appl. Physiol. 54:45-50; 1983.

17. Chasiotis, D.; Hultman, E.; Sahlin, K. Acidotic depression of cyclic AMP accumulation and phosphorylase b to a transformation in skeletal muscle of man. J. Physiol. Lond. 335:197-204; 1983.

18. Chasiotis, D.; Harris, R.C.; Hultman, E. The cyclic-AMP concentration in plasma and in muscle in response to exercise and beta-blockade in man. Acta Physiol. Scand. 117:293-298; 1983.

19. Cheetham, M.E.; Boobis, L.H.; Brooks, S.; Williams, C. Human muscle metabolism during sprint running. J. Appl. Physiol. 61:54-60; 1986.

19a. Chesley, A.; Dyck, D.J.; Spriet, L.L. High physiological levels of epinephrine do not enhance muscle glycogenolysis during tetanic stimulation. J. Appl. Physiol. 77:956-962; 1994.

20. Colowick, S.P. The hexokinases. In: Boyer, P.D., ed. The enzymes. New York: Academic Press; 1973: 1-48. (Vol. 9).

21. Cori, C.F. Regulation of enzyme activity in muscle during work. In: Gaebler, O.H., ed. Enzymes: units of biological structure and function. New York: Academic Press; 1956: 573-583.

22. Costill, D.L.; Coyle, E.F.; Fink, W.J.; Lesmes, G.R.; Witzmann, F.A. Adaptations in skeletal muscle following strength training. J. Appl. Physiol. 46:96-99; 1979.

23. Costill, D.L.; Barnett, A.; Sharp, R.; Fink, W.J.; Katz, A. Leg muscle pH following sprint running. Med. Sci. Sports Exerc. 15:325-329; 1983.

24. Crim, M.C.; Calloway, D.H.; Margen, S. Creatine metabolism in men: creatine pool size and turnover in relation to creatine intake. J. Nutr. 106:371-381; 1976.

25. Dobson, G.P.; Yamamoto, E.; Hochachka, P.W. Phosphofructokinase control in muscle: nature and reversal of pH-dependent ATP inhibition. Am. J. Physiol. 250:R71-R76; 1986.

26. Edwards, R.H.T.; Dawson, M.J.; Wilkie, D.R.; Gordon, R.E.; Shaw, D. Clinical use of nuclear magnetic resonance in the investigation of myopathy. Lancet i:725-731; 1982.

27. Entman, M.S.; Keslensky, S.S.; Chu, A.; Van Winkle, W.B. The sarcoplasmic reticulum-glycogenolytic complex in mammalian fast twitch skeletal muscle. J. Biol. Chem. 255:6245-6252; 1980.

28. Essen, B. Studies on the regulation of metabolism in human skeletal muscle using intermittent exercise as an experimental model. Acta Physiol. Scand. 454(Suppl.):1-64; 1978.

29. Gollnick, P.D.; Hermansen, L. Biochemical adaptation to exercise: anaerobic metabolism. In: Wilmore, J.H., ed. Exercise and sport science reviews. New York: Academic Press; 1973: 1-43. (Vol. 1).

30. Graham, T.; Bangsbo, J.; Saltin, B. Skeletal muscle ammonia production and repeated, intense exercise in humans. Can. J. Physiol. Pharmacol. 71:484-490; 1993.

31. Greenhaff, P.L.; Gleeson, M.; Maughan, R.J. The effects of dietary manipulation on blood acid-base status and the performance of high-intensity exercise. Eur. J. Appl. Physiol. 56:331-337; 1987.

32. Greenhaff, P.L.; Gleeson, M.; Maughan, R.J. The effects of a glycogen loading regimen on acid-base status and blood lactate concentration before and after a fixed period of high intensity exercise in man. Eur. J. Appl. Physiol. 57:254-259; 1988.

33. Greenhaff, P.L.; Ren, J.-M.; Soderlund, K.; Hultman, E. Energy metabolism in single human muscle fibers during contraction without and with epinephrine infusion. Am. J. Physiol. 260:E713-E718; 1991.

34. Greenhaff, P.L.; Nevill, M.E.; Soderlund, K.; Bodin, K.; Boobis, L.H.; Williams, C.; Hultman, E. The metabolic responses of human type I and II muscle fibres during maximal treadmill sprinting. J. Physiol. 478:149-155; 1994.

35. Greenhaff, P.L.; Soderlund, K.; Ren, J.-M.; Hultman, E. Energy metabolism in single human muscle fibers during intermittent contraction with occluded circulation. J. Physiol. 460:443-453; 1993.

36. Greenhaff, P.L.; Casey, A.; Short, A.H.; Soderlund, K.; Hultman, E. Influence of oral creatine supplementation of muscle torque during repeated bouts of maximal voluntary exercise in man. Clin. Sci. 84:565-571; 1993.

37. Greenhaff, P.L.; Bodin, K.; Harris, R.C.; Hultman, E.; Jones, D.A.; McIntyre, D.B.; Soderlund, K.; Turner, D.L. The influence of oral creatine supplementation on muscle phosphocreatine resynthesis following intense contraction in man. J. Physiol. 467:75P; 1993 (Abstract).

38. Harris, R.C.; Hultman, E.; Nordesjo, L.-O. Glycogen, glycolytic intermediates and high-energy phosphates determined in biopsy samples of musculus quadriceps femoris of man at rest. Methods and variance of values. Scand. J. Clin. Lab. Invest. 33:109-120; 1974.

39. Harris, R.C.; Edwards, R.H.T.; Hultman, E.; Nordesjo, L.-O.; Nylind, B.; Sahlin, K. The time course of phosphorylcreatine resynthesis during recovery of the quadriceps muscle in man. Pflugers Arch. 367:137-142; 1976.

40. Harris, R.C.; Soderlund, K.; Hultman, E. Elevation of creatine in resting and exercised muscle of normal subjects by creatine supplementation. Clin. Sci. 83:367-374; 1992.

41. Harris, R.C.; Viru, M.; Greenhaff, P.L.; Hultman, E. The effect of oral creatine supplementation on running performance during maximal short-term exercise in man. J. Physiol. 467:74P; 1993 (Abstract).

42. Hermansen, L. Anaerobic energy release. Med. Sci. Sports 1:32-38; 1969.

43. Hue, L.; Rider, M.H. Role of fructose 2,6-bisphosphate in the control of glycolysis in mammalian tissues. Biochem. J. 245:313-324; 1987.

44. Hultman, E.; Sjoholm, H. Energy metabolism and contraction force of human skeletal muscle in situ during electrical stimulation. J. Physiol. Lond. 345:525-532; 1983.

45. Hultman, E.; Sjoholm, H. Substrate availability. In: Knuttgen, H.G.; Vogel, J.A.; Poortmans, J., eds. Biochemistry of exercise. Champaign, IL: Human Kinetics; 1983: 63-75. (Vol. V).

46. Hultman, E.; Bergstrom, J.; McLennan-Anderson, N. Breakdown and resynthesis of phosphorylcreatine and adenosine triphosphate in connection with muscular work in man. Scand. J. Clin. Lab. Invest. 19:56-66; 1967.

47. Jacobs, I. Lactate concentrations after short, maximal exercise at various glycogen levels. Acta Physiol. Scand. 111:465-469; 1981.

48. Jacobs, I.; Bar-Or, O.; Karlsson, J.; Dotan, R.; Tesch, P.; Kaiser, P.; Inbar, O. Changes in muscle metabolites in females with 30-s exhaustive exercise. Med. Sci. Sports Exerc. 14:457-460; 1982.

49. Jacobs, I.; Tesch, P.; Bar-Or, O.; Karlsson, J.; Dotan, R. Lactate in human skeletal muscle after 10 and 30 s of supramaximal exercise. J. Appl. Physiol. 55:365-367; 1983.

50. Jansson, E.; Esbjornsson, M.; Holm, I.; Jacobs, I. Increase in the proportion of fast-twitch muscle fibers by sprint training in males. Acta Physiol. Scand. 140:359-363; 1990.

51. Jones, N.L.; McCartney, N.; Graham, T.; Spriet, L.L.; Kowalchuk, J.M.; Heigenhauser, G.J.F.; Sutton, J.R. Muscle performance and metabolism in maximal isokinetic cycling at slow and fast speeds. J. Appl. Physiol. 59:132-136; 1985.

52. Karlsson, J.; Saltin, B. Lactate, ATP and CP in working muscles during exhaustive exercise in man. J. Appl. Physiol. 29:598-602; 1970.

53. Karlsson, J.; Funderburk, C.F.; Essen, B.; Lind, A.R. Constituents of human muscle in isometric fatigue. J. Appl. Physiol. 38:208-211; 1975.

54. Katz, A.; Broberg, S.; Sahlin, K.; Wahren, J. Leg glucose uptake during maximal dynamic exercise in humans. Am. J. Physiol. 251:E71-E77; 1986.

55. Katz, A.; Sahlin, K.; Henriksson, J. Carbohydrate metabolism in human skeletal muscle during exercise is not regulated by G-1,6-P_2. J. Appl. Physiol. 65: 487-489; 1988.

56. Kavanagh, M.F.; Jacobs, I. Breath-by-breath oxygen consumption during performance of the Wingate test. Can. J. Sport Sci. 13:91-93; 1988.

57. Lee, A.D.; Katz, A. Transient increase in glucose 1,6-bisphosphate in human skeletal muscle during isometric contraction. Biochem. J. 258:915-918; 1988.

58. MacDougall, J.D.; Ward, G.R.; Sale, D.G.; Sutton, J.R. Biochemical adaptation of human skeletal muscle to heavy resistance training and immobilization. J. Appl. Physiol. 43:700-703; 1977.

59. Margaria, R.; Cerretelli, P.; Mangili, E. Balance and kinetics of anaerobic energy release during strenuous exercise in man. J. Appl. Physiol. 19:623-628; 1964.

60. Margaria, R.; Oliva, D.; Di Prampero, P.E.; Cerretelli, P. Energy utilization in intermittent exercise of supramaximal intensity. J. Appl. Physiol. 26:752-756; 1969.

61. Maughan, R.J.; Poole, D.C. The effects of a glycogen-loading regimen on the capacity to perform anaerobic exercise. Eur. J. Appl. Physiol. 46:211-219; 1981.

62. McCartney, N.; Spriet, L.L.; Heigenhauser, G.J.F.; Kowalchuk, J.M.; Sutton, J.R.; Jones, N.L. Muscle power and metabolism in maximal intermittent exercise. J. Appl. Physiol. 60:1164-1169; 1986.

63. McCully, K.K.; Vandenborne, K.; DeMeirleir, K.; Posner, J.D.; Leigh, J.S. Muscle metabolism in track athletes, using ^{31}P magnetic resonance spectroscopy. Can. J. Physiol. Pharmacol. 70:1353-1359; 1992.

64. Medbø, J.I. Letter to the editor—response. J. Appl. Physiol. 73:1208-1209; 1992.

65. Medbø, J.I.; Tabata, I. Relative importance of aerobic and anaerobic energy release during short-lasting exhausting bicycle exercise. J. Appl. Physiol. 67:1881-1886; 1989.

66. Medbø, J.I.; Burgers, S. Effect of training on the anaerobic capacity. Med. Sci. Sports Exerc. 22:501-507; 1990.

67. Medbø, J.I.; Mohn, A.-C.; Tabata, I.; Bahr, R.; Vaage, O.; Sejersted, O.M. Anaerobic capacity determined by maximal accumulated O_2 deficit. J. Appl. Physiol. 64:50-60; 1988.

68. Miller, R.G.; Boska, M.D.; Moussavi, R.S.; Carson, P.J.; Weiner, M.W. ^{31}P Nuclear magnetic resonance studies of high energy phosphates and pH in human muscle fatigue. J. Clin. Invest. 81:1190-1196; 1988.

69. Minatogwa, Y.; Hue, L. Fructose 2,6-bisphosphate in rat skeletal muscle during contraction. Biochem. J. 223:73-79; 1984.

70. Nevill, M.E.; Boobis, L.H.; Brooks, S.; Williams, C. Effect of training on muscle metabolism during treadmill sprinting. J. Appl. Physiol. 67:2376-2382; 1989.

71. Newsholme, E.A.; Start, C. Regulation in metabolism. Toronto: Wiley; 1973.

72. Newsholme, E.A.; Leech, A.R. Biochemistry for the medical sciences. Toronto: Wiley; 1983.

73. Parkhouse, W.S. Regulation of skeletal muscle metabolism by enzyme binding. Can. J. Physiol. Pharmacol. 70:150-156; 1992.

74. Ren, J.-M.; Hultman, E. Regulation of glycogenolysis in human skeletal muscle. J. Appl. Physiol. 67:2243-2248; 1989.

75. Ren, J.-M.; Hultman, E. Regulation of phosphorylase *a* activity in human skeletal muscle. J. Appl. Physiol. 69:919-923; 1990.

76. Ren, J.-M.; Chasiotis, D.; Bergstrom, M.; Hultman, E. Skeletal muscle glucolysis, glycogenolysis and glycogen phosphorylase during electrical stimulation in man. Acta Physiol. Scand. 133:101-107; 1988.

77. Ren, J.-M.; Broberg, S.; Sahlin, K.; Hultman, E. Influence of reduced glycogen level on glycogenolysis during short-term stimulation in man. Acta Physiol. Scand. 139:467-474; 1990.

78. Sahlin, K. Intracellular pH and energy metabolism in human skeletal muscle. Acta Physiol. Scand. 455(Suppl.):1-56; 1978.

79. Sahlin, K.; Harris, R.C.; Hultman, E. Creatine kinase equilibrium and lactate content compared with muscle pH in tissue samples obtained after isometric exercise. Biochem. J. 152:173-180; 1975.

80. Sahlin, K.; Harris, R.C.; Hultman, E. Resynthesis of creatine phosphate in human muscle after exercise in relation to intramuscular pH and availability of oxygen. Scand. J. Clin. Lab. Invest. 39:551-558; 1979.

81. Saltin, B. 1990. Anaerobic capacity: Past, present and prospective. In: Taylor, A.W.; Gollnick, P.D.; Green, H.J.; Ianuzzo, C.D.; Noble, E.G.; Metivier, G.; Sutton, J.R., eds. Biochemistry of exercise. Champaign, IL: Human Kinetics; 1990: 387-412. (Vol. VII).

82. Saltin, B.; Gollnick, P.D.; Eriksson, B.-O.; Piehl, K. Metabolic and circulatory adjustments at onset of maximal work. In: Gilbert, A.; Guille, P., eds. Onset of exercise. Toulouse: University of Toulouse Press; 1971: 63-76.

83. Scott, C.B.; Roby, F.B.; Lohman, T.G.; Bunt, J.C. The maximally accumulated oxygen deficit as an indicator of anaerobic capacity. Med. Sci. Sports Exerc. 23:618-624; 1991.

84. Serresse, O.; Lortie, G.; Bouchard, C.; Boulay, M.R. Estimation of the contribution of the various energy systems during maximal work of short duration. Int. J. Sports Med. 9:456-460; 1988.

85. Sipifa, I.; Rapola, J.; Simall, O.; Vannas, A. Supplementary creatine as a treatment for gyrate atrophy of the choroid and retina. N. Engl. J. Med. 304:867-870; 1981.

86. Sinoway, L.; Prophet, S.; Gorman, I.; Mosher, T.; Shenberger, J.; Dolecki, M.; Briggs, R.; Zelis, R. Muscle acidosis during static exercise is associated with calf vasoconstriction. J. Appl. Physiol. 66:429-436; 1989.

87. Smith, J.C.; Hill, D.W. Contribution of energy systems during a Wingate power test. Br. J. Sports Med. 25:196-199; 1991.

88. Soderlund, K.; Hultman, E. Effects of delayed freezing on content of phosphagens in human skeletal muscle biopsy samples. J. Appl. Physiol. 61:832-835; 1986.

89. Soderlund, K.; Hultman, E. ATP content in single fibers from human skeletal muscle after electrical stimulation and during recovery. Acta Physiol. Scand. 139:459-466; 1990.

90. Soderlund, K.; Hultman, E. ATP and phosphocreatine changes in single human muscle fibers after intense electrical stimulation. Am. J. Physiol. 261:E737-E741; 1991.

91. Soderlund, K.; Greenhaff, P.L.; Hultman, E. Energy metabolism in type I and type II human muscle fibers during short term electrical stimulation at different frequencies. Acta Physiol. Scand. 144:15-22; 1992.

92. Spriet, L.L.; Soderlund, K.; Bergstrom, M.; Hultman, E. Anaerobic energy release in skeletal muscle during electrical stimulation in men. J. Appl. Physiol. 62:611-615; 1987.

93. Spriet, L.L.; Soderlund, K.; Bergstrom, M.; Hultman, E. Skeletal muscle glycogenolysis, glycolysis, and pH during electrical stimulation in men. J. Appl. Physiol. 62:616-621; 1987.

94. Spriet, L.L.; Lindinger, M.I.; McKelvie, R.S.; Heigenhauser, G.J.F.; Jones, N.L. Muscle glycogenolysis and H^+ concentration during maximal intermittent cycling. J. Appl. Physiol. 66:8-13; 1989.

95. Symons, J.D.; Jacobs, I. High intensity exercise performance is not impaired by low intramuscular glycogen. Med. Sci. Sports Exerc. 21:550-557; 1989.

96. Taylor, D.J.; Styles, P.; Matthews, P.M.; Arnold, D.A.; Gadian, D.J.; Bore, P.; Radda, G.K. Energetics of human muscle: Exercise-induced ATP depletion. Mag. Resonance Med. 3:44-54; 1986.

97. Tesch, P.; Thorsson, A.; Fujitsuka, N. Creatine phosphate in fiber types of skeletal muscle before and after exhaustive exercise. J. Appl. Physiol. 66:1756-1759; 1989.

98. Thomsen, C.; Jensen, K.E.; Astrup, A.; Bulow, J.; Henrikssen, O. Changes of high-energy phosphorous compounds in skeletal muscle during glucose-induced thermogenesis in man. A ^{31}P NMR spectroscopy study. Acta Physiol. Scand. 137:335-339; 1989.

99. Thorstensson, A.; Sjodin, B.; Karlsson, J. Enzyme activities and muscle strength after sprint training in man. Acta Physiol. Scand. 94:313-318; 1975.

100. Trivedi, B.; Danforth, W.H. Effect of pH on the kinetics of frog muscle phosphofructokinase. J. Biol. Chem. 241:4110-4112; 1966.

101. Ui, M. A role of phosphofructokinase in pH-dependent regulation of glycolysis. Biochim. Biophys. Acta 124:310-322; 1966.

102. Uyeda, K. Phosphofructokinase. Adv. Enzymol. Rel. Areas Mol. Biol. 48:193-244; 1979.

103. Wilson, J.R.; McCully, K.K.; Mancini, D.M.; Boden, B.; Chance, B. Relationship of muscular fatigue to pH and diprotonated P_i in humans: a ^{31}P-NMR study. J. Appl. Physiol. 64:2333-2339; 1988.

104. Withers, R.T.; Sherman, W.M.; Clark, D.G.; Esselbach, P.C.; Nolan, S.R.; Mackay, M.H.; Brinkman, M. Muscle metabolism during 30, 60 and 90 s of maximal cycling on air-braked ergometer. Eur. J. Appl. Physiol. 63:354-362; 1991.

Chapter 2

Skeletal Muscle Carbohydrate Metabolism During Exercise

MARK HARGREAVES

Since the early years of this century, the importance of carbohydrates as an energy source during exercise has been recognized (33, 34, 60, 129). Indeed, the studies of Christensen and Hansen, based on respiratory exchange ratio measurements during prolonged exercise, emphasized the vital role of carbohydrate availability and utilization for endurance performance. Studies using radiolabeled glucose (156) and direct measurement of arteriovenous glucose differences across exercising limbs (177, 201) demonstrated that skeletal muscle glucose uptake increased during exercise. The application of the percutaneous needle biopsy technique to exercise studies in the 1960s confirmed the importance of muscle glycogen availability for exercise performance (14, 95) and established the theoretical basis for glycogen loading (13). Over the last 25 years, there has been considerable interest in the effects of exercise on skeletal muscle carbohydrate metabolism, the important regulatory mechanisms and the implications for fatigue, exercise performance, and the nutritional preparation for exercise.

Muscle glycogen and blood glucose are important substrates for ATP resynthesis within contracting skeletal muscle during exercise. The importance of their availability during prolonged exercise is demonstrated by the observation that fatigue is often associated with muscle glycogen depletion and/or hypoglycemia (36, 45, 51, 95, 175). The lack of carbohydrate results in reduced pyruvate levels (175), a substrate for both acetyl CoA formation and for reactions that supply tricarboxylic acid (TCA) cycle intermediates, which are necessary for the continued oxidation of free fatty and amino acids. Muscle IMP levels are increased at the point of fatigue (175), implying impaired ATP resynthesis. Indeed, muscle ATP levels were reduced by 10-15% (175); however, other investigators have seen no such fall in muscle ATP levels during prolonged exercise (10). Carbohydrate supplementation during prolonged exercise results in maintenance of intramuscular levels of TCA cycle intermediates and an attenuation of muscle IMP accumulation (182). Aspects of the metabolic bases of fatigue will be discussed in chapter 7.

Further evidence of the importance of carbohydrates during exercise is provided by the observation that the sole use of lipid as a fuel source cannot usually support exercise intensities in excess of 50-60% of maximal oxygen uptake ($\dot{V}O_2$ max) (54). In addition, patients who lack glycogen phosphorylase (McArdle's disease) and are, therefore, unable to utilize muscle glycogen have maximal exercise capacities that are only about 50% of expected normal values (131). Such patients also exhibit an exaggerated adenine nucleotide degradation and IMP accumulation during exercise (174). Taken together, these observations indicate that muscle glycogen and blood glucose are essential substrates for ATP resynthesis during exercise. In addition to this role, the breakdown of muscle glycogen and blood glucose can result in the production of lactate, a potential substrate for both gluconeogenesis in the liver (206) and oxidation in contracting skeletal (192) and cardiac muscle (68). Studies of prolonged exercise in dogs have suggested that there is a gradual shift in muscle carbohydrate utilization from oxidative to nonoxidative metabolism, resulting in an increased release of metabolic intermediates and gluconeogenic precursors such as lactate, pyruvate, and glutamine (208). Such a shift represents a potential mechanism by which muscle glycogen can contribute to blood glucose homeostasis, via the release of lactate. In humans, however, net lactate release is usually lowest in the latter stages of prolonged exercise (3, 4, 6), although there are observations of lactate release from inactive muscle during and after prolonged exercise (1, 3, 6). Nevertheless, it has been suggested that a portion of the carbohydrate utilized during exercise may enter the lactate pool before undergoing complete oxidation (193).

Muscle Glycogen Breakdown During Exercise

Using both biochemical measurement and histochemical estimation of muscle glycogen in mixed muscle and specific muscle fiber types, researchers have assessed the effects of exercise of varying intensity and duration on muscle glycogenolysis. Based on a number of these studies, the general pattern of muscle glycogenolysis during exercise is summarized in Figure 2.1. Muscle glycogen breakdown is most rapid during the early stages of exercise, its rate of utilization being exponentially related to exercise intensity (73, 176). As exercise continues, the rate of muscle glycogen utilization declines as a result of the decrease in muscle glycogen availability. It may also reflect, in part, alterations in glycogen phosphorylase activity and/or increased availability of alternative fuels such as glucose and free fatty acids. During prolonged exercise at intensities of 60-75% $\dot{V}O_2$ max, muscle glycogenolysis occurs primarily in the type I muscle fibers (69, 73, 198), although there may be some glycogen degradation in type IIa fibers (198). In the latter stages of such exercise, there is evidence of glycogenolysis in the other subgroups of type II muscle fibers (198). As exercise intensity increases, there is increased glycogenolysis in type I fibers, together with progressive recruitment of type II fibers (199), so that at exercise intensities approaching and exceeding $\dot{V}O_2$ max, muscle glycogenolysis occurs in all muscle fiber types, but at a higher rate in type II fibers (70). Thus, the greater muscle glycogenolysis with increasing exercise intensity is likely to be the result of increased involvement of the type II fibers, which have a glycogenolytic capacity greater than that of type I fibers (28, 83). In addition, the increased circulating epinephrine levels at higher intensities (137) probably also play a role.

Recent studies in rats (138, 139) have raised the possibility that muscle glycogenolysis occurs not only in contracting skeletal muscle during exercise, but also in noncontracting muscle. These authors have observed significant glycogen loss within inactive muscle during prolonged treadmill exercise in rats (138, 139) and have suggested that the glycogen

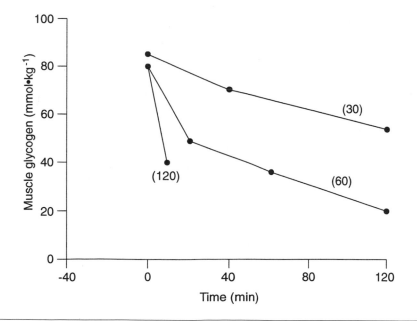

Figure 2.1 Muscle glycogen degradation in vastus lateralis during cycling exercise. Numbers in parentheses refer to exercise intensity (% $\dot{V}O_2$ max). Data from Gollnick et al. (73).

mobilized is released from the muscle as lactate and made available for gluconeogenesis and/or oxidation (139). As mentioned earlier, there is evidence of lactate release from inactive forearm muscle during prolonged leg exercise in humans, particularly in the latter stages of exercise when there was no net lactate release from the exercising legs (3). In contrast, during prolonged arm exercise, no net lactate release was observed from the "relatively inactive" legs, although there was a net lactate release from the legs during recovery from arm exercise (6). The forearm release of lactate could not be entirely accounted for by forearm glucose uptake (3), implying that muscle glycogen was mobilized from inactive forearm muscle. Relatively few studies have examined muscle glycogen levels in noncontracting muscle during exercise in humans. The early work of Bergstrom and Hultman (14) reported no change in the glycogen level of resting muscle, despite almost complete glycogen depletion in contracting muscle. This was confirmed by Ball-Burnett et al. (10), who observed no change in the glycogen level of mixed muscle or specific muscle fiber types within a nonexercising leg in subjects performing 2 hours of one-legged cycling exercise with the contralateral limb. Furthermore, no significant change in deltoid muscle glycogen content was observed in subjects during 2 hours of leg exercise (55% $\dot{V}O_2$ max), which resulted in a 60-65% decline in vastus lateralis glycogen content (127). In contrast, vastus lateralis glycogen content in an inactive leg has been observed to decline by approximately 20% during 4 hours of cycling (20% $\dot{V}O_2$ max), whereas muscle glycogen declined by 50% in the contralateral, exercising leg (17). The quantitative importance of glycogenolysis in inactive muscle, if it occurs to a significant extent, remains to be fully clarified.

Regulation of Skeletal Muscle Glycogenolysis

The rapid increase in muscle glycogen utilization during exercise occurs as the result of activation of glycogen phosphorylase and phosphofructokinase (PFK), the key enzymes for glycogenolysis and glycolysis, respectively. Glycogen phosphorylase catalyzes the first step in the breakdown of glycogen. Together with hexokinase, which catalyzes the phosphorylation of glucose taken up from the bloodstream, glycogen phosphorylase is responsible for supplying glucose units to the glycolytic pathway. The factors influencing glucose delivery to the glycolytic pathway will be discussed later. The subsequent metabolism of hexose monophosphates and formation of triose phosphates is determined by PFK activity, which is sensitive to a large number of metabolic intermediates (191). These include its substrate, fructose 6-phosphate (F-6-P); hexose bisphosphates (e.g., glucose 1,6-bisphosphate, G-1,6-P_2); the adenine nucleotides ATP, ADP, and AMP; hydrogen ions; citrate; and ammonium ions (191). The major regulator of PFK activity is the energy state of the muscle cell (191), with input from substrate supply. During high-intensity exercise (95%

$\dot{V}O_2$ max), a reduction in F-6-P supply as a result of low muscle glycogen availability is compensated for by increases in ADP and AMP (as reflected by increased muscle IMP levels), so that glycolytic rate is maintained (181). Lowering of muscle glycogen prior to less intense (75% $\dot{V}O_2$ max), but more prolonged, exercise also results in lower muscle levels of hexose phosphates and higher muscle IMP levels during exercise; however, muscle pyruvate and lactate levels were also reduced, implying reduced glycolysis (183). These metabolic alterations were associated with reduced muscle levels of the major TCA cycle intermediates, citrate, malate, and fumarate (183). This emphasizes the important role of glycolysis in skeletal muscle energy metabolism during exercise. Not only does it serve as a supplementary source of ATP when oxidative ATP production is unable to match metabolic demand, it also has a vital role in the generation of substrate for those reactions that supply TCA cycle intermediates (191). G-1,6-P$_2$ is a potent activator of PFK; however, there is no evidence that this hexose bisphosphate is an important regulator of skeletal muscle carbohydrate metabolism during dynamic exercise (120). Although increases in [H$^+$] inhibit PFK activity *in vitro*, it seems that alterations in other allosteric modulators of PFK are sufficient to ensure adequate PFK activity during intense exercise, despite a large increase in intramuscular [H$^+$] (184). During exercise, the activity of the pyruvate dehydrogenase complex is increased (45), thereby enhancing the capacity for pyruvate oxidation.

Glycogen phosphorylase has been studied extensively over the years, and much is known about its regulation (112). In the resting state, the enzyme exists primarily in the inactive *b* form, the activity of which can be increased by AMP and IMP or inhibited by ATP and glucose 6-phosphate (G-6-P). In response to muscle contraction or hormonal stimulation by epinephrine, phosphorylase *b* is phosphorylated by phosphorylase kinase to produce the active *a* form. Dephosphorylation, catalyzed by phosphatase I in response to insulin stimulation, results in inactivation of phosphorylase but activation of glycogen synthase (112). During exercise, the activity of glycogen phosphorylase is increased, while that of glycogen synthase is decreased (29). The activity of glycogen phosphorylase is subject to a number of potential regulatory mechanisms, which include calcium and cyclic AMP mediated transformation of phosphorylase *b* to *a*, allosteric effects of muscle metabolites, and substrate availability.

Local Factors.   The increase in cytosolic calcium during excitation-contraction coupling activates phosphorylase kinase, thereby stimulating conversion of phosphorylase *b* to *a* (84), by binding to the calmodulin subunit of phosphorylase kinase (147). Further activation is achieved from calcium binding to troponin C, which, in turn, activates phosphorylase kinase (147). This increase in phosphorylase *a* activity is transient and rapidly reversed, despite ongoing contractile activity (29, 40, 169). It has been suggested that this reversal of phosphorylase activity may be linked to glycogen breakdown itself, because there is evidence that phosphorylase is associated with a sarcoplasmic reticulum complex that contains not only glycogen, but also the regulatory enzymes phosphorylase kinase and phosphatase (61). The breakdown of glycogen would liberate phosphoryl-ase into the cytosol, thereby uncoupling it from phosphorylase kinase and calcium ions (61). There is partial support for such a hypothesis (43), although these authors observed a similar degree of phosphorylase inactivation, despite large differences in the amount of glycogen degraded. Other possible mechanisms include exercise-induced conformational changes in phosphorylase and/or phosphorylase kinase (43) and a de-crease in muscle pH (31) as a result of rapid glycogenolysis with the onset of exercise.

Despite the reversal of phosphorylase a activity, glycogenolysis contin-ues during exercise, especially at high intensities. This may be due to either an adequate residual level of phosphorylase a activity and/or increased phosphorylase b activity. Increases in muscle ADP, AMP, IMP, and inor-ganic phosphate (P_i) that occur during moderate- to high-intensity exercise are activators of phosphorylase b (7, 29, 112), and an increased activity of phosphorylase b may be sufficient for stimulation of muscle glycogenol-ysis. Such metabolic alterations are likely to be of greater importance in type II fibers during more intense exercise (28). Other possibilities include reactivation of phosphorylase by increased epinephrine (161, 169), or that P_i availability, rather than the percentage of phosphorylase a, is the major determinant of glycogenolysis (158).

The importance of P_i, one of the substrates for phosphorylase, in the regulation of phosphorylase activity has been studied extensively in recent years (29, 30, 159, 160). It was demonstrated that at rest and during epinephrine infusion, the rate of glycogenolysis was relatively low, despite a high proportion of phosphorylase in the a form (29, 30). This finding was explained by a low muscle [P_i]. During exercise, when muscle P_i levels increased due to creatine phosphate degradation, the rate of glyco-genolysis was significantly enhanced (29). More recent studies from the same laboratory have indicated that significant phosphorylase b to a con-version and increased muscle [P_i] are not the sole determinants of muscle glycogenolysis (159, 160), and that the rate of glycogenolysis is closely correlated with the rate of ATP turnover (160). Thus, other factors are likely to be within contracting skeletal muscle that ensure that glycogenol-ysis is closely matched to ATP demand.

Substrate Availability.   Muscle glycogen is the other substrate for phos-phorylase, and there is evidence that glycogen availability can influence phosphorylase activity and the rate of glycogenolysis in contracting skele-tal muscle (96). Glycogen can bind to phosphorylase and, in so doing, increase its activity (112). In keeping with this effect is the observation in most studies (67, 72, 74, 96, 97, 166, 178), but not all (157, 185), that the rate of muscle glycogenolysis during exercise is directly related to the preexercise muscle glycogen concentration. Thus, increases in preexercise muscle glycogen result in enhanced muscle glycogen utilization during subsequent exercise (Table 2.1). This stimulatory effect on muscle glycogenolysis does not appear to have negative effects on endurance performance, which is enhanced by increased muscle glycogen availability (13, 114).

Alterations in the availability of blood-borne substrates, in particular glucose and free fatty acids (FFA), may also influence muscle glycogenolysis during exercise. In exercising rats, elevations in blood glucose have been shown to decrease muscle glycogen breakdown in some studies (9, 130, 212) but not all (80, 179). In man, intravenous infusion of glucose, resulting in elevated arterial glucose levels (13-30 mmol $\cdot$ L^{-1}), decreased muscle glycogen use by 20-25% (14). In contrast, when blood glucose was maintained at 10-12 mmol $\cdot$ L^{-1} by intravenous glucose infusion, no alteration in glycogen utilization was observed (53). Oral carbohydrate supplementation during prolonged exercise increases blood glucose and enhances endurance exercise performance (36, 51, 52, 182). A reduction in net glycogen utilization with carbohydrate ingestion has been observed in subjects during prolonged exercise at 50% $\dot{V}O_2$ max, in combination with 30-s intermittent high-intensity (100% $\dot{V}O_2$ max) exercise bouts (87). It is possible that during the low-intensity exercise and rest periods between sprints, the increased blood glucose with carbohydrate feeding promoted glycogen resynthesis (44, 130), thereby reducing the net glycogen use over 4 hours. During more intense (70-75% $\dot{V}O_2$ max), continuous cycling exercise, however, no effect of carbohydrate ingestion on muscle glycogen utilization has been observed (51, 86). Thus, the ergogenic benefit of carbohydrate ingestion during prolonged, strenuous exercise appears to be due to its ability to maintain blood glucose levels and a high rate of

Table 2.1 Influence of Preexercise Muscle Glycogen Availability on Glycogen Utilization

	Pre	Post	Δ
HCHO	124.7 ± 10.8	62.0 ± 8.5	62.7 ± 7.9
LCHO	90.3 ± 6.0*	40.6 ± 4.2*	49.1 ± 6.6*

These values were obtained before and after 40 min of exercise at 65% $\dot{V}O_2$ max. Muscle glycogen levels were manipulated by having subjects consume diets containing either 80% CHO (HCHO) or 10-25% CHO (LCHO). Values are means ± SE ($n=7$). *denotes different from HCHO, P<0.05. Data from Hargreaves et al. (90a).

carbohydrate oxidation at a time when muscle glycogen levels are low (36, 51), rather than by reducing the rate of muscle glycogen utilization during exercise.

Reduced blood glucose levels during exercise may increase the reliance on muscle glycogen as the carbohydrate source for muscle. The onset of exercise in the presence of hyperinsulinemia results in a rapid fall in blood glucose and an increase in muscle glycogen utilization (47, 89). This increase in muscle glycogenolysis is absent if the insulin level at the onset of exercise is lower (89) or if the blood glucose level remains within the normal range (88). The hyperinsulinemia will also inhibit adipose tissue lipolysis and reduce plasma FFA availability. Thus, it is difficult to attribute the increased muscle glycogenolysis to reduced blood glucose availability entirely, because reduced FFA availability has been shown to increase muscle glycogen utilization during exercise (15). On the other hand, increasing plasma FFA levels results in reduced muscle glycogen utilization during exercise in rats (98, 163) and humans (47, 200). The reduction in muscle glycogen use is believed to be due to a citrate-mediated inhibiton of PFK activity, as a result of increased FFA uptake and oxidation by muscle (153, 162). The reduction in glycolytic rate results in the accumulation of G-6-P (162), which is an inhibitor of phosphorylase (112). In contrast, a twofold increase in plasma FFA within the physiological range had no effect on muscle glycogen utilization during 60 min of dynamic knee-extension exercise at 80% of the knee extensor W_{max} (90). Whether this result is due to the use of a different exercise model is difficult to ascertain. Nevertheless, the potential for a reduction in glycogen utilization due to increased FFA availability and oxidation has resulted in interest in caffeine as a potential ergogenic aid, because one of the metabolic effects of caffeine ingestion is to increase plasma FFA levels (48). Indeed, studies have demonstrated increased endurance performance with caffeine ingestion (48, 81, 186) and reduced muscle glycogen utilization during exercise (62, 186). It has been suggested that increased utilization of intramuscular triglycerides (62) and/or plasma FFA following caffeine ingestion might inhibit muscle glycogenolysis via increases in muscle citrate and the acetyl-CoA/CoA-SH ratio (186). Another possibility is a direct inhibitory effect of caffeine on phosphorylase activity (112, 186).

Hormonal Regulation.   In addition to local muscular factors and alterations in substrate availability, there is important hormonal regulation of phosphorylase activity and muscle glycogenolysis. Epinephrine increases phosphorylase activity (30) via cyclic AMP mediated activation of phosphorylase kinase. Removal of the adrenal medulla from rats results in reduced epinephrine levels and attenuation of muscle glycogenolysis during moderate- (164, 180) and high-intensity (133) exercise. Normalization of plasma epinephrine levels by epinephrine infusion increases muscle glycogenolysis (8, 170). In the perfused, stimulated rat hindlimb, epinephrine increases muscle glycogenolysis via increases in phosphorylase *a* activity (169). Infusion of epinephrine has been shown to increase muscle glycogenolysis during exercise in dogs (105) and humans (108, 187), due to an increase in phosphorylase activity (187). Studies utilizing β-adrenergic blockade to elucidate the role of epinephrine in the regulation of muscle glycogenolysis during exercise have produced conflicting results. Some have observed decreased glycogenolysis (27, 79, 104), whereas others have observed increased muscle glycogen use (111, 141). Other potential effects of β-blockade, such as impaired adipose tissue and muscle lipolysis, reduced hepatic glycogenolysis, and alterations in cardiac output and leg blood flow, make examination of the direct effects of β-blockade on muscle glycogenolysis difficult. Of interest, specific $β_2$-adrenergic blockade reduces muscle glycogen breakdown during prolonged exercise (197). Although the effects of epinephrine on muscle glycogenolysis are generally believed to be mediated via β-adrenergic receptors, a possible α-adrenergic mechanism has also been suggested (168). In addition to effects on glycogen metabolism in contracting muscle during exercise, it has been suggested that epinephrine also stimulates glycogenolysis in noncontracting muscle (1, 138), resulting in lactate release. Taken together, these results demonstrate that circulating epinephrine is an important regulator of muscle glycogenolysis, which, along with local changes associated with muscle contractile activity, will ensure that the rate of muscle glycogenolysis is increased during exercise (92, 105, 169).

Muscle Glucose Uptake During Exercise

Exercise is a potent stimulus for skeletal muscle glucose uptake, the increase in glucose uptake by contracting skeletal muscle being greater than that elicited by maximal insulin stimulation (107). At rest, skeletal muscle accounts for approximately 15-20% of the total peripheral glucose utilization, while during cycling exercise at 55-60% $\dot{V}O_2$ max, leg muscle glucose uptake can account for as much as 80-85% of total body glucose utilization (124) and may be even greater at higher intensities (115). The increase in glucose uptake arises from both an increase in glucose delivery to contracting muscle, as a result of elevated skeletal muscle blood flow, and an increase in glucose extraction, as measured by the arteriovenous glucose difference (3, 4, 91, 115, 119, 201). Increased glucose extraction by contracting muscle is due to enhanced membrane glucose transport and activation of the glycolytic and oxidative pathways responsible for glucose disposal. During the latter stages of prolonged exercise, glucose delivery may become a limiting factor as arterial blood glucose levels decline (3, 4, 119). The magnitude of the increase in muscle glucose uptake is influenced by both exercise intensity and duration

(Figure 2.2). Glucose uptake increases in proportion to exercise intensity (115, 201), and at low- to moderate-intensity exercise this is accompanied by an increase in glucose utilization because there is no accumulation of free glucose within contracting muscle (115). At higher exercise intensities, however, an increase in muscle [glucose] suggests that glucose phosphorylation and subsequent utilization is inhibited (115). The likely explanation for this is an increase in muscle G-6-P, derived from muscle glycogenolysis, which is an inhibitor of hexokinase. Under such conditions, the preferential utilization of muscle glycogen is an advantage because the glycolytic ATP yield per glucosyl unit derived from glycogen (three) is greater than that from glucose (two).

Regulation of Skeletal Muscle Glucose Uptake

Although an increase in glucose and insulin delivery to contracting skeletal muscle occurs during exercise, the contribution of these factors to increased muscle glucose uptake is relatively small (222). Thus, local factors within contracting muscle play a major role in enhancing muscle glucose uptake during exercise (222).

Local Factors.   Glucose transport across the muscle cell membrane occurs by facilitated diffusion in a process that is not energy dependent

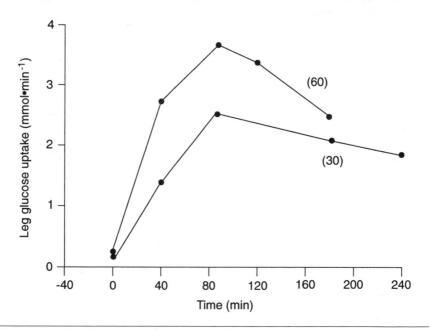

Figure 2.2   Leg glucose uptake during cycling exercise. Numbers in parentheses refer to exercise intensity (% $\dot{V}O_2$ max). Data from Ahlborg et al. (3, 4).

and exhibits Michaelis-Menten saturation kinetics, thereby suggesting the presence of a membrane carrier or transporter (100). Kinetic studies in perfused rat muscle and muscle membrane vesicle preparations have demonstrated that contractile activity increases the V_{max} of glucose transport (100, 122, 149, 150, 194). Numerous studies utilizing cytochalasin B binding, Western blot analysis, and immunohistochemistry have demonstrated that this is due to an increase in the number of glucose transporters in the plasma membrane, as a result of translocation from an intracellular storage site (57-59, 66, 75-78, 99, 122, 151, 172). Because the increase in muscle glucose transport and uptake is often larger than the increase in plasma membrane glucose transporter number, it has been suggested that there is also an increase in the intrinsic activity of glucose transporters (76, 78, 122, 194), although not all authors share this view (172). There exists a family of facilitative glucose transporters with similar structure, but different tissue localization (113, 125). The isoforms GLUT1 and GLUT4 have been located in skeletal muscle, although much of the GLUT1 is believed to originate from nerves and blood vessels within muscle (85, 151). Contractile activity results in an increase in plasma membrane GLUT4 content, but no change in intracellular GLUT1 distribution (57, 59, 75, 77, 151). Skeletal muscle GLUT4 levels are closely related to oxidative capacity (77, 94) and are increased by endurance exercise training in rats (143, 171) and humans (101, 101a).

The increase in sarcoplasmic calcium during excitation-contraction coupling is likely to be involved in the activation of glucose transport because small elevations in muscle calcium have been shown to enhance glucose transport (100, 216). Hypoxia also increases muscle glucose transport via calcium release (26), by a mechanism similar to that seen with contractile activity, because the effects of these two stimuli are not additive (26, 103). Such effects of calcium may be mediated via translocation and activation of protein kinase C (35, 165), although the relationships between excitation-contraction coupling, phosphoinositol metabolism, and glucose transport are not fully clear. Under most circumstances, the membrane transport of glucose is considered rate limiting for muscle glucose uptake (100). There may be situations, however, where glucose phosphorylation and disposal become the limiting factors (e.g., during moderate- to high-intensity exercise increased muscle G-6-P levels, derived from accelerated glycogenolysis, will inhibit glucose phosphorylation and utilization; 115, 119).

The metabolic state within contracting muscle is also likely to influence muscle glucose uptake. Hypoxia is a stimulus for glucose transport and uptake (26, 103, 202), and hypoxia and exercise are believed to stimulate glucose transport by a common mechanism. Breathing hypoxic gas mixtures results in increased glucose disposal during exercise in humans (46), although muscle glucose utilization may not be enhanced because muscle glucose accumulation has been observed under such conditions (117).

During both hypoxia and exercise/contractile activity, an inverse relationship between intramuscular creatine phosphate levels and muscle glucose transport/uptake has been observed (103, 115, 202), implying a coupling of glucose uptake to the metabolic state of the muscle. Glucose uptake during exercise at 55% $\dot{V}O_2$ peak is higher in individuals with a low muscle respiratory capacity compared with those with a high respiratory capacity (38). The metabolic perturbations (e.g., alterations in creatine phosphate, ADP, AMP) as a result of such exercise will be greater in the individuals with a low muscle respiratory capacity.

Hormonal Regulation.   The role of insulin in the regulation of glucose uptake has been the subject of considerable interest over the years. It was thought that a certain "permissive" amount of insulin was required for the increase in muscle glucose uptake with exercise/contraction to occur (12) despite the fact that plasma insulin levels fall during exercise. In contrast, it has been demonstrated that contractile activity can increase muscle glucose uptake (148, 204, 205) and plasma membrane glucose transporter number (78) in the absence of insulin. The effects of exercise on glucose transport are mediated solely by a process associated with contraction (42). Furthermore, several studies have observed that the effects of insulin and contraction in muscle are additive (42, 142, 149, 150, 203), implying that insulin and exercise activate glucose transport via different mechanisms. This is in keeping with the finding that while both insulin and exercise stimulate translocation of the GLUT4 isoform, they appear to activate different pools of transporters or differentially activate the same pool (58, 59, 150, 151). Insulin binding to rat (19, 196) and human (18) skeletal muscle and muscle insulin receptor tyrosine kinase activity (196) are unaltered by acute exercise. Thus, insulin does not appear to be essential for an increase in muscle glucose transport and uptake during exercise. This is not to say, however, that insulin is without effect on glucose uptake during whole-body exercise. Exercise increases the sensitivity of skeletal muscle to the action of insulin (207), which, together with increased insulin inflow due to enhanced muscle blood flow (55), may overcome, in part, a reduction in plasma insulin levels. It has been demonstrated that the effects of insulin and exercise on muscle glucose uptake are synergistic (55, 207) and that the increased glucose delivery associated with exercise can enhance the glucose disposal associated with a maximal insulin stimulus (25). The presence of hyperinsulinemia at the onset of exercise results in a rapid fall in blood glucose (47, 89), presumably as a consequence of increased glucose uptake by contracting muscle. Insulin deficiency attenuates glucose uptake by approximately 50% in exercising dogs (209) and in the long term reduces the capacity for glucose transport during *in vitro* muscle contraction (205). Furthermore, insulin will influence muscle glucose uptake via its inhibitory effects of adipose tissue lipolysis and perhaps muscle glycogenolysis also (214).

Although the interaction between insulin and exercise has been well studied, the role of epinephrine in exercise-induced alterations in muscle glucose uptake is less clear. Under resting conditions, epinephrine or isoproterenol has been shown to decrease (16, 219) and increase (32, 168) muscle glucose uptake and/or transport. Epinephrine increases plasma membrane glucose transport (16), although this was associated with reduced membrane glucose transport (16), suggesting that epinephrine inhibited transporter activity. Both β- (219) and α- (168) adrenergic mechanisms have been proposed as mediating these responses. In stimulated, perfused rat muscle, epinephrine had variable effects on muscle glucose uptake (168), which were related, in part, to alterations in muscle oxygen uptake. These effects were impaired by α-adrenergic blockade but enhanced by β-adrenergic blockade (168). During exercise in humans, epinephrine and isoproterenol infusion reduced muscle glucose uptake by contracting leg (108) and forearm (93) muscle, respectively. This could be due to either direct effects of catecholamines on muscle glucose uptake mechanisms and/or to indirect effects (i.e., increased lipolysis and muscle glycogenolysis). Epinephrine will activate glycogen phosphorylase, thereby increasing muscle glycogenolysis and muscle G-6-P levels (155), which will inhibit glucose utilization and uptake.

Substrate Availability.   A temporal relationship has been demonstrated between intramuscular glycogen levels and muscle glucose uptake during exercise. Studies in the exercising rat have suggested that muscle glucose uptake is dependent upon a reduction in muscle glycogen (107, 148). Furthermore, glycogen loss in noncontracting skeletal muscle during exercise is associated with increased muscle glucose transport (140), although possible humoral stimuli cannot be excluded entirely. A significant inverse relationship between muscle glycogen levels and glucose uptake has been observed during exercise in humans (91). While this result may simply reflect independent effects of exercise on muscle glycogenolysis and glucose uptake, which are not causally related, the strong association suggests a potential regulatory influence of muscle glycogen availability. Exercise and dietary manipulation of muscle glycogen levels prior to exercise has produced alterations in muscle glucose uptake during subsequent exercise. Lowering of muscle glycogen is associated with increased glucose extraction from the blood during exercise (72). Furthermore, leg glucose uptake was directly related to the percentage of glycogen-empty fibers (estimated histochemically) and inversely related to muscle G-6-P levels (72). In perfused, contracting rat skeletal muscle, increased preexercise muscle glycogen availability reduces glucose uptake (97, 166), whereas low preexercise muscle glycogen levels enhance glucose uptake (97). The likely effect of increased muscle glycogen availability is to increase the rate of glycogen breakdown and increase muscle G-6-P levels (97, 119), thereby impairing glucose disposal. In addition, the alterations in glucose transport observed with different preexercise muscle glycogen levels (97) suggest that this process is also influenced by glycogen availability and/or the rate of glycogenolysis during exercise. A regulatory influence of muscle glycogen on glucose uptake would limit muscle glucose uptake early in exercise, at a time when muscle glycogen is readily available.

Availability of blood-borne substrates will also influence muscle glucose uptake during exercise. The decline in muscle glucose uptake during the latter stages of prolonged exercise (3, 4) is likely to be due, in part, to a reduction in arterial blood glucose levels (3, 4). Increased blood glucose availability increases leg glucose uptake and oxidation during exercise in dogs (221). Ingestion of glucose during prolonged exercise at 30% $\dot{V}O_2$ max in humans results in enhanced leg glucose uptake (2). Whether this occurs at higher exercise intensities, when glycogenolysis is proceeding at a more rapid rate, has not been well studied. We have recently observed that increased blood glucose and insulin levels, as a result of carbohydrate ingestion, enhance glucose uptake during 2 hours of exercise at 70% $\dot{V}O_2$ max (137a). Also of note are the observations that well-trained cyclists are capable of taking up and oxidizing large amounts of glucose (36, 39, 51) during the latter stages of prolonged, strenuous exercise, when muscle glycogen levels are very low, provided blood glucose levels are maintained by carbohydrate ingestion or intravenous glucose infusion. It is interesting that carbohydrate ingestion appears to be less effective in improving performance when muscle glycogen availability is adequate (211).

There has also been considerable interest in the effects of alterations in plasma FFA availability on muscle glucose uptake during exercise. About 30 years ago, Randle and co-workers proposed the "glucose-fatty acid cycle," in which increased uptake and oxidation of FFA, due to elevated plasma FFA levels, result in a citrate-mediated inhibition of PFK activity and glycolysis (152, 153). The resultant increase in muscle G-6-P levels inhibits hexokinase activity, glucose phosphorylation, and glucose uptake (153). Two studies in perfused rat skeletal muscle showed no effect of increased palmitate or ketones on muscle glucose uptake, either at rest or during electrical stimulation (11, 169). In contrast, addition of oleate to the perfusion medium has been shown to inhibit glucose uptake during contractile activity (162), accompanied by increased muscle citrate, G-6-P, and glucose levels. It has been suggested that the glucose-fatty acid cycle operates only in red muscle during recovery from exercise (223). In man, increased FFA availability is associated with reduced glucose utilization under resting conditions (64), although no effect of FFA on plasma glucose oxidation has also been reported (213). During moderate-intensity (44% $\dot{V}O_2$ max) exercise, elevation of FFA had no effect on carbohydrate oxidation (154). More recently, a doubling of plasma FFA within the physiological range was associated with a 30-35% reduction in muscle glucose uptake during 1 hour of knee-extension exercise at 80% W_{max} (90). No changes were observed in muscle FFA uptake or oxidation, muscle G-6-P levels, or muscle citrate release during exercise, suggesting that the observed effect on glucose uptake may have been due to direct inhibition of glucose transport by FFA, rather than operation of the "classical" glucose-fatty acid cycle (90). A recent preliminary report has observed no effect of oleate on insulin-stimulated 3-O-methyl glucose uptake by human skeletal muscle *in vitro* (220), although palmitate inhibits insulin-stimulated glucose transport in rat soleus muscle (85a). The effects of alterations in FFA availability on muscle glucose metabolism during exercise, their significance, and the underlying mechanisms require further clarification. Nevertheless, increased circulating FFA may limit muscle glucose uptake during the latter stages of prolonged exercise, when muscle glycogen and arterial glucose levels are low. Under such conditions, inhibition of FFA mobilization by nicotinic acid results in a rapid fall in blood glucose levels (72).

Lactate Metabolism During Exercise

Over the years, there has been great interest in lactate metabolism during exercise and the potential role of lactate in fatigue, ventilatory control, and intermediary metabolism. For many years, lactate was considered simply a metabolic waste product of glycolysis during moderate- to high-intensity exercise. There is increasing evidence, however, that lactate is an important metabolic intermediate, serving as both a gluconeogenic precursor for the liver (206) and an oxidative substrate for contracting skeletal (192) and cardiac (68) muscle. This has resulted in the development of the lactate shuttle hypothesis (21, 22), for which there is growing experimental support. There has been great debate in the literature on the underlying mechanisms responsible for lactate production and accumulation during exercise and the validity of various experimental approaches to the study of lactate metabolism during exercise. Most interest has focused on the influence of oxygen availability on lactate production and whether hypoxia is a necessary prerequisite for lactate production (41, 116, 118, 189). Factors other than oxygen availability that are likely to influence lactate production include the rate of muscle glycogenolysis and subsequent pyruvate formation, diet, training status, and circulating catecholamines. Given the interest in lactate metabolism during exercise, considerable literature exists in which more detailed discussion of lactate metabolism during exercise can be found (21, 22, 41, 71, 116, 118, 173, 188-190, 210).

Factors Influencing Skeletal Muscle Carbohydrate Metabolism During Exercise

As mentioned earlier, the major factors that influence the magnitude of muscle glycogenolysis and glucose uptake during exercise are likely to be exercise intensity and duration. The general pattern of muscle carbohydrate metabolism, however, will be affected by other factors, which include mode of exercise, training status, preceding diet, environmental conditions, and gender.

Exercise Mode

It has been suggested that glycogen utilization during running exercise is lower than that during cycling exercise at similar relative exercise intensities (50). This probably reflects differences in the recruitment patterns of the leg muscles during the two activities and a greater metabolic stress on vastus lateralis (the muscle sampled) during cycling exercise. Overall carbohydrate oxidation rates, estimated from respiratory exchange ratio measurements, are similar during running and cycling at similar relative exercise intensities (50, 95). During arm exercise, there is a greater lactate release and estimated muscle glycogenolysis than during leg exercise at the same relative intensity (5). This may reflect differences in the cardiovascular and hormonal responses to the two forms of exercise. The addition of arm exercise to leg exercise has been shown to reduce leg glucose uptake (167), although this may not occur at higher exercise intensities (124).

Training

It is well documented that endurance training results in a reduction in muscle glycogen utilization (102, 110) and glucose uptake and oxidation (37, 110), with a concomitant increase in lipid metabolism (102). The metabolic adaptations to training will be discussed in more detail in chapter 6.

Diet

Consumption of a high carbohydrate diet is associated with an increased rate of carbohydrate oxidation during exercise (13, 33, 67, 134), increased muscle glycogenolysis (67, 74) (Table 2.1), and an increase in leg glucose uptake (134). In contrast, carbohydrate oxidation and muscle glycogenolysis are reduced following consumption of a low carbohydrate diet (13, 67, 109), whereas effects on muscle glucose uptake are less clear (109, 134). These effects of diet are likely to be mediated by alterations in the levels of insulin, glucagon, and catecholamines (67), and by changes in substrate (muscle glycogen, blood glucose, plasma FFA) availability and its effects on muscle glycogenolysis and glucose uptake, as described in previous sections of this chapter. In rats, fasting is associated with increased fat mobilization and utilization and decreased muscle glycogen utilization during exercise (56). In contrast, muscle glycogen utilization does not appear to be significantly influenced by fasting in humans (132, 145), although the data of Knapik et al. (126) suggest there may be a slight reduction. These authors also observed a reduction in glucose disposal during exercise following a 3.5 day fast (126).

Environment

Heat stress increases muscle glycogen breakdown (63, 65) (Table 2.2), muscle and blood lactate accumulation (63, 65, 218), and blood glucose levels (63, 215) during exercise. It has been suggested that these responses are due, in part, to reduced blood flow and oxygen delivery to contracting muscle (65); however, the effects of heat stress on muscle blood flow are somewhat equivocal (144). Additional possibilities include increased circulating epinephrine levels (63) and a Q_{10} effect due to elevated muscle temperature (63, 128). Following a period of heat acclimation, muscle glycogen utilization and lactate accumulation are reduced during exercise in the heat (63, 121, 123, 218). Furthermore, no increase in muscle glycogenolysis during exercise in the heat is observed in well-trained, heat acclimatized subjects (215). The reduction in muscle glycogen utilization is not accompanied by alterations in the exchange of blood-borne substrates (123) and is most likely due to a reduction in plasma epinephrine levels (63). Muscle glycogen utilization during low-intensity exercise at 9 °C is greater than at 21 °C (106), most likely due to shivering thermogenesis increasing glycogen use (135). At higher exercise intensities, with increased metabolic heat production, no difference is observed in muscle glycogenolysis during exercise at the two temperatures (106).

Exercise under hypoxic conditions is associated with increased glucose disposal (23, 46), increased glycolysis (82), and elevated blood and muscle lactate levels (24, 82). Following a period of altitude acclimatization, glycogenolysis, glycolysis, and lactate accumulation are reduced (82, 217). These adaptations are believed to reflect a number of possible changes with acclimatization that include increased FFA levels (217), improved metabolic control (82), and reduced epinephrine levels (136).

Gender

Relatively few studies have compared the metabolic responses of males and females during exercise due, in part, to the difficulties in matching

Table 2.2 Metabolic Responses During Exercise and Heat Stress

	20°C	40°C
Oxygen uptake (L·min^{-1})	2.94 ± 0.50	2.94 ± 0.60
RER	0.88 ± 0.01	0.91 ± 0.01*
Blood glucose (mmol·L^{-1})	4.6 ± 0.1	5.5 ± 0.2*
Blood lactate (mmol·L^{-1})	1.8 ± 0.3	3.7 ± 0.5*
Plasma epinephrine (pg·mL^{-1})	323 ± 44	489 ± 72*
Muscle lactate (mmol·kg^{-1})	12.0 ± 2.0	20.7 ± 2.2*
Δ glycogen (mmol·kg^{-1})	166 ± 20	218 ± 18*

These values were obtained during 40 min of cycling at 70% $\dot{V}O_2$ max in either a 20°C or 40°C environment. Oxygen uptake and RER values represent average of four measurements during exercise; Δ glycogen is the difference between pre- and post-exericse muscle glycogen values; remaining values obtained after 40 min of exercise. Muscle metabolites measured on dry muscle. Values are means ± SE (n=12). *denotes different from 20°C, P<0.05. Some data from Febbraio et al. (63).

male and female subjects for $\dot{V}O_2$ max, training status, body composition, and exercise intensity. It has been observed that carbohydrate oxidation and muscle glycogen utilization during exercise are lower in female subjects than in male subjects (146, 195), in keeping with the suggestion that females have a greater capacity for lipid oxidation, although this may not necessarily be the case (49). Other investigators have observed no differences between male and female runners in the metabolic responses to treadmill running (20). Possible gender differences in skeletal muscle carbohydrate metabolism and their potential significance require further clarification.

Summary

Muscle glycogen and blood-borne glucose are important substrates for ATP resynthesis in contracting skeletal muscle during prolonged exercise. In addition, their metabolism can produce lactate, an important gluconeogenic and oxidative substrate. The magnitude of muscle glycogenolysis and glucose uptake during exercise will be determined primarily by exercise intensity and duration. Further influences include exercise mode, training status, diet, environmental conditions, and gender. The regulation of skeletal muscle carbohydrate metabolism involves the interplay between local exercise-induced alterations in muscle calcium, inorganic phosphate and metabolites, hormonal control, and substrate availability, so that muscle glycogenolysis and glucose uptake are enhanced to meet the increased metabolic demands of exercise.

References

1. Ahlborg, G. Mechanism for glycogenolysis in nonexercising human muscle during and after exercise. Am. J. Physiol. 248:E540-E545; 1985.

2. Ahlborg, G.; Felig, P. Influence of glucose ingestion on fuel-hormone response during prolonged exercise. J. Appl. Physiol. 41:683-688; 1976.

3. Ahlborg, G.; Felig, P. Lactate and glucose exchange across the forearm, legs, and splanchnic bed during and after prolonged leg exercise. J. Clin. Invest. 69:45-54; 1982.

4. Ahlborg, G.; Felig, P.; Hagenfeldt, L.; Hendler, R.; Wahren, J. Substrate turnover during prolonged exercise in man: splanchnic and leg metabolism of glucose, free fatty acids, and amino acids. J. Clin. Invest. 53:1080-1090; 1974.

5. Ahlborg, G.; Jensen-Urstad, M. Metabolism in exercising arm vs. leg muscle. Clin. Physiol. 11:459-468; 1991.

6. Ahlborg, G.; Wahren, J.; Felig, P. Splanchnic and peripheral glucose and lactate metabolism during and after prolonged arm exercise. J. Clin. Invest. 77:690-699; 1986.

7. Aragon, J.J.; Tornheim, K.; Lowenstein, J.M. On a possible role of IMP in the regulation of phosphorylase activity in skeletal muscle. FEBS Lett. 117:K56-K64; 1980.

8. Arnall, D.A.; Marker, J.C.; Conlee, R.K.; Winder, W.W. Effect of infusing epinephrine on liver and muscle glycogenolysis during exercise in rats. Am. J. Physiol. 250:E641-E649; 1986.

9. Bagby, G.J.; Green, H.J.; Katsuta, S.; Gollnick, P.D. Glycogen depletion in exercising rats infused with glucose, lactate or pyruvate. J. Appl. Physiol. 45:425-429; 1978.

10. Ball-Burnett, M.; Green, H.J.; Houston, M.E. Energy metabolism in human slow and fast twitch fibres during prolonged cycle exercise. J. Physiol. 437:257-267; 1991.

11. Berger, M.; Hagg, S.; Goodman, M.; Ruderman, N.B. Glucose metabolism in perfused skeletal muscle: effects of starvation, diabetes, fatty acids, acetoacetate, insulin and exercise on glucose uptake and disposition. Biochem. J. 158:191-202; 1976.

12. Berger, M.; Hagg, S.; Ruderman, N.B. Glucose metabolism in perfused skeletal muscle: interaction of insulin and exercise on glucose uptake. Biochem. J. 146:231-238; 1975.

13. Bergstrom, J.; Hermansen, L.; Hultman, E.; Saltin, B. Diet, muscle glycogen and physical performance. Acta Physiol. Scand. 71:140-150; 1967.

14. Bergstrom, J.; Hultman, E. A study of the glycogen metabolism during exercise in man. Scand. J. Clin. Lab. Invest. 19:218-228; 1967.

15. Bergstrom, J.; Hultman, E.; Jorfeldt, L.; Pernow, B.; Wahren, J. Effect of nicotinic acid on physical working capacity and on metabolism of muscle glycogen in man. J. Appl. Physiol. 26:170-176; 1969.

16. Bonen, A.; Megeney, L.A.; McCarthy, S.C.; McDermott, J.C.; Tan, M.H. Epinephrine administration stimulates GLUT4 translocation but reduces glucose transport in muscle. Biochem. Biophys. Res. Comm. 187:685-691; 1992.

17. Bonen, A.; Ness, G.W.; Belcastro, A.N.; Kirby, R.L. Mild exercise impedes glycogen repletion in muscle. J. Appl. Physiol. 58:1622-1629; 1985.

18. Bonen, A.; Tan, M.H.; Clune, P.; Kirby, R.L. Effects of exercise on insulin binding to human muscle. Am. J. Physiol. 248:E403-E408; 1985.

19. Bonen, A.; Tan, M.H.; Watson-Wright, W.M. Effects of exercise on insulin binding and glucose metabolism in muscle. Can. J. Physiol. Pharmacol. 62:1500-1504; 1984.

20. Brewer, J.C.; Williams, C.; Patton, A. The influence of high carbohydrate diets on endurance running performance. Eur. J. Appl. Physiol. 57:698-706; 1988.

21. Brooks, G.A. The lactate shuttle during exercise and recovery. Med. Sci. Sports Exerc. 18:360-368; 1986.

22. Brooks, G.A. Current concepts in lactate exchange. Med. Sci. Sports Exerc. 23:895-906; 1991.

23. Brooks, G.A.; Butterfield, G.E.; Wolfe, R.R.; Groves, B.M.; Mazzeo, R.S.; Sutton, J.R.; Wolfel, E.E.; Reeves, J.T. Increased dependence on blood glucose after acclimatization to 4,300 m. J. Appl. Physiol. 70:919-927; 1991.

24. Brooks, G.A.; Butterfield, G.E.; Wolfe, R.R.; Groves, B.M.; Mazzeo, R.S.; Sutton, J.R.; Wolfel, E.E.; Reeves, J.T. Decreased reliance on lactate during exercise after acclimatization to 4,300 m. J. Appl. Physiol. 71:333-341; 1991.

25. Bourey, R.E.; Coggan, A.R.; Kohrt, W.M.; Kirwan, J.P.; King, D.S.; Holloszy, J.O. Effect of exercise on glucose disposal: response to a maximal insulin stimulus. J. Appl. Physiol. 69:1689-1694; 1990.

26. Cartee, G.D.; Douen, A.G.; Ramlal, T.; Klip, A.; Holloszy, J.O. Stimulation of glucose transport in skeletal muscle by hypoxia. J. Appl. Physiol. 70:1593-1600; 1991.

27. Chasiotis, D.; Brandt, R.; Harris, R.C.; Hultman, E. Effects of β-blockade on glycogen metabolism in human subjects during exercise. Am. J. Physiol. 245:E166-E170; 1983.

28. Chasiotis, D.; Edstrom, L.; Sahlin, K.; Hultman, E. Activation of glycogen phosphorylase by electrical stimulation of isolated fast-twitch and slow-twitch muscles from rats. Acta Physiol. Scand. 123:43-47; 1985.

29. Chasiotis, D.; Sahlin, K.; Hultman, E. Regulation of glycogenolysis in human muscle at rest and during exercise. J. Appl. Physiol. 53:708-715; 1982.

30. Chasiotis, D.; Sahlin, K.; Hultman, E. Regulation of glycogenolysis in human muscle in response to epinephrine infusion. J. Appl. Physiol. 54:45-50; 1983.

31. Chasiotis, D.; Hultman, E.; Sahlin, K. Acidotic depression of cyclic AMP accumulation and phosphorylase b to a transformation in skeletal muscle of man. J. Physiol. (London) 335:197-204; 1983.

32. Chiasson, J.-L.; Shikama, H.; Chu, D.T.W.; Exton, J.H. Inhibitory effect of epinephrine on insulin-stimulated glucose uptake by rat skeletal muscle. J. Clin. Invest. 68:706-713; 1981.

33. Christensen, E.H.; Hansen, O. Arbeitsfahigkeit und ernahrung. Skand. Arch. Physiol. 81:160-171; 1939.

34. Christensen, E.H.; Hansen, O. Hypoglykamie, arbeitsfahigkeit und ermu-dung. Skand. Arch. Physiol. 81:172-179; 1939.

35. Cleland, P.J.F.; Appleby, G.J.; Rattigan, S.; Clark, M.G. Exercise-induced translocation of protein kinase C and production of diacylglycerol and phosphatidic acid in rat skeletal muscle in vivo: relationship to changes in glucose transport. J. Biol. Chem. 264:17704-17711; 1989.

36. Coggan, A.R.; Coyle, E.F. Reversal of fatigue during prolonged exercise by carbohydrate infusion or ingestion. J. Appl. Physiol. 63:2388-2395; 1987.

37. Coggan, A.R.; Kohrt, W.M.; Spina, R.J.; Bier, D.M.; Holloszy, J.O. Endurance training decreases plasma glucose turnover and oxidation during moderate-intensity exercise in men. J. Appl. Physiol. 68:990-996; 1990.

38. Coggan, A.R.; Kohrt, W.M.; Spina, R.J.; Kirwan, J.P.; Bier, D.M.; Holloszy, J.O. Plasma glucose kinetics during exercise in subjects with high and low lactate thresholds. J. Appl. Physiol. 73:1873-1880; 1992.

39. Coggan, A.R.; Spina, R.J.; Kohrt, W.M.; Bier, D.M.; Holloszy, J.O. Plasma glucose kinetics in a well-trained cyclist fed glucose throughout exercise. Int. J. Sports Nutr. 1:279-288; 1991.

40. Conlee, R.K.; McLane, J.A.; Rennie, M.J.; Winder, W.W.; Holloszy, J.O. Reversal of phosphorylase activation in muscle despite continued contractile activity. Am. J. Physiol. 237:R291-R296; 1979.

41. Connett, R.J.; Honig, C.R.; Gayeski, T.E.J.; Brooks, G.A. Defining hypoxia: a systems view of VO_2, glycolysis, energetics, and intracellular PO_2. J. Appl. Physiol. 68:833-842; 1990.

42. Constable, S.H.; Favier, R.J.; Cartee, G.D.; Young, D.A.; Holloszy, J.O. Muscle glucose transport: interactions of in vitro contractions, insulin and exercise. J. Appl. Physiol. 64:2329-2332; 1988.

43. Constable, S.H.; Favier, R.J.; Holloszy, J.O. Exercise and glycogen depletion: effects on the ability to activate muscle phosphorylase. J. Appl. Physiol. 60:1518-1523; 1986.

44. Constable, S.H.; Young, J.C.; Higuchi, M.; Holloszy, J.O. Glycogen resynthe-sis in leg muscles of rats during exercise. Am. J. Physiol. 247:R880-R883; 1984.

45. Constantin-Teodosiu, D.; Cederblad, G.; Hultman, E. PDC activity and ace-tyl group accumulation in skeletal muscle during prolonged exercise. J. Appl. Physiol. 73:2403-2407; 1992.

46. Cooper, D.M.; Wasserman, D.H.; Vranic, M.; Wasserman, K. Glucose turn-over in response to exercise during high- and low-FIO_2 breathing in man. Am. J. Physiol. 251:E209-E214; 1986.

47. Costill, D.L.; Coyle, E.; Dalsky, G.; Evans, W.; Fink, W.; Hoopes, D. Effects of elevated plasma FFA and insulin on muscle glycogen usage during exercise. J. Appl. Physiol. 43:695-699; 1977.

48. Costill, D.L.; Dalsky, G.P.; Fink, W.J. Effects of caffeine ingestion on metabo-lism and exercise performance. Med. Sci. Sports. 10:155-158; 1978.

49. Costill, D.L.; Fink, W.J.; Getchell, L.; Ivy, J.L.; Witzmann, F. Lipid metabolism in skeletal muscle of endurance-trained males and females. J. Appl. Physiol. 47:787-791; 1979.

50. Costill, D.L.; Sparks, K.; Gregor, R.; Turner, C. Muscle glycogen utilization during exhaustive running. J. Appl. Physiol. 31:353-356; 1971.

51. Coyle, E.F.; Coggan, A.R.; Hemmert, M.K.; Ivy, J.L. Muscle glycogen utilization during prolonged strenuous exercise when fed carbohydrate. J. Appl. Physiol. 61:165-172; 1986.

52. Coyle, E.F.; Hagberg, J.M.; Hurley, B.F.; Martin, W.H.; Ehsani, A.A.; Holloszy, J.O. Carbohydrate feeding during prolonged strenuous exercise can delay fatigue. J. Appl. Physiol. 55:230-235; 1983.

53. Coyle, E.F.; Hamilton, M.T.; Gonzalez-Alonso, J.; Montain, S.J.; Ivy, J.L. Carbohydrate metabolism during intense exercise when hyperglycemic. J. Appl. Physiol. 70:834-840; 1991.

54. Davies, C.T.M.; Thompson, M.W. Aerobic performance of female and male ultramarathon athletes. Eur. J. Appl. Physiol. 41:233-245; 1979.

55. DeFronzo, R.A.; Ferrannini, E.; Sato, Y.; Felig, P.; Wahren, J. Synergistic interaction between exercise and insulin on peripheral glucose uptake. J. Clin. Invest. 68:1468-1474; 1981.

56. Dohm, G.L.; Tapscott, E.B.; Barakat, H.A.; Kasperek, G.J. Influence of fasting in rats on glycogen depletion during exercise. J. Appl. Physiol. 55:830-833; 1983.

57. Douen, A.G.; Ramlal, T.; Cartee, G.D.; Klip, A. Exercise modulates the insulin-induced translocation of glucose transporters in rat skeletal muscle. FEBS Letters 261:256-260; 1990.

58. Douen, A.G.; Ramlal, T.; Klip, A.; Young, D.A.; Cartee, G.D.; Holloszy, J.O. Exercise-induced increase in glucose transporters in plasma membranes of rat skeletal muscle. Endocrinology 124:449-454; 1989.

59. Douen, A.G.; Ramlal, T.; Rastogi, S.; Bilan, P.J.; Cartee, G.D.; Vranic, M.; Holloszy, J.O.; Klip, A. Exercise induces recruitment of the "insulin-responsive glucose transporter": evidence for distinct intracellular insulin- and exercise-recruitable transporter pools in skeletal muscle. J. Biol. Chem. 265:13427-13430; 1990.

60. Edwards, H.T.; Margaria, R.; Dill, D.B. Metabolic rate, blood sugar and the utilization of carbohydrate. Am. J. Physiol. 108:203-209; 1934.

61. Entman, M.L.; Keslensky, S.S.; Chu, A.; Van Winkle, W.B. The sarcoplasmic reticulum-glycogenolytic complex in mammalian fast-twitch skeletal muscle. J. Biol. Chem. 255:6245-6252; 1980.

62. Essig, D.; Costill, D.L.; Van Handel, P.J. Effects of caffeine ingestion on utilization of muscle glycogen and lipid during leg ergometer cycling. Int. J. Sports Med. 1:86-90; 1980.

63. Febbraio, M.A.; Snow, R.J.; Hargreaves, M.; Stathis, C.G.; Martin, I.K.; Carey, M.F. Muscle metabolism during exercise and heat stress in trained men: effect of acclimation. J. Appl. Physiol. 76:589-597; 1994.

64. Ferrannini, E.; Barrett, E.J.; Bevilacqua, S.; DeFronzo, R.A. Effect of fatty acids on glucose production and utilization in man. J. Clin. Invest. 72:1737-1747; 1983.

65. Fink, W.J.; Costill, D.L.; Van Handel, P.J. Leg muscle metabolism during exercise in the heat and cold. Eur. J. Appl. Physiol. 34:183-190; 1975.

66. Fushiki, T.; Wells, J.A.; Tapscott, E.B.; Dohm, G.L. Changes in glucose transporters in muscle in response to exercise. Am. J. Physiol. 256:E580-E587; 1989.

67. Galbo, H.; Holst, J.J.; Christensen, N.J. The effect of different diets and of insulin on the hormonal response to prolonged exercise. Acta Physiol. Scand. 107:19-32; 1979.

68. Gertz, E.W.; Wisneski, J.A.; Stanley, W.C.; Neese, R.A. Myocardial substrate utilization during exercise in humans: dual carbon-labeled carbohydrate isotope experiments. J. Clin. Invest. 82:2017-2025; 1988.

69. Gollnick, P.D.; Armstrong, R.B.; Saubert, C.W.; Sembrowich, W.L.; Shepherd, R.E.; Saltin, B. Glycogen depletion patterns in human skeletal muscle fibers during prolonged work. Pflugers Arch. 344:1-12; 1973.

70. Gollnick, P.D.; Armstrong, R.B.; Sembrowich, W.L.; Shepherd, R.E.; Saltin, B. Glycogen depletion pattern in human skeletal muscle fibers after heavy exercise. J. Appl. Physiol. 34:615-618; 1973.

71. Gollnick, P.D.; Bayly, W.M.; Hodgson, D.R. Exercise intensity, training, diet, and lactate concentration in muscle and blood. Med. Sci. Sports Exerc. 18:334-340; 1986.

72. Gollnick, P.D.; Pernow, B.; Essen, B.; Jansson, E.; Saltin, B. Availability of glycogen and plasma FFA for substrate utilization in leg muscle of man during exercise. Clin. Physiol. 1:27-42; 1981.

73. Gollnick, P.D.; Piehl, K.; Saltin, B. Selective glycogen depletion pattern in human muscle fibers after exercise of varying intensity and at varying pedalling rates. J. Physiol. 241:45-57; 1974.

74. Gollnick, P.D.; Piehl, K.; Saubert, C.W.; Armstrong, R.B.; Saltin, B. Diet, exercise, and glycogen in human muscle fibers. J. Appl. Physiol. 33:421-425; 1972.

75. Goodyear, L.J.; Hirshman, M.F.; Horton, E.S. Exercise-induced translocation of skeletal muscle glucose transporters. Am. J. Physiol. 261:E795-E799; 1991.

76. Goodyear, L.J.; Hirshman, M.F.; King, P.A.; Horton, E.D.; Thompson, C.M.; Horton, E.S. Skeletal muscle plasma membrane glucose transport and glucose transporters after exercise. J. Appl. Physiol. 68:193-198; 1990.

77. Goodyear, L.J.; Hirshman, M.F.; Smith, R.J.; Horton, E.S. Glucose transporter number, activity, and isoform content in plasma membranes of red and white skeletal muscle. Am. J. Physiol. 261:E556-E561; 1991.

78. Goodyear, L.J.; King, P.A.; Hirshman, M.F.; Thompson, C.M.; Horton, E.D.; Horton, E.S. Contractile activity increases plasma membrane glucose transporters in absence of insulin. Am. J. Physiol. 258:E667-E672; 1990.

79. Gorski, J.; Pietrzyk, K. The effect of β-adrenergic receptor blockade on intramuscular glycogen mobilization during exercise in the rat. Eur. J. Appl. Physiol. 48:201-205; 1982.

80. Gorski, J.; Zendzian-Piotrowska, M.; Gorska, M.; Rutkiewicz, J. Effect of hyperglycemia on muscle glycogen mobilization during muscle contractions in the rat. Eur. J. Appl. Physiol. 61:408-412; 1990.

81. Graham, T.E.; Spriet, L.L. Performance and metabolic responses to a high caffeine dose during prolonged exercise. J. Appl. Physiol. 71:2292-2298; 1991.

82. Green, H.J.; Sutton, J.R.; Wolfel, E.E.; Reeves, J.T.; Butterfield, G.E.; Brooks, G.A. Altitude acclimatization and energy metabolic adaptations in skeletal muscle during exercise. J. Appl. Physiol. 73:2701-2708; 1992.

83. Greenhaff, P.L.; Soderlund, K.; Ren, J.-M.; Hultman, E. Energy metabolism in single human muscle fibres during intermittent contraction with occluded circulation. J. Physiol. 460:443-453; 1993.

84. Gross, S.R.; Meyer, S.E. Regulation of phosphorylase b to a conversion in muscle. Life Sci. 14:401-414; 1974.

85. Handberg, A.; Kayser, L.; Høyer, P.E.; Vinten, J. A substantial part of GLUT1 in crude membranes from muscle originates from perineural sheaths. Am. J. Physiol. 262:E721-E727; 1992.

85a. Hardy, R.W.; Ladenson, J.H.; Henriksen, E.J.; Holloszy, J.O.; McDonald, J.M. Palmitate stimulates glucose transport in rat adipocytes by a mechanism involving translocation of the insulin sensitive glucose transporter (GLUT4). Biochem. Biophys. Res. Comm. 177:343-349; 1991.

86. Hargreaves, M.; Briggs, C.A. Effect of carbohydrate ingestion on exercise metabolism. J. Appl. Physiol. 65:1553-1555; 1988.

87. Hargreaves, M.; Costill, D.L.; Coggan, A.; Fink, W.J.; Nishibata, I. Effect of carbohydrate feedings on muscle glycogen utilization and exercise performance. Med. Sci. Sports Exerc. 16:219-222; 1984.

88. Hargreaves, M.; Costill, D.L.; Fink, W.J.; King, D.S.; Fielding, R.A. Effect of preexercise carbohydrate feedings on endurance cycling performance. Med. Sci. Sports Exerc. 19:33-36; 1987.

89. Hargreaves, M.; Costill, D.L.; Katz, A.; Fink, W.J. Effect of fructose ingestion on muscle glycogen use during exercise. Med. Sci. Sports Exerc. 17:360-363; 1985.

90. Hargreaves, M.; Kiens, B.; Richter, E.A. Effect of increased plasma free fatty acid concentrations on muscle metabolism in exercising men. J. Appl. Physiol. 70:194-201; 1991.

90a. Hargreaves, M.; McConell, G.; Proietto, J. Influence of muscle glycogen on glycogenolysis and glucose uptake during exercise. J. Appl. Physiol. 78:288-292; 1995.

91. Hargreaves, M.; Meredith, I.; Jennings, G.L. Muscle glycogen and glucose uptake during exercise in humans. Exp. Physiol. 77:641-644; 1992.

92. Hargreaves, M.; Richter, E.A. Regulation of skeletal muscle glycogenolysis during exercise. Can. J. Sport Sci. 13:197-203; 1988.

93. Hartling, O.J.; Trap-Jensen, J.P. Stimulation of β-adrenoceptors in the exercising human forearm. Clin. Physiol. 2:363-371; 1982.

94. Henriksen, E.J.; Bourey, R.E.; Rodnick, K.J.; Koranyi, L.; Permutt, M.A.; Holloszy, J.O. Glucose transporter protein content and glucose transport capacity in rat skeletal muscles. Am. J. Physiol. 259:E593-E598; 1990.

95. Hermansen, L.; Hultman, E.; Saltin, B. Muscle glycogen during prolonged severe exercise. Acta Physiol. Scand. 71:129-139; 1967.

96. Hespel, P.; Richter, E.A. Mechanism linking glycogen concentration and glycogenolytic rate in perfused contracting rat skeletal muscle. Biochem. J. 284:777-780; 1992.

97. Hespel, P.; Richter, E.A. Glucose uptake and transport in contracting, perfused rat muscle with different pre-contraction glycogen concentrations. J. Physiol. 427:347-359; 1990.

98. Hickson, R.C.; Rennie, M.J.; Conlee, R.K.; Winder, W.W.; Holloszy, J.O. Effects of increased plasma fatty acids on glycogen utilization and endurance. J. Appl. Physiol. 43:829-833; 1977.

99. Hirshman, M.F.; Wallberg-Henriksson, H.; Wardzala, L.J.; Horton, E.D.; Horton, E.S. Acute exercise increases the number of plasma membrane glucose transporters in rat skeletal muscle. FEBS Lett. 238:235-239; 1988.

100. Holloszy, J.O.; Constable, S.H.; Young, D.A. Activation of glucose transport in muscle by exercise. Diabetes/Metabolism Reviews 1:409-423; 1986.

101. Houmard, J.A.; Egan, P.C.; Neufer, P.D.; Friedman, J.E.; Wheeler, W.S.; Israel, R.G.; Dohm, G.L. Elevated skeletal muscle glucose transporter levels in exercise trained middle-aged men. Am. J. Physiol. 261:E437-E443; 1991.

101a. Houmard, J.A.; Shinebarger, M.H.; Dolan, P.L.; Leggett-Frazier, N.; Bruner, R.K.; McCammon, M.R.; Israel, R.G.; Dohm, G.L. Exercise training increases GLUT4 protein concentration in previously sedentary middle-aged men. Am. J. Physiol. 264:E896-E901; 1993.

102. Hurley, B.F.; Nemeth, P.M.; Martin, W.H.; Hagberg, J.M.; Dalsky, G.P.; Holloszy, J.O. Muscle triglyceride utilization during exercise: effect of training. J. Appl. Physiol. 60:562-567; 1986.

103. Idstrom, J.-P.; Rennie, M.J.; Schersten, T.; Bylund-Fellenius, A.-C. Membrane transport in relation to net uptake of glucose in the perfused rat hindlimb: stimulatory effects of insulin, hypoxia and contractile activity. Biochem. J. 233:131-137; 1986.

104. Issekutz, B. Effect of β-adrenergic blockade on lactate turnover in exercising dogs. J. Appl. Physiol. 57:1754-1759; 1984.

105. Issekutz, B. Effect of epinephrine on carbohydrate metabolism in exercising dogs. Metabolism 34:457-464; 1985.

106. Jacobs, I.; Romet, T.T.; Kerrigan-Brown, D. Muscle glycogen depletion during exercise at 9°C and 21°C. Eur. J. Appl. Physiol. 54:35-39; 1985.

107. James, D.E.; Kraegen, E.W.; Chisholm, D.J. Muscle glucose metabolism in exercising rats: comparison with insulin stimulation. Am. J. Physiol. 248:E575-E580; 1985.

108. Jansson, E.; Hjemdahl, P.; Kaijser, L. Epinephrine-induced changes in muscle carbohydrate metabolism during exercise in male subjects. J. Appl. Physiol. 60:1466-1470; 1986.

109. Jansson, E.; Keijser, L. Effect of diet on the utilization of blood-borne and intramuscular substrates during exercise in man. Acta Physiol. Scand. 115:19-30; 1982.

110. Jansson, E.; Kaijser, L. Substrate utilization and enzymes in skeletal muscle of extremely endurance-trained men. J. Appl. Physiol. 62:999-1005; 1987.

111. Juhlin-Dannfelt, A.C.; Terblanche, S.E.; Fell, R.D.; Young, J.C.; Holloszy, J.O. Effects of β-adrenergic receptor blockade on glycogenolysis during exercise. J. Appl. Physiol. 53:549-554; 1982.

112. Johnson, L.N. Glycogen phosphorylase: control by phosphorylation and allosteric effectors. FASEB J. 6:2274-2282; 1992.

113. Kahn, B.B. Facilitative glucose transporters: regulatory mechanisms and dysregulation in diabetes. J. Clin. Invest. 89:1367-1374; 1992.

114. Karlsson, J.; Saltin, B. Diet, muscle glycogen, and endurance performance. J. Appl. Physiol. 31:203-206; 1971.

115. Katz, A.; Broberg, S.; Sahlin, K.; Wahren, J. Leg glucose uptake during maximal dynamic exercise in humans. Am. J. Physiol. 251:E65-E70; 1986.

116. Katz, A.; Sahlin, K. Regulation of lactic acid production during exercise. J. Appl. Physiol. 65:509-518; 1988.

117. Katz, A.; Sahlin, K. Effect of hypoxia on glucose metabolism in human skeletal muscle during exercise. Acta Physiol. Scand. 136:377-382; 1989.

118. Katz, A.; Sahlin, K. Role of oxygen in regulation of glycolysis and lactate production in human skeletal muscle. Ex. Sport Sci. Rev. 18:1-28; 1990.

119. Katz, A.; Sahlin, K.; Broberg, S. Regulation of glucose utilization in human skeletal muscle during moderate dynamic exercise. Am. J. Physiol. 260:E411-E415; 1991.

120. Katz, A.; Sahlin, K.; Henriksson, J. Carbohydrate metabolism in human skeletal muscle during exercise is not regulated by G-1,6-P_2. J. Appl. Physiol. 65:487-489; 1988.

121. King, D.S.; Costill, D.L.; Fink, W.J.; Hargreaves, M.; Fielding, R.A. Muscle metabolism during exercise in the heat in unacclimatized and acclimatized humans. J. Appl. Physiol. 59:1350-1354; 1985.

122. King, P.A.; Hirshman, M.F.; Horton, E.D.; Horton, E.S. Glucose transport in skeletal muscle membrane vesicles from control and exercised rats. Am. J. Physiol. 257:C1128-C1134; 1989.

123. Kirwan, J.P.; Costill, D.L.; Kuipers, H.; Burrell, M.J.; Fink, W.J.; Kovaleski, J.E.; Fielding, R.A. Substrate utilization in leg muscle of men after heat acclimation. J. Appl. Physiol. 63:31-35; 1987.

124. Kjær, M.; Kiens, B.; Hargreaves, M.; Richter, E.A. Influence of active muscle mass on glucose homeostasis during exercise in humans. J. Appl. Physiol. 71:552-557; 1991.

125. Klip, A.; Paquet, M.R. Glucose transport and glucose transporters in muscle and their metabolic regulation. Diabetes Care 13:228-243; 1990.

126. Knapik, J.J.; Meredith, C.N.; Jones, B.H.; Suek, L.; Young, V.R.; Evans, W.J. Influence of fasting on carbohydrate and fat metabolism during rest and exercise in men. J. Appl. Physiol. 64:1923-1929; 1988.

127. Koivisto, V.A.; Harkonen, M.; Karonen, S.-L.; Groop, P.H.; Elovainio, R.; Ferrannini, E.; Sacca, L.; DeFronzo, R.A. Glycogen depletion during prolonged exercise: influence of glucose, fructose, or placebo. J. Appl. Physiol. 58:731-737; 1985.

128. Kozlowski, S.; Brzezinska, Z.; Kruk, B.; Kaciuba-Uscilko, H.; Greenleaf, J.E.; Nazar, K. Exercise hyperthermia as a factor limiting physical performance: temperature effect on muscle metabolism. J. Appl. Physiol. 59:766-773; 1985.

129. Krogh, A.; Lindhard, J. The relative value of fat and carbohydrate as sources of muscular energy. Biochem. J. 14:290-363; 1920.

130. Kuipers, H.; Costill, D.L.; Porter, D.A.; Fink, W.J.; Morse, W.M. Glucose feeding and exercise in trained rats: mechanism of glycogen sparing. J. Appl. Physiol. 61:859-863; 1986.

131. Lewis, S.F.; Haller, R.G. The pathophysiology of McArdle's disease: clues to regulation in exercise and fatigue. J. Appl. Physiol. 61:391-401; 1986.

132. Loy, S.F.; Conlee, R.K.; Winder, W.W.; Nelson, A.G.; Arnall, D.A.; Fisher, A.G. Effects of 24-hour fast on cycling endurance time at two different intensities. J. Appl. Physiol. 61:654-659; 1986.

133. Marker, J.C.; Arnall, D.A.; Conlee, R.K.; Winder, W.W. Effect of adrenodemedullation on metabolic responses to high-intensity exercise. Am. J. Physiol. 251:R552-R559; 1986.

134. Martin, B.; Robinson, S.; Robertshaw, D. Influence of diet on leg glucose uptake during heavy exercise. Am. J. Clin. Nutr. 31:62-67; 1978.

135. Martineau, L.; Jacobs, I. Muscle glycogen utilization during shivering thermogenesis in humans. J. Appl. Physiol. 65:2046-2050; 1988.

136. Mazzeo, R.S.; Bender, P.R.; Brooks, G.A.; Butterfield, G.E.; Groves, B.M.; Sutton, J.R.; Wolfel, E.E.; Reeves, J.T. Arterial catecholamine responses during exercise with acute and chronic high altitude exposure. Am. J. Physiol. 261:E419-E424; 1991.

137. Mazzeo, R.S.; Marshall, P. Influence of plasma catecholamines on the lactate threshold during graded exercise. J. Appl. Physiol. 67:1319-1322; 1989.

137a. McConell, G.; Fabris, S.; Proietto, J.; Hargreaves, M. Effect of carbohydrate ingestion on glucose kinetics during exercise. J. Appl. Physiol. 77:1537-1541; 1994.

138. McDermott, J.C.; Elder, G.C.B.; Bonen, A. Adrenal hormones enhance glycogenolysis in nonexercising muscle during exercise. J. Appl. Physiol. 63:1275-1283; 1987.

139. McDermott, J.C.; Elder, G.C.B.; Bonen, A. Non-exercising muscle metabolism during exercise. Pflugers Arch. 418:301-307; 1991.

140. Megeney, L.A.; Elder, G.C.B.; Tan, M.H.; Bonen, A. Increased glucose transport in nonexercising muscle. Am. J. Physiol. 262:E20-E26; 1992.

141. Nazar, K.; Brezezinska, Z.; Kowalski, W. Mechanism of impaired capacity for prolonged muscular work following β-adrenergic blockade in dogs. Pflugers Arch. 336:72-78; 1972.

142. Nesher, R.; Karl, I.E.; Kipnis, D.M. Dissociation of effects of insulin and contraction on glucose transport in rat epitrochlearis muscle. Am. J. Physiol. 249:C226-C232; 1985.

143. Neufer, P.D.; Shinebarger, M.H.; Dohm, G.L. Effect of training and detraining on skeletal muscle glucose transporter (GLUT4) content in rats. Can. J. Physiol. Pharmacol. 70:1286-1290; 1992.

144. Nielsen, B.; Savard, G.; Richter, E.A.; Hargreaves, M.; Saltin, B. Muscle blood flow and metabolism during exercise and heat stress. J. Appl. Physiol. 69:1040-1046; 1990.

145. Nieman, D.C.; Carlson, K.A.; Brandstater, M.E.; Naegele, R.T.; Blankenship, J.W. Running endurance in 27-h-fasted humans. J. Appl. Physiol. 63:2502-2509; 1987.

146. Nygaard, E.; Honnens, B.; Tungelund, K.; Chritensen, T.; Galbo, H. Fat as a fuel in energy-turnover of man and woman. Acta Physiol. Scand. 120:51a; 1984.

147. Picton, C.; Klee, C.B.; Cohen, P. The regulation of muscle phosphorylase kinase by calcium ions, calmodulin and troponin C. Cell Calcium 2:281-294; 1981.

148. Ploug, T.; Galbo, H.; Richter, E.A. Increased muscle glucose uptake during contractions: no need for insulin. Am. J. Physiol. 247:E726-E731; 1984.

149. Ploug, T.; Galbo, H.; Vinten, J.; Jørgensen, M.; Richter, E.A. Kinetics of glucose transport in rat muscle; effects of insulin and contractions. Am. J. Physiol. 253:E12-E20; 1987.

150. Ploug, T.; Galbo, H.; Ohkuwa, T.; Tranum-Jensen, J.; Vinten, J. Kinetics of glucose transport in rat skeletal muscle membrane vesicles: effects of insulin and contractions. Am. J. Physiol. 262:E700-E711; 1992.

151. Ploug, T.; Wojtaszewski, J.; Kristiansen, S.; Hespel, P.; Galbo, H.; Richter, E.A. Glucose transport and transporters in muscle giant vesicles: differential effects of insulin and contractions. Am. J. Physiol. 264:E270-E278; 1993.

152. Randle, P.J.; Garland, P.B.; Hales, C.N.; Newsholme, E.A. The glucose-fatty acid cycle: its role in insulin sensitivity and the metabolic disturbances of diabetes mellitus. Lancet 1:785-789; 1963.

153. Randle, P.J.; Newsholme, E.A.; Garland, P.B. Regulation of glucose uptake by muscle: 8. Effects of fatty acids, ketone bodies and pyruvate, and of alloxan diabetes and starvation, on the uptake and metabolic rate of glucose in rat heart and diaphragm muscles. Biochem. J. 93:652-665; 1964.

154. Ravussin, E.; Bogardus, C.; Scheidegger, K.; LaGrange, B.; Horton, E.D.; Horton, E.S. Effect of elevated FFA on carbohydrate and lipid oxidation during prolonged exercise in humans. J. Appl. Physiol. 60:893-900; 1986.

155. Raz, I.; Katz, A.; Spencer, M.K. Epinephrine inhibits insulin-mediated glycogenesis but enhances glycolysis in human skeletal muscle. Am. J. Physiol. 260:E430-E435; 1991.

156. Reichard, G.A.; Issekutz, B.; Kimbel, P.; Putnam, R.C.; Hochella, N.J.; Weinhouse, S. Blood glucose metabolism in man during muscular work. J. Appl. Physiol. 16:1001-1005; 1961.

157. Ren, J.-M.; Broberg, S.; Sahlin, K.; Hultman, E. Influence of reduced glycogen level on glycogenolysis during short-term stimulation in man. Acta Physiol. Scand. 139:467-474; 1990.

158. Ren, J.-M.; Gulve, E.A.; Cartee, G.D.; Holloszy, J.O. Hypoxia causes glycogenolysis without an increase in percent phosphorylase a in rat skeletal muscle. Am. J. Physiol. 263:E1086-E1091; 1992.

159. Ren, J.-M.; Hultman, E. Regulation of glycogenolysis in human skeletal muscle. J. Appl. Physiol. 67:2243-2248; 1989.

160. Ren, J.-M.; Hultman, E. Regulation of phosphorylase a activity in human skeletal muscle. J. Appl. Physiol. 69:919-923; 1990.

161. Rennie, M.J.; Fell, R.D.; Ivy, J.L.; Holloszy, J.O. Adrenaline reactivation of muscle phosphorylase activity after deactivation during phasic contractile activity. Biosci. Rep. 2:323-331; 1982.

162. Rennie, M.J.; Holloszy, J.O. Inhibition of glucose uptake and glycogenolysis by availability of oleate in perfused skeletal muscle. Biochem. J. 168:161-170; 1977.

163. Rennie, M.J.; Winder, W.W.; Holloszy, J.O. A sparing effect of increased plasma fatty acids on muscle and liver glycogen content in the exercising rat. Biochem. J. 156:647-655; 1976.

164. Richter, E.A.; Christensen, N.J.; Galbo, H. Control of exercise-induced muscular glycogenolysis by adrenal medullary hormones in rats. J. Appl. Physiol. 50:21-26; 1981.

165. Richter, E.A.; Cleland, P.J.F.; Rattigan, S.; Clark, M.G. Contraction-associated translocation of protein kinase C in rat skeletal muscle. FEBS Lett. 217:232-236; 1987.

166. Richter, E.A.; Galbo, H. High glycogen levels enhance glycogen breakdown in isolated contracting skeletal muscle. J. Appl. Physiol. 61:827-831; 1986.

167. Richter, E.A.; Kiens, B.; Saltin, B.; Christensen, N.J.; Savard, G. Skeletal muscle glucose uptake during dynamic exercise in humans: role of muscle mass. Am. J. Physiol. 254:E555-E561; 1988.

168. Richter, E.A.; Ruderman, N.B.; Galbo, H. Alpha and beta adrenergic effects on metabolism in contracting, perfused muscle. Acta Physiol. Scand. 116:215-222; 1982.

169. Richter, E.A.; Ruderman, N.B.; Gavras, H.; Belur, E.R.; Galbo, H. Muscle glycogenolysis during exercise: dual control by epinephrine and contractions. Am. J. Physiol. 242:E25-E32; 1982.

170. Richter, E.A.; Sonne, B.; Christensen, N.J.; Galbo, H. Role of epinephrine for muscular glycogenolysis and pancreatic hormonal secretion in running rats. Am. J. Physiol. 240:E526-E532; 1981.

171. Rodnick, K.J.; Henriksen, E.J.; James, D.E.; Holloszy, J.O. Exercise training, glucose transporters, and glucose transport in rat skeletal muscles. Am. J. Physiol. 262:C9-C14; 1992.

172. Rodnick, K.J.; Slot, J.W.; Studelska, D.R.; Hanpeter, D.E.; Robinson, L.J.; Geuze, H.J.; James, D.E. Immunocytochemical and biochemical studies of GLUT4 in rat skeletal muscle. J. Biol. Chem. 267:6278-6285; 1992.

173. Roth, D.A. The sarcolemmal lactate transporter: transmembrane determinants of lactate flux. Med. Sci. Sports Exerc. 23:925-934; 1991.

174. Sahlin, K.; Areskog, N.-H.; Haller, R.G.; Henriksson, K.G.; Jorfeldt, L.; Lewis, S.F. Impaired oxidative metabolism increases adenine nucleotide breakdown in McArdle's disease patients. J. Appl. Physiol. 69:1231-1235; 1990.

175. Sahlin, K.; Katz, A.; Broberg, S. Tricarboxylic acid cycle intermediates in human muscle during prolonged exercise. Am. J. Physiol. 259:C834-C841; 1990.

176. Saltin, B.; Karlsson, J. Muscle glycogen utilization during work of different intensities. In: Saltin, B.; Pernow, B., eds. Muscle metabolism during exercise. New York: Plenum Press; 1971: 289-299.

177. Sanders, C.A.; Levinson, G.E.; Abelmann, W.H.; Freinkel, N. Effect of exercise on the peripheral utilization of glucose. N. Engl. J. Med. 271:220-225; 1964.

178. Sherman, W.M.; Costill, D.L.; Fink, W.J.; Miller, J.M. Effect of exercise-diet manipulation on muscle glycogen and its subsequent utilization during performance. Int. J. Sports Med. 2:114-118; 1981.

179. Slentz, C.A.; Davis, J.M.; Settles, D.L.; Pate, R.R.; Settles, S.J. Glucose feedings and exercise in rats: glycogen use, hormone responses, and performance. J. Appl. Physiol. 69:989-994; 1990.

180. Sonne, B.; Mikines, K.J.; Richter, E.A.; Christensen, N.J.; Galbo, H. Role of liver nerves and adrenal medulla in glucose turnover in running rats. J. Appl. Physiol. 59:1640-1646; 1985.

181. Spencer, M.K.; Katz, A. Role of glycogen in control of glycolysis and IMP formation in human muscle during exercise. Am. J. Physiol. 260:E859-E864; 1991.

182. Spencer, M.K.; Yan, Z.; Katz, A. Carbohydrate supplementation attenuates IMP accumulation in human muscle during prolonged exercise. Am. J. Physiol. 261:C71-C76; 1991.

183. Spencer, M.K.; Yan, Z.; Katz, A. Effect of low glycogen on carbohydrate and energy metabolism in human muscle during exercise. Am. J. Physiol. 262:C975-C979; 1992.

184. Spriet, L.L. Phosphofructokinase activity and acidosis during short-term tetanic contractions. Can. J. Physiol. Pharmacol. 69:298-304; 1991.

185. Spriet, L.L.; Berardinucci, L.; Marsh, D.R.; Campbell, C.B.; Graham, T.E. Glycogen content has no effect on skeletal muscle glycogenolysis during short-term tetanic stimulation. J. Appl. Physiol. 68:1883-1888; 1990.

186. Spriet, L.L.; MacLean, D.A.; Dyck, D.J.; Hultman, E.; Cederblad, G.; Graham, T.E. Caffeine ingestion and muscle metabolism during prolonged exercise in humans. Am. J. Physiol. 262:E891-E898; 1992.

187. Spriet, L.L.; Ren, J.-M.; Hultman, E. Epinephrine infusion enhances muscle glycogenolysis during prolonged electrical stimulation. J. Appl. Physiol. 64:1439-1444; 1988.

188. Stainsby, W.N.; Brechue, W.F.; O'Drobinak, D.M. Regulation of muscle lactate production. Med. Sci. Sports Exerc. 23:907-911; 1991.

189. Stainsby, W.N.; Brooks, G.A. Control of lactic acid metabolism in contracting muscles and during exercise. Ex. Sport Sci. Rev. 18:29-63; 1990.

190. Stanley, W.C. Myocardial lactate metabolism during exercise. Med. Sci. Sports Exerc. 23:920-924; 1991.

191. Stanley, W.C.; Connett, R.J. Regulation of muscle carbohydrate metabolism during exercise. FASEB J. 5:2155-2159; 1991.

192. Stanley, W.C.; Gertz, E.W.; Wisneski, J.A.; Morris, D.L.; Neese, R.; Brooks, G.A. Lactate metabolism in exercising human skeletal muscle: evidence for lactate extraction during net lactate release. J. Appl. Physiol. 60:1116-1120; 1986.

193. Stanley, W.C.; Wisneski, J.A.; Gertz, E.W.; Neese, R.A.; Brooks, G.A. Glucose and lactate interrelations during moderate-intensity exercise in humans. Metabolism 37:850-858; 1988.

194. Sternlicht, E.; Barnard, R.J.; Grimditch, G.K. Exercise and insulin stimulate skeletal muscle glucose transport through different mechanisms. Am. J. Physiol. 256:E227-E230; 1989.

195. Tarnopolsky, L.J.; MacDougall, J.D.; Atkinson, S.A.; Tarnopolsky, M.A.; Sutton, J.R. Gender differences in substrate for endurance exercise. J. Appl. Physiol. 68:302-308; 1990.

196. Treadway, J.L.; James, D.E.; Burcel, E.; Ruderman, N.B. Effect of exercise on insulin receptor binding and kinase activity in skeletal muscle. Am. J. Physiol. 256:E138-E144; 1989.

197. Trudeau, F.; Peronnet, F.; Beliveau, L.; Brisson, G. Metabolic and endocrine responses to prolonged exercise in rats under β_2-adrenergic blockade. Can. J. Physiol. Pharmacol. 67:192-196; 1989.

198. Vøllestad, N.K.; Vaage, O.; Hermansen, L. Muscle glycogen depletion patterns in type I and subgroups of type II fibres during prolonged severe exercise in man. Acta Physiol. Scand. 122:433-441; 1984.

199. Vøllestad, N.K.; Blom, P.C.S. Effect of varying exercise intensity on glycogen depletion in human muscle fibres. Acta Physiol. Scand. 125:395-405; 1985.

200. Vukovich, M.D.; Costill, D.L.; Hickey, M.S.; Trappe, S.W.; Cole, K.J.; Fink, W.J. Effect of fat emulsion infusion and fat feeding on muscle glycogen utilization during cycle exercise. J. Appl. Physiol. 75:1513-1518; 1993.

201. Wahren, J.; Felig, P.; Ahlborg, G.; Jorfeldt, L. Glucose metabolism during leg exercise in man. J. Clin. Invest. 50:2715-2725; 1971.

202. Walker, P.M.; Idstrom, J.-P.; Schersten, T.; Bylund-Fellenius, A.-C. Glucose uptake in relation to metabolic state in perfused rat hindlimb at rest and during exercise. Eur. J. Appl. Physiol. 48:163-176; 1982.

203. Wallberg-Henriksson, H.; Constable, S.H.; Young, D.A.; Holloszy, J.O. Glucose transport into rat skeletal muscle: interaction between exercise and insulin. J. Appl. Physiol. 65:909-913; 1988.

204. Wallberg-Henriksson, H.; Holloszy, J.O. Contractile activity increases glucose uptake by muscle in severely diabetic rats. J. Appl. Physiol. 57:1045-1049; 1984.

205. Wallberg-Henriksson, H.; Holloszy, J.O. Activation of glucose transport in diabetic muscle: responses to contraction and insulin. Am. J. Physiol. 249:C233-C237; 1985.

206. Wasserman, D.H.; Connolly, C.C.; Pagliassotti, M.J. Regulation of hepatic lactate balance during exercise. Med. Sci. Sports Exerc. 23:912-919; 1991.

207. Wasserman, D.H.; Geer, R.J.; Rice, D.E.; Bracy, D.; Flakoll, P.J.; Brown, L.L.; Hill, J.O.; Abumrad, N.N. Interaction of exercise and insulin action in humans. Am. J. Physiol. 260:E37-E45; 1991.

208. Wasserman, D.H.; Lacy, D.B.; Bracy, D.; Williams, P.E. Metabolic regulation in peripheral tissues and transition to increased gluconeogenic mode during prolonged exercise. Am. J. Physiol. 263:E345-E354; 1992.

209. Wasserman, D.H.; Mohr, T.; Kelly, P.; Lacy, D.B.; Bracy, D. Impact of insulin deficiency on glucose fluxes and muscle glucose metabolism during exercise. Diabetes 41:1229-1238; 1992.

210. Wasserman, K.; Beaver, W.L.; Whipp, B.J. Mechanisms and patterns of blood lactate increase during exercise in man. Med. Sci. Sports Exerc. 18:344-352; 1986.

211. Widrick, J.J.; Costill, D.L.; Fink, W.J.; Hickey, M.S.; McConell, G.K.; Tanaka, H. Carbohydrate feedings and exercise performance: influence of muscle glycogen concentration. J. Appl. Physiol. 74:2998-3005; 1993.

212. Winder, W.W.; Arogyasami, J.; Yang, H.T.; Thompson, K.G.; Nelson, L.A.; Kelly, K.P.; Han, D.H. Effects of glucose infusion in exercising rats. J. Appl. Physiol. 64:2300-2305; 1988.

213. Wolfe, B.M.; Klein, S.; Peters, E.J.; Schmidt, B.F.; Wolfe, R.R. Effect of elevated free fatty acids on glucose oxidation in normal humans. Metabolism 37:323-329; 1988.

214. Yamatani, K.; Shi, Z.Q.; Giacca, A.; Gupta, R.; Fisher, S.; Lickley, H.L.A.; Vranic, M. Role of FFA-glucose cycle in glucoregulation during exercise in total absence of insulin. Am. J. Physiol. 263:E646-E653; 1992.

215. Yaspelkis, B.B.; Scroop, G.C.; Wilmore, K.M.; Ivy, J.L. Carbohydrate metabolism during exercise in hot and thermoneutral environments. Int. J. Sports Med. 14:13-19; 1993.

216. Youn, J.H.; Gulve, E.A.; Holloszy, J.O. Calcium stimulates glucose transport in skeletal muscle by a pathway independent of contraction. Am. J. Physiol. 260:C555-C561; 1991.

217. Young, A.J.; Evans, W.J.; Cymerman, A.; Pandolf, K.B.; Knapik, J.J.; Maher, J.T. Sparing effect of chronic high-altitude exposure on muscle glycogen utilization. J. Appl. Physiol. 52:857-862; 1982.

218. Young, A.J.; Sawka, M.N.; Levine, L.; Cadarette, B.S.; Pandolf, K.B. Skeletal muscle metabolism during exercise is influenced by heat acclimation. J. Appl. Physiol. 59:1929-1935; 1985.

219. Young, D.A.; Wallberg-Henriksson, H.; Cranshaw, J.; Chen, M.; Holloszy, J.O. Effect of catecholamines on glucose uptake and glycogenolysis in rat skeletal muscle. Am. J. Physiol. 248:C406-C409; 1985.

220. Zierath, J.R.; Galuska, D.; Thorne, A.; Nolte, L.; Smedegaard Kristensen, J.; Wallberg-Henriksson, H. Elevated oleate levels have no effect on insulin-stimulated glucose transport in human skeletal muscle. Acta Physiol. Scand. 146 (Suppl. 608):88; 1992.

221. Zinker, B.A.; Lacy, D.B.; Bracy, D.; Jacobs, J.; Wasserman, D.H. Regulation of glucose uptake and metabolism by working muscle. An in vivo analysis. Diabetes 42:956-965; 1993.

222. Zinker, B.A.; Lacy, D.B.; Bracy, D.P.; Wasserman, D.H. Role of glucose and insulin loads to the exercising limb in increasing glucose uptake and metabolism. J. Appl. Physiol. 74:2915-2921; 1993.

223. Zorzano, A.T.; Balon, T.W.; Brady, L.J.; Rivera, P.; Garetto, L.P.; Young, J.C.; Goodman, M.N.; Ruderman, N.B. Effects of starvation and exercise on concentrations of citrate, hexose phosphates and glycogen in skeletal muscle and heart: evidence for selective operation of the glucose-fatty acid cycle. Biochem. J. 232:585-591; 1985.

————— Chapter 3 —————

Hepatic Fuel Metabolism During Exercise

MICHAEL KJÆR

During physical exercise, an increased release of glucose from the liver is important to maintain blood glucose homeostasis and thereby avoid hypoglycemia. In 1961 scientists, using an isotope dilution technique with infusion of [U-14C]-glucose, demonstrated, in one human subject, that whole-body glucose turnover was increased during physical activity (61). The decrease in blood glucose specific activity during exercise provided indirect evidence that hepatic glucose production was accelerated 3-6 times that of resting values during muscular work (61). Later, measurements of splanchnic glucose output during exercise in humans taken with arterial and hepatic venous catherization showed an increase in glucose production during exercise of up to 20 μmol/kg/min at whole-body oxygen uptake rates of 2.2-2.3 L O_2/min (67). Although the catheter-technique, when used in humans, does not distinguish between the contributions of substances from liver and gut, measurement of splanchnic glucose output provides a good indicator of glucose production from the liver, as long as subjects are postabsorptive. The experiment by Rowell et al. (67) demonstrated that liver glucose production during exercise in humans was increased threefold from resting values. In several later studies, hepatic glucose output was found to increase two- to threefold during moderate exercise and up to seven- to tenfold during more vigorous leg exercise in both humans (1, 4, 8, 9, 12, 13, 17-19, 29, 31, 41, 43-45, 47-49, 53, 57, 72, 87, 88) and other species (73-76, 79, 80, 82, 90, 93, 94). During steady state exercise in the rat, the rate of glucose turnover, and thereby of hepatic glucose output, is directly related to work intensity in both trained (11) and untrained animals (73, 75). In accordance with this, in postabsorptive humans the exercise-induced rise in splanchnic glucose production is correlated with an increase in work output (87) (Figure 3.1). Summarizing data obtained from experiments in humans indicates that splanchnic glucose output rises linearly with exercise intensity up to 50-60% $\dot{V}O_2$ max, whereas at higher workloads the glucose output increases exponentially with the relative exercise intensity (%$\dot{V}O_2$ max), despite a gradual decrease in hepato-splanchnic blood flow (68).

During moderate exercise (<60% $\dot{V}O_2$ max), the blood glucose level remains relatively constant, despite a marked exercise-induced rise in peripheral uptake of glucose in contracting muscle (47), and a major drop in blood glucose is not observed unless exercise is prolonged for several hours (1, 20). This indicates that the exercise-induced rise in hepatic glucose output matches the increased glucose uptake by contracting skeletal muscle as long as sufficient stores of glycogen are present in the liver. In contrast, if exercise becomes more intense (> 60% $\dot{V}O_2$ max), blood glucose is usually found to increase in humans, indicating that the hepatic glucose output exceeds the peripheral glucose uptake (13, 29, 43, 44, 47). This confirms the hypothesis that mechanisms other than feedback regulation to maintain euglycemia are involved in the mobilization of glucose from the liver during exercise.

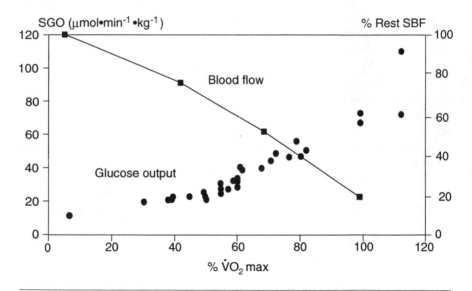

Figure 3.1 Hepatic glucose production (splanchnic glucose output=SGO) at rest and during exercise related to the relative work intensity (%$\dot{V}O_2$ max). The basal value is the mean of values obtained from 84 subjects, and during exercise (running and bicycling) each value represents the mean of 5-10 subjects. Data are taken from references 1,4,8,9,12,13,17-19,29,31,41,43-45,47-49,53,57,72,87, and 88. Determination of splanchnic glucose output was done using either an isotope dilution technique with infusion of radiolabeled glucose or an arterial and hepatic venous catherization, with measurement of arterial and hepatic venous glucose concentration and simultaneous determination of hepato-splanchnic blood flow.

In addition to the glucose-mobilizing role of the liver, carbon- and nitrogen-bound compounds are extracted from the bloodstream. Some of these compounds serve as substrates for formation of glucose via gluconeogenesis, whereas others are metabolized into urea, built into proteins, or cause an acceleration of ketogenesis. Although not all processes are thoroughly investigated, they are all likely to be accelerated markedly during physical activity (15, 21, 71, 88, 89, 93).

Hepatic Glucose Output During Exercise: Glycogenolysis and Gluconeogenesis

With the transition from rest to exercise, liver glucose production increases due to an enhancement of both glycogenolysis and gluconeogenesis. During moderate and heavy exercise of short duration (less than 30 min), almost the entire increase in splanchnic glucose output is caused by an accelerated hepatic glycogenolysis (87, 88, 92). The contribution of glycogenolysis is demonstrated by an exercise-induced reduction in liver glycogen content in both the rat (76) and in humans (33) (Figure 3.2).

The contribution of gluconeogenesis to hepatic glucose output during the first 60 min of light exercise is only 5-15%, as estimated from the total

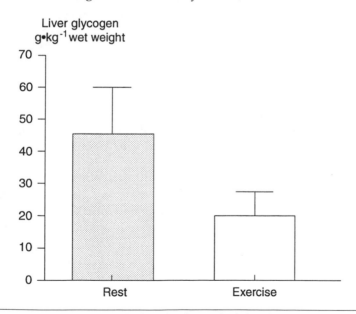

Figure 3.2   Fourteen overnight-fasted subjects had their liver glycogen concentration determined in liver biopsies after they completed 1 hour of heavy exercise on a bicycle ergometer. Concentrations were significantly lower (p<0.001) compared with liver glycogen concentration determined in 33 normal postabsorptive resting subjects who underwent a liver biopsy at the same time of the day as the exercising subjects. Data taken from Hultman and Nilsson (33). Values are mean ± SE.

hepatic uptake of gluconeogenic substances in dogs (92, 98). However, when exercise is continued for more than 60 min, the relative contribution of gluconeogenesis increases to 20-25% (92, 98). In humans, the uptake of gluconeogenic precursors increases with exercise duration, accounting for almost half the total splanchnic glucose production after 4 hours of exercise (1). Further evidence for increased gluconeogenesis during exercise is obtained from experiments that found that gluconeogenic enzyme activity is elevated by exercise (22). Taken together, these findings indicate that the relative contribution of glycogenolysis and gluconeogenesis in the liver is determined by both duration and intensity of exercise, and that the role of gluconeogenesis increases with duration and decreases with intensity of the physical activity.

The absorptive state of the organism influences the relative importance of gluconeogenesis. In subjects who fasted for 60 hours, almost all of the increase in splanchnic glucose output during mild exercise is due to uptake of gluconeogenic precursors (9). It should be noted, however, that in fasted subjects overall peripheral glucose uptake is markedly diminished compared with postabsorptive control subjects, indicating a decrease in the overall requirement for glucose output (9, 53). Furthermore, the delivery of gluconeogenic precursors was, in that study, found to be markedly increased in the fasted compared with the postabsorptive state (9). In contrast, if subjects receive glucose or fructose before or during exercise, a diminished splanchnic uptake of gluconeogenic precursors is observed, most likely resulting in a reduced contribution of gluconeogenesis (2, 3, 6). However, in those experiments the intake of glucose induced hormonal changes favoring a reduced overall hepatic glucose output, making it difficult to draw conclusions regarding the role of glucose per se on gluconeogenesis during exercise. Thus, the relative contribution of gluconeogenesis to the total glucose output from the liver during exercise increases with the time since the last intake of carbohydrates, and it is, at least partly, due to a gradual reduction in liver glycogen content as exercise proceeds (33).

The increase in liver gluconeogenesis during prolonged exercise is important for the conversion of glycerol, lactate, and amino acids into glucose in order to delay depletion of liver and muscle glycogen, and the gluconeogenic capacity is increased with physical training (34). When gluconeogenesis is blocked in rats by administration of mercaptopicolinic acid, exercise endurance time is diminished by approximately 30% in both trained and untrained animals (40). This inhibition of gluconeogenesis resulted in a 20% lower glucose output from the liver and a more marked hepatic glycogen breakdown during exercise in experimental running rats compared with sham-operated and treated controls (77). In humans, gluconeogenic substrate uptake has been reduced by an infusion of ethanol, and this resulted in a marked reduction in hepatic glucose output after 180 min of mild exercise (41). In contrast, if one increases the output of gluco-neogenic precursors by performing a given absolute workload with the arms instead of the legs, hepatic gluconeogenesis is increased more during arm exercise compared with leg exercise (5).

The liver glycogen content influences the magnitude of glucose output during exercise. This is based on findings in rats in which liver glycogen levels were increased and decreased by fructose feeding and food restriction, respectively (75, 76). During treadmill running a correlation was found between the rise in hepatic glucose output and liver glycogen levels, indicating that liver glycogen concentration is an important determinant of liver glycogenolysis and, therefore, of glucose production (75, 76). Furthermore, in running rats who were either controls or fasted then fed, whereby they obtained supranormal liver glycogen levels, hepatic glycogenolysis during exercise was directly related to hepatic glycogen content (82). In trained rats, and probably also in trained man, liver glycogen contents are larger compared with physically untrained counterparts (27). In accordance with the aforementioned findings, hepatic glucose output during exercise was greater in trained than in untrained rats (11) and greater in endurance trained athletes than in untrained healthy control subjects when groups were compared at identical relative workloads (45). Therefore, the glycogenolytic activity and thereby the glucose mobilization from the liver during exercise is dependent on the glycogen content of the liver.

Feedback Regulation of Hepatic Glucose Output During Exercise

Feedback mechanisms have been claimed to be very important for a precise matching of hepatic glucose output to the increased glucose requirements of contracting muscles. It has been suggested that a major regulating mechanism is a change in blood glucose levels per se, reflecting changes in the need for substrate mobilization. In support of this, infusion of glucose during exercise, in order to mimic the exercise-induced increase in hepatic glucose production in control experiments, resulted in an abolition of the endogenous glucose production during moderate exercise in both humans (60% $\dot{V}O_2$ max) (38, 39) and rats (79). The fact that glucose infusion in those experiments resulted in only a very moderate change in plasma glucose (4-5 mg%) indicates that hepatic glucose production is very sensitive to feedback signals and, furthermore, that signals that contribute to an exercise-induced increase in glucose production can be inhibited by glucose infusion. Also in the running dog, infusion of glucose reduced endogenous glucose production, but the hepatic glucose production was not totally abolished, especially not at the onset of exercise (37). This indicates that feedback signals are active during muscle contraction, but are not solely responsible for the exercise-induced increase in mobilization of glucose. To further support the suggestion that feedback signals might not be the only mechanisms responsible for a rise in hepatic glucose production during exercise, human experiments with plasma glucagon and insulin kept at constant and basal levels have been carried out. They demonstrated that splanchnic glucose production increased and reached a plateau after approximately 10 min of mild exercise, despite the fact that plasma glucose underwent an ongoing decrease from 5 to 4 mmol · L^{-1} throughout the 20-min exercise period (48).

In rats, infusion of phlorizin during exercise has been used to increase renal loss of glucose and thereby increase glucose clearance (80). In experiments where infusion of phlorizin increased glucose loss but did not decrease blood glucose level from rest, a compensatory increase in splanchnic glucose output was seen in rats during mild exercise compared with saline-infused running control rats (80). These findings indicate that metabolic feedback mechanisms, unrelated to glycemia per se, might also be involved in regulation of hepatic glucose production during mild exercise.

Afferent nervous activity from contracting muscles potentially could be important for hepatic glucose production. In cats, electrical stimulation of the central end of cut muscle nerves (n. femoralis) resulted in both an increase in plasma glucose and a rise in hepatic glucose output (84a). In humans, however, reducing the afferent neural feedback by partial lumbar epidural sensory blockade did not influence glucose production during leg cycling (46). Although afferent neural reflex mechanisms can result in increased glucose mobilization during exercise, they probably are secondary to more important regulatory mechanisms in healthy humans. In patients, however, neural feedback mechanisms might be of major importance if other mechanistic pathways are restricted. In myophosphorylase deficient humans (McArdle's disease) with absent muscle glycogenolysis, mobilization of extramuscular fuel during exercise (i.e., splanchnic glucose output) is enhanced compared with results obtained in healthy control subjects. This difference cannot be explained by blood-error signals and, therefore, indicates the importance of neural feedback from metabolism in working skeletal muscle in these patients (84). When glucose was infused into patients to mimic the normal increase in splanchnic glucose output seen in control subjects during exercise, the endogenous splanchnic glucose production was abolished (84).

Feed-Forward Regulation of Hepatic Glucose Output During Exercise

Contradicting the feedback hypothesis on regulation of hepatic glucose production during exercise, an early study found that plasma glucose concentration does not decrease, but rather increases, during intense exercise (60). This has been found to be caused by an exercise-induced rise in hepatic glucose production that exceeds the rise in peripheral glucose uptake in both running rats (73) and bicycling and running humans (13,

43-45, 47, 57). This mismatch between glucose production and peripheral glucose uptake is more pronounced with increasing work intensity (19, 44, 47, 87) and early in exercise compared with late in exercise (45, 73). This indicates that mobilization of hepatic glucose in response to exercise is an event determined, at least in part, by activity in motor centers in the central nervous system (central command) and that glucose production is subject to feed-forward rather than feedback regulation (Figure 3.3).

In humans, experiments have been carried out where central command was enhanced by partial neuromuscular blockade (tubocurarine), and it has been demonstrated that the initial increase in glucose production was greater in curare-treated subjects than in control subjects, although absolute workloads (and peripheral glucose uptake) were identical in the two situations (45) (Figure 3.4). Further indicating that hepatic glucose production can rise independently of feedback signals, glucose infused at a high rate (twice the liver glycogenolysis rate in a control study) resulting in a large increase in plasma glucose decreased liver glycogen breakdown by only 30-40% in exercising rats (101). More direct evidence for the role of feed-forward mechanisms in hepatic glucose production was derived from experiments on rats whose hypothalamic centers were blocked or stimulated. When the ventromedial area of the hypothalamus (VMH) was blocked with infusion of an α-adrenergic antagonist, the normal exercise-induced increase in the rats' plasma glucose during swimming exercise was blocked (69). And when bilateral anaesthetic ablation of the VMH was established in rats, the increase in hepatic glucose production and plasma glucose during running was attenuated when compared with results from control rats (83). In addition, when electrical stimulation of the posterior hypothalamic locomotor region was performed in decorticated and anesthetized cats, where feedback from contracting muscle was prevented by neuromuscular blockade and anesthesia, respectively, an increase in hepatic glucose production similar to that seen during voluntary exercise was found (81). These results strongly support the findings in human studies that activation of motor centers in the brain, in parallel with activation of locomotion, induces an increase in glucose mobilization from the liver, either directly via nerves or indirectly via changes in glucoregulatory hormones.

In tetraplegic individuals whose legs were electrically stimulated by computer in bicycle exercise, peripheral glucose uptake rose by approximately 50% and plasma glucose declined by 0.7 mM. During exercise these subjects did not have any increase in hepatic glucose production from resting levels (52). This indicates that when both central command and neural feedback from muscles are lacking during exercise, neither the change in blood glucose concentration nor any other blood-borne signals from the contracting muscles were sufficient to cause an increase in hepatic glucose production (52). A similar experiment with functional electrical stimulation recently has been carried out in healthy subjects whose lower limbs were paralyzed

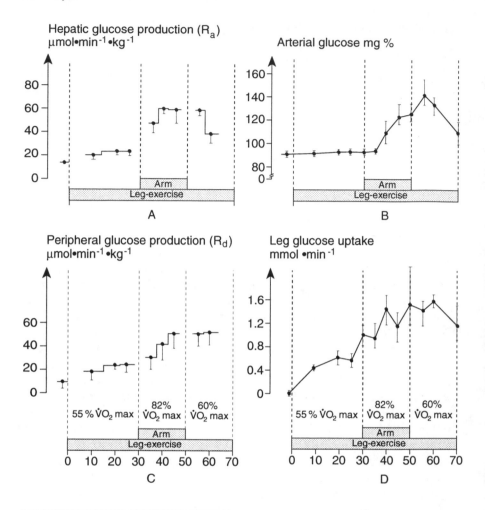

Figure 3.3 Blood glucose concentrations, whole-body glucose turnover determined with a primed constant rate tracer infusion technique (3-³H-glucose), and glucose uptake in an exercising leg determined directly from glucose concentrations in femoral arterial and venous blood and determination of blood flow using a thermo-dilution technique. This was determined at rest and during 70 min of continuous bicycling with legs only or arms and legs in 7 healthy young subjects. The legs carried out the same absolute work output (155 ± 10 Watts, mean ± SE) throughout the study. Calculated glucose uptake over 2 exercising legs showed that this accounted for approximately 82% of whole-body glucose uptake during leg exercise only. During arm and leg exercise, leg glucose uptake averaged 68% of whole-body glucose uptake. During intense exercise hepatic glucose production was always significantly (p<0.05) higher compared with peripheral glucose uptake. Values are mean ± SE. Relative workload is given as percentage of $\dot{V}O_2$ max during leg bicycling. Reprinted with permission from Kjær et al. (1991).

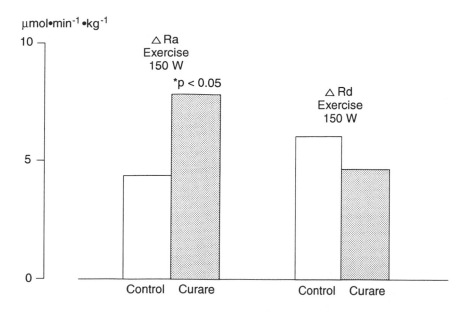

Figure 3.4   Glucose turnover during bicycling at 56% $\dot{V}O_2$ max. Eight subjects were studied with, as well as without, partial neuromuscular blockade (curare) to vary the motor center activity needed for a given workload. Mean values for changes in hepatic glucose production (Ra) and peripheral glucose uptake (Rd) during the initial 5 min of the work period are given. *(p<0.05) denotes difference between curare-treated and untreated control subjects, as well as between exercise-induced changes in Ra and Rd in curare treatments. Reprinted with permission from Kjær (1989).

temporarily with epidural anesthesia. In those subjects it was possible to perform electrically induced bicycling at an oxygen uptake rate of 1.9 L/ min (51). In accordance with the findings in tetraplegic subjects, plasma glucose was stable during voluntary $\dot{V}O_2$ matched control (no blockade) exercise with the legs, whereas plasma glucose gradually dropped when exercise was induced electrically in the absence of central command and reduced peripheral neural feedback (51). This indicates that central command and/or neural feedback is needed for a sufficient exercise-induced increase in hepatic glucose production in humans.

Whereas hepatic glucose production seems to be sensitive to inhibition by a rise in plasma glucose above normal postabsorptive resting levels, glucose production apparently is relatively insensitive to minor decreases in plasma glucose (48, 52). Furthermore, findings indicate that factors linked to exercise intensity level, and thereby to the level of motor activity, are setting the magnitude of glucose production during physical activity (45, 81, 83). In addition to this, it is possible that an unidentified factor produced by contracting muscle can directly increase hepatic glucose production during exercise. In accordance with this, during sleep, which is associated with muscle inactivity and reduced metabolic rate and glucose uptake, a drop in hepatic glucose production was found that could not be explained by known glucoregulatory (i.e., hormonal) mechanisms (16). In an attempt to investigate this question, Hua and Mikines recently perfused rat muscle and liver combined in series. In that preparation, with no endocrine glands present, no substances released from contracting muscle could be identified that were responsible for the exercise-induced increase in glucose production (Hua and Mikines, unpublished observation).

Hormonal and Neural Regulation of Hepatic Glucose Output During Exercise

The regulation of hepatic glucose output during exercise is likely to involve a complex interaction between both hormonal and neural control mechanisms.

Pancreatic Hormones.   An essential hormonal factor for the increase in hepatic glucose production during exercise is the decrease in plasma insulin (85). In exercising dogs, a rapid depression of the plasma insulin level by infusion of mannoheptulose resulted in a sudden rise in hepatic glucose production (35). The isolated role of a decrease in insulin during exercise has been studied by preventing the normal exercise-induced fall in insulin by infusing insulin intraportally, by infusing glucose to maintain euglycemia, and by infusing glucagon to obtain the normal increase during exercise. In that experiment, the insulin fall was responsible for an estimated 50-60% of the exercise-induced increase in hepatic glucose production (94). In the same experiment, the stimulatory effect was most pronounced on glycogenolysis, whereas gluconeogenesis was stimulated mainly when glucose was allowed to fall and counterregulatory hormonal responses were present (94). This seems logical because counterregulatory hormones are known to stimulate gluconeogenic precursor delivery.

In both exercising dogs and sheep, a somatostatin-induced suppression of glucagon resulted in a reduction of liver glucose production and a subsequent drop in plasma glucose (10, 36). Furthermore, in rats, treatment with glucagon antibodies resulted in a diminished glycogen breakdown in the liver in response to exercise (65). In exercising dogs, it has been shown that when both endogenous insulin and glucagon secretion are blocked by somatostatin, and insulin and glucagon are infused into the portal vein, a rise in glucagon concentration is the major factor responsible for the rise in hepatic glucogenolysis and gluconeogenesis during muscular activity (90, 93). In that study it was also demonstrated that the enhancing effect of a rise in glucagon on the hepatic glucose output during exercise was even more pronounced when it was accompanied by a fall in insulin (93). One difficult factor is that a lack of glucagon results in a drop in glucose and, therefore, activation of a counterregulatory hormonal response. To overcome this problem, counterregulation was prevented by infusing glucose to maintain euglycemia, and it was then shown that the exercise-induced increase in glucagon was responsible for 60% of the glucose output (93). Although glucagon might be an important regulator of hepatic glucose output during exercise in the dog, in humans glucagon concentration does not increase unless exercise is prolonged more than 1 hour. This indicates that an increase in glucagon is not of major importance for a rise in hepatic glucose production in humans in the early stages of exercise, but it might be of secondary importance late in exercise when blood glucose drops (26, 78).

In human experiments where plasma insulin and glucagon were held constant, conflicting results for the role of insulin and glucagon have been obtained. In some studies the glucose production was abolished (30, 56), whereas most studies found an increase (9, 31, 32, 48, 103). In one study in humans it was shown that a simultanous increase in plasma glucagon and decrease in plasma insulin had the greatest effect on hepatic glucose production, indicating interaction between the two hormones (56). In addition, if a drop in plasma insulin is prevented during exercise in dogs, the rise in hepatic glucose output, although diminished, is more sensitive to other stimuli (e.g., a drop in plasma glucose). This compensating mechanism involves acceleration primarily of gluconeogenesis, but also of glycogenolysis (99). In dogs, the ratio between glucagon and insulin probably shows the strongest correlation with a rise in liver glucose production during exercise (86). Despite the demonstration of a role for both the exercise-induced fall in insulin and the rise in plasma glucagon, these mechanisms cannot fully explain the increased hepatic glucose output during exercise in humans.

Sympathoadrenergic Activity.   In experiments in humans, the exercise-induced rise in hepatic glucose production was paralleled by a rise in plasma epinephrine and norepinephrine. If exercise was carried out in hypoxia, the rise in glucose production during exercise was more pronounced compared with that in exercise at a similar workload carried out in normoxia (18). This was accompanied by a more pronounced catecholamine response in hypoxia, whereas responses of pancreatic hormones were identical in the two experimental conditions (18). Furthermore, in experiments using leg exercise as well as combined arm and leg exercise, a positive correlation was found between plasma catecholamine concentration and hepatic glucose production (47). These findings are compatible with, but not conclusive for, the idea that sympathoadrenergic activity regulates glucose output from the liver during exercise. Both infusion of physiological doses of epinephrine and stimulation of liver nerves are known to result in an increased liver glucose output in resting humans and dogs (28, 59). In the rat, removal of the adrenal medulla resulted in a reduced hepatic glycogenolysis in response to swimming (64), and in adrenodemedullated rats, the exercise-induced increase in hepatic glucose production in response to treadmill running was diminished compared with rats with intact epinephrine secretion (74). These experiments in rats indicate that epinephrine is important for the exercise-induced rise in hepatic glucose output. However, some experiments in rats have been unable to show any effect of epinephrine on the liver glycogen breakdown during exercise (7, 14, 55, 100). The difference in study conclusions can be due to either the use of different exercise protocols including a large variety of intensities or the fact that adrenodemedullation caused a rise in plasma insulin disfavoring liver glycogenolysis. Finally, it is possible that the role of epinephrine on glycogen breakdown is mainly on muscle glycogenolysis, thereby providing more gluconeogenic precursors to the liver. The latter is in accordance with findings of higher plasma lactate levels and increased glycogen breakdown in muscles in rats with intact epinephrine production compared with adrenodemedullated animals during exercise (64). Furthermore, in fasted exercising rats depending very much on gluconeogenesis, the role of epinephrine seems to be more pronounced compared with rats that were postabsorptive (101). Experiments in dogs indicate that although a normal rise in hepatic glucose output is maintained in adrenalectomized cortisol substituted dogs, epinephrine may play a minor role in liver glucose output in the late stage during prolonged exercise (58). This is compatible with the idea that a role for epinephrine is to increase the gluconeogenic precursor level in the blood.

The role of liver nerves has been investigated in animal models. Surgical or chemical denervation of the liver did not diminish the increment in hepatic glucose production during exercise in rats (63, 74). Furthermore, in dogs the exercise-induced increase in liver glycogenolysis and gluconeogenesis was not influenced by hepatic surgical denervation (97). These findings indicate that liver nerves are not essential for the increase in liver glucose output during exercise. In humans the sympathetic liver nerve innervation is more abundant than it is in most animals, and because at the onset of exercise sympathetic liver nerve activity and hepatic glucose output increase more rapidly than production of most hormones, liver nerves might be important for the regulation of hepatic glucose production during exercise in humans. In a human study in which changes in plasma glucagon and insulin were prevented, the exercise-induced increase in glucose production was diminished if α- and β-adrenergic blockade was added (32). In addition, a comparable increase in glucose production during exercise was found between surgically adrenalectomized human subjects and control subjects (31). This provided indirect evidence for the conclusion that sympathetic liver nerves, rather than adrenomedullary secretory activity, are important for the exercise-induced rise in hepatic glucose production. The importance of sympathetic liver nerves has, however, been disputed by findings from other experiments in which α and β blockade was unable to block the normal rise in liver glucose production during exercise in humans (56, 72). In recent studies, the role of sympathoadrenergic activity has been addressed more directly in healthy subjects who underwent local anesthesia of the sympathetic coeliac ganglion that innervates the liver, the pancreas, and the adrenal medulla. Levels of pancreatic hormones and plasma glucose were held constant during rest, and during exercise at 40 and 75% $\dot{V}O_2$ max, normal exercise-induced changes in peripheral glucagon and insulin levels were assured by venous infusion of somatostatin and pancreatic hormones. During coeliac ganglion blockade, the exercise-induced increase in epinephrine was reduced by 40-90% and the plasma glucose decreased and glucose production increased as in control experiments without blockade (48). This was also the case when epinephrine was infused in substituting doses, whereas epinephrine enhanced the glucose production during exercise when infused in supraphysiological doses. This indicates that, although high physiological doses of epinephrine can enhance glucose output in exercising humans, normally neither epinephrine nor sympathetic liver nerve activity are major stimuli (48). Further support for the lack of importance of liver nerves is obtained from experiments in liver transplant patients. In accordance with findings from animal studies, the exercise-induced increase in glucose production in liver transplant patients was identical to that of healthy control subjects and kidney transplant patients who received a similar hormonal and immunosuppressive drug treatment as the liver transplant patients (49) (Figure 3.5). Liver transplant patients were investigated approximately 8 months after surgery, and no sign of hepatic sympathetic nerve reinnervation was found in any of the patients as judged from the content of norepinephrine in liver biopsies (50). These findings indicate that sympathetic liver nerves do not play an important role in the exercise-induced rise in glucose production in man.

Other Factors.   Because surgical denervation in rats diminished the exercise-induced rise in glucagon and the fall in insulin (54), it has been proposed that parasympathetic nerves to the liver influence the hepatic metabolism during exercise. If vagal activity to the liver has any functional importance, it is probably indirect via pancreatic hormones. It has not been possible to demonstrate any exercise endurance limiting effect of vagotomy (23), and no systematic influence of vagotomy on the exercise-induced rate of liver glycogen breakdown has been found (23, 54).

The hormones cortisol and growth hormone may play a minor role in stimulation of hepatic glucose production during exercise. Endurance time in running rats has been prolonged after corticosterone injection, probably due to stimulation of gluconeogenetic enzymes and increases in the gluconeogenic supply to the liver, rather than acceleration of hepatic glycogenolysis (70).

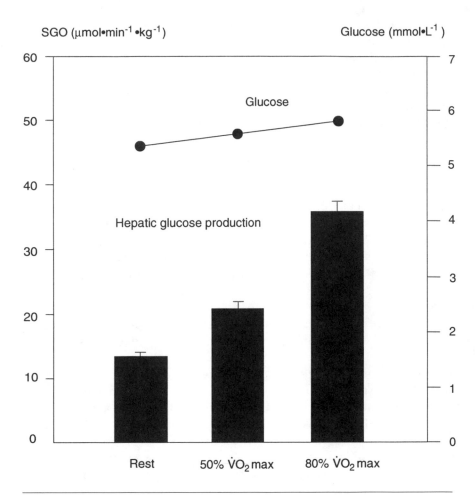

SGO (µmol•min⁻¹•kg⁻¹)

Glucose (mmol•L⁻¹)

Figure 3.5   Hepatic glucose production (splanchnic glucose output=SGO) in four postabsorptive liver transplant subjects during bicycle exercise for 20 min at 50% of maximal oxygen uptake (% $\dot{V}O_2$ max) and 20 min at 80% $\dot{V}O_2$ max, determined with infusion of 3-³H-glucose. Blood glucose concentrations were measured in arterialized hand vein blood; mean values are presented.

Hepatic Uptake of Gluconeogenic Precursors During Exercise

Hepatic Amino Acid Metabolism

An increased release of amino acids from muscle as a result of increased proteolysis during muscular work has been demonstrated with both arterio-venous catherization (1, 21, 25) and isotope dilution methods (103). These amino acids provide an important source for gluconeogenesis, and in humans splanchnic uptake of amino acids increases with exercise (Figure 3.6), the quantitatively most important one being alanine uptake, which increases by 15-20% during moderate exercise (25). This increased uptake is a consequence of a rise in splanchnic fractional extraction during exercise (1). During exercise in humans only splanchnic balance has been measured, but true hepatic balance has been determined by needle puncture of the portal vein in resting subjects undergoing abdominal surgery (25). Measurements of the arterio-portal gradient for amino acids support the notion that measuring splanchnic balance may *under*estimate true hepatic uptake of amino acids because some amino acids are released from the gut during rest (92). Compatible with this, Wasserman et al. (98) using arterial, hepatic venous, and portal catheters, demonstrated that the amino acid glutamine in running dogs was taken up by the liver five- to sixfold more during exercise than during rest, whereas a transient release of glutamine from the gut during exercise was observed. This supports the hypothesis that not only muscle, but also gut proteolysis, contributes to an increased supply of amino acids to the liver for gluconeogenesis. In addition to this, an increased proteolysis inside the liver itself can also contribute to formation of amino acids (42).

It is not clear what regulates the magnitude of amino acids involved in gluconeogenesis in humans, but an important role for the exercise-induced rise in glucagon has recently been demonstrated in exercising

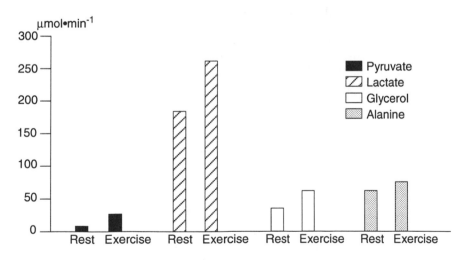

Figure 3.6 Splanchnic exchange of gluconeogenic substrates in 8 healthy control subjects at rest and after 40 min of bicycle exercise at 55-60% $\dot{V}O_2$ max. Calculations were performed using measurements of arterial and hepatic venous substrate concentrations, and estimation of hepatic blood flow was obtained using continuous infusion of indocyanine-green dye. Data are taken from Wahren, Hagenfeldt, and Felig (88).

dogs (93), and in humans the amount of alanine taken up by the liver has been found to correlate with the hepatic venous concentration of glucagon (71).

Despite the large channeling of amino acids into gluconeogenesis whereby carbon compounds are built into glucose, it is clear that pathways for nitrogen metabolism (e.g., urea formation) also need to be accelerated to take care of excess nitrogen formed by the breakdown of amino acids and to absorb ammonia released by working muscles (24). In dogs, the liver urea formation is increased 1.5-2 times during moderate exercise (98), and during extreme exercise plasma levels of urea have been found to rise markedly, indirectly indicating an increased production (62). During very mild exercise (30% $\dot{V}O_2$ max), however, it has not been possible to detect any rise in whole-body urea turnover with the isotope dilution method (102). This indicates that either exercise intensity was too low or there were limitations in the method for detecting exercise-induced effects.

Despite the fact that most studies agree on an acceleration of urea formation during exercise, the uptake of nitrogen compounds in the liver during exercise is larger than can be explained by increased urea formation, and alternative pathways have to exist. It is interesting that a recent study has demonstrated that acute exercise results in incorporation of infused radiolabeled amino acids by the liver into acute-phase proteins (fibrinogen and fibronectin) (15).

Splanchnic Lipolysis and Ketogenesis

Lipolysis in adipose tissue is markedly accelerated during muscular work, and major amounts of glycerol and free fatty acids (FFA) are released to the bloodstream. Both the uptake of glycerol, serving as a precursor for gluconeogenesis, and the uptake of FFA are increased during exercise (1, 88). The uptake of glycerol is increased twofold during prolonged exercise (Figure 3.6), and in healthy subjects this is explained by the increased arterial plama concentration rather than an increase in fractional extraction (1, 89).

During exercise the release of ketone bodies (acetoacetate and β-hydroxybutyrate) from the liver is also accelerated and correlated to the rise in FFA supply to the liver (71, 87, 89). In fact, when the rise in plasma FFA is prevented by blocking the decrease in insulin, no rise in output of ketogenic substances from the liver is found during exercise (95). It has been demonstrated in other experiments that the exercise-induced drop in insulin increases ketogenesis by increasing the extraction of FFA during exercise (96). In addition to a drop in insulin, the rise in plasma glucagon also accounts for the rise in ketogenesis during exercise (96).

In addition to increased hepatic uptake of FFA during exercise, intrahepatic fat stores might also be activated. Wahren et al. (89) found that radiolabeled oleic acid was taken up in the liver and released from the liver at increased rates during exercise, which is compatible with the idea that intrahepatic fat depots were mobilized. However, catherization of the hepatic vein in that experiment did not exclude the possibility that the mobilization of fat was actually derived from the gut rather than from the liver. In accordance with this idea, an increase in gut release and in liver uptake, respectively, of FFA during exercise was found in the running dog (95). Mobilization of splanchnic (i.e., gut) fat depots during exercise is probably regulated by local sympathetic nervous activity. This theory is supported by experiments on humans in which sympathetic nerves to the splanchnic area were blocked by local anesthesia of the coeliac ganglion. In these subjects, plasma glycerol and FFA concentrations during exercise were lower than those in control experiments without blockade (48). Even high rates of epinephrine infusion during exercise did not fully equalize this difference. Furthermore, electrical stimulation of sympathetic nerves to the canine omentum has been shown to elicit fat mobilization (66), supporting the hypothesis that sympathetic nerve activity is responsible for the mobilization of fat from the splanchnic area during exercise.

Hepatic Lactate Balance

Lactate as a glycolytic end product in muscle is a major precursor for hepatic gluconeogenesis during exercise (1, 88), and in humans a pronounced splanchnic uptake of lactate has been demonstrated during prolonged exercise (1, 88) (Figure 3.6). In running dogs true hepatic lactate balance has been determined, and Wasserman et al. (91) found that, whereas at the onset of exercise lactate was released from the liver as a result of increased glycogenolysis, when exercise duration progresses the liver switches to an uptake of lactate (91). The latter is due to increased delivery of lactate, which results in a rise in lactate uptake probably due to a mass action effect, resulting in an increase in gluconeogenesis.

The increase in plasma epinephrine during exercise may, as mentioned earlier, indirectly stimulate hepatic gluconeogenesis by increasing the muscular glycogenolysis (73, 76). When epinephrine was infused in high physiological doses during exercise, blood lactate concentrations during exercise increased more than during control experiments, despite similar peripheral glucose uptake rates in the two situations. A more pronounced counterregulatory response at the end of prolonged exercise thereby can accelerate the release of lactate from muscle and provide substrate for increased gluconeogenesis, which is necessary to produce glucose from the liver in order to match peripheral glucose uptake.

Summary

The role of the liver as a metabolic organ during exercise primarily involves the increase in production and mobilization of glucose into the bloodstream, but also includes chemical pathways for amino acid and fat metabolism that are accelerated during muscular work. Liver glucose production increases during exercise in a curvilinear fashion with work intensity. During light to moderate exercise glucose output rises two- to threefold, and during intense exercise it rises seven- to tenfold above resting values. The magnitude of liver glucose output during exercise is dependent on the liver glycogen content, which varies with the degree of fasting, the intake of food prior to exercise, and the degree of training in the individual. During exercise the glucose production is derived mainly from breakdown of liver glycogen (glycogenolysis), and only a small part (10-20%) is accounted for by gluconeogenesis. With increasing exercise duration (several hours) the contribution of gluconeogenesis rises to about 50% of the total liver glucose production. This rise occurs in parallel with a decline in liver glycogen stores and an increase in supply of gluconeogenic precursors to the liver.

During light and prolonged exercise, feedback signals from contracting muscles, mediated both neurally and via the bloodstream, adjust the stimulus for glucose production to maintain euglycemia in the blood. A rise in blood glucose directly inhibits glucose production during exercise, whereas a drop in blood glucose via stimulation of counterregulatory hormones (e.g., glucagon) indirectly enhances liver glucose production during physical activity. In contrast, during intense exercise and at the onset of exercise, central mechanisms coupled to the degree of motor center activity, leading to a very pronounced hormonal response (e.g., rise in plasma epinephrine), are responsible for an increase in glucose mobilization that exceeds the peripheral glucose uptake, resulting in a rise in blood glucose level during intense exercise.

A decrease in the plasma level of insulin is important for a rise in hepatic glucose production during exercise in both humans and other species. However, this cannot fully explain the rise in liver glucose output, especially during mild exercise. A rise in plasma glucagon has been shown to be important in some species, but in humans plasma glucagon increases only during prolonged exercise and thereby cannot explain early rises in hepatic glucose production. Epinephrine can explain a minor part of the rise in glucose production during intense exercise, and it may become important late in prolonged exercise by increasing the muscular release and thereby the hepatic supply of gluconeogenic precursors. Sympathetic liver innervation has been demonstrated to be without any role in hepatic glucose production during exercise in both humans and other species, and growth hormone and cortisol contribute only minimally to the exercise-induced rise in liver glucose output.

Hormonal mechanisms can so far only partially explain the stimulation of glucose production during exercise in humans. Factors other than the ones currently identified must contribute to the exercise-induced rise in liver glucose production in humans.

Amino acid uptake in the liver is accelerated during exercise to meet increased supply from muscle and gut proteolysis. Besides an increased gluconeogenic activity, urea formation, and probably formation of acute-phase proteins, is also intensified during exercise. Splanchnic fat depots may be mobilized by sympathetic nerve activity during exercise, and they probably reflect release of free fatty acids and glycerol from the gut that is taken up by the liver which not only accelerates gluconeogenesis, but also increases the ketogenesis during physical activity.

Acknowledgments

This work was supported by grants from Danish Medical Research Council (J.nr. SSF 12-9360), The Danish National Research Foundation (J. nr. 504-14), The NOVO Foundation, Danish Sports Research Council, and P. Carl Petersens Foundation.

References

1. Ahlborg, G.; Felig, P.; Hagenfeldt, L.; Hendler, R.; Wahren, J. Substrate turnover during prolonged exercise in man. J. Clin. Invest. 53:1080-1090; 1974.

2. Ahlborg, G.; Felig, P. Influence of glucose ingestion on fuel-hormone response during prolonged exercise. J. Appl. Physiol. 41:683-688; 1976.

3. Ahlborg, G.; Felig, P. Substrate utilization during prolonged exercise preceded by ingestion of glucose. Am. J. Physiol. 233:E188-E194; 1977.

4. Ahlborg, G.; Felig, P. Lactate and glucose exchange across the forearm, legs, and splanchnic bed during and after prolonged leg exercise. J. Clin. Invest. 69:45-54; 1982.

5. Ahlborg, G.; Wahren, J.; Felig, P. Splanchnic and peripheral glucose and lactate metabolism during and after prolonged arm exercise. J. Clin. Invest. 77:690-699; 1986.

6. Ahlborg, G.; Björkman, O. Splanchnic and muscle fructose metabolism during and after exercise. J. Appl. Physiol. 69:1244-1251; 1990.

7. Arnall, D.A.; Marker, J.C.; Conlee, R.K.; Winder, W.W. Effect of infusing epinephrine on liver and muscle glycogenolysis during exercise in rats. Am. J. Physiol. 250:E641-E649; 1986.

8. Björkman, O.; Felig, P.; Hagenfeldt, L.; Wahren, J. Influence of hypoglucagonemia on splanchnic glucose output during leg exercise in man. Clin. Physiol. 1:43-57; 1981.

9. Björkman, O.; Eriksson, L.S. Splanchnic glucose metabolism during leg exercise in 60-hour-fasted human subjects. Am. J. Physiol. 245:E443-E448; 1983.

10. Brockman, R.P. Effect of somatostatin on plasma glucagon and insulin, and glucose turnover in exercising sheep. J. Appl. Physiol. 47:273-278; 1979.

11. Brooks, G.A.; Donovan, C.M. Effect of endurance training on glucose kinetics during exercise. Am. J. Physiol. 244:E505-E512; 1983.

12. Brooks, G.A.; Butterfield, G.E.; Wolfe, R.R.; Groves, B.M.; Mazzeo, R.S.; Sutton, J.R.; Wolfel, E.E.; Reeves, J.T. Increased dependence on blood glucose after acclimatization to 4.300 m. J. Appl. Physiol. 70:919-927; 1991.

13. Calles, J.; Cunningham, J.J.; Nelson, L.; Brown, N.; Nadel, E.; Sherwin, R.S.; Felig, P. Glucose turnover during recovery from intense exercise. Diabetes 32:734-738; 1983.

14. Carlson, K.I.; Marker, J.C.; Arnall, D.A.; Terry, M.L.; Yang, H.T.; Lindsay, L.G.; Bracken, M.E.; Winder, W.W. Epinephrine is unessential for stimulation of liver glycogenolysis during exercise. J. Appl. Physiol. 58:544-548; 1985.

15. Carraro, F.; Hartl, W.H.; Stuart, C.A.; Layman, D.K.; Jahoor, F.; Wolfe, R.R. Whole body and plasma protein synthesis in exercise and recovery in human subjects. Am. J. Physiol. 258:E821-E831; 1990.

16. Clore, J.N.; Nestler, J.E.; Blackard, W.G. Sleep-associated fall in glucose disposal and hepatic glucose output in normal humans: putative signaling mechanism linking peripheral and hepatic events. Diabetes 38:285-290; 1989.

17. Coggan, A.R.; Kohrt, W.M.; Spina, R.J.; Bier, D.M.; Holloszy, J.O. Endurance training decreases plasma glucose turnover and oxidation during moderate-intensity exercise in men. J. Appl. Physiol. 68:990-996; 1990.

18. Cooper, D.M.; Wasserman, D.W.; Vranic, M.; Wasserman, K. Glucose turnover in response to exercise during high- and low-FIO$_2$ breathing in man. Am. J. Physiol. 251:E209-E214; 1986.

19. Cooper, D.M.; Barstow, T.J.; Bergner, A.; Lee, W.-N.P. Blood glucose turnover during high- and low-intensity exercise. Am. J. Physiol. 257:E405-E412; 1989.

20. Coyle, E.; Coggan, A.; Hemmert, M.; Ivy, J. Muscle glycogen utilization during prolonged strenuous exercise when fed carbohydrate. J. Appl. Physiol. 61:165-172; 1986.

21. Dohm, G.L.; Kasperek, G.J.; Topscott, E.B.; Beecher, G.R. Effect of exercise on synthesis and degradation of muscle protein. Biochem. J. 188:255-262; 1980.

22. Dohm, G.L.; Kasperek, G.J.; Barakat, H.A. Time course of changes in gluconeogenic enzyme activities during exercise and recovery. Am. J. Physiol. 249:E6-E11; 1985.

23. Doiron, B.; Cardin, S.; Brisson, G.R.; Lavoie, J.M. Effects of selective hepatic vagotomy on running endurance in rats. J. Appl. Physiol. 69:2197-2201; 1990.

24. Eriksson, L.S.; Broberg, S.; Björkman, O.; Wahren, J. Ammonia metabolism during exercise in man. Clin. Physiol. 5:325-336; 1985.

25. Felig, P.; Wahren, J. Amino acid metabolism in exercising man. J. Clin. Invest. 50:2703-2714; 1971.

26. Galbo, H.; Christensen, N.J.; Holst, J.J. Glucose-induced decrease in glucagon and epinephrine responses to exercise in man. J. Appl. Physiol. 42:525-530; 1977.

27. Galbo, H.; Richter, E.A.; Holst, J.J.; Christensen, N.J. Diminished hormonal responses to exercise in trained rats. J. Appl. Physiol. 43:953-958; 1977.

28. Garceau, D.; Yamaguchi, N.; Goyer, R.; Guitard, F. Correlation between endogenous noradrenaline and glucose released from the liver upon hepatic sympathetic nerve stimulation in anesthetized dogs. Can. J. Physiol. Pharmacol. 62:1086-1091; 1984.

29. Hargreaves, M.; Proietto, J. Glucose kinetics during exercise in trained men. Acta Physiol. Scand. 150:221-225; 1994.

30. Hirsch, I.B.; Marker, J.C.; Smith, L.J.; Spina, R.J.; Holloszy, J.O.; Cryer, P.E. Insulin and glucagon in prevention of hypoglycemia during exercise in humans. Am. J. Physiol. 260:E695-E704; 1991.

31. Hoelzer, D.R.; Dalsky, G.P.; Clutter, W.E.; Shah, S.D.; Holloszy, J.O.; Cryer, P.E. Glucoregulation during exercise: Hypoglycemia is prevented by redundant glucoregulatory systems, sympathochromaffin activation, and changes in islet hormone secretion. J. Clin. Invest. 77:212-221; 1986.

32. Hoelzer, D.R.; Dalsky, G.P.; Schwartz, N.S.; Clutter, W.E.; Shah, S.D.; Holloszy, J.O.; Cryer, P.E. Epinephrine is not critical to prevention of hypoglycemia during exercise in humans. Am. J. Physiol. 251:E104-E110; 1986.

33. Hultman, E.; Nilsson, L.H. Liver glycogen in man. Effect of different diets and muscular exercise. Advan. Exp. Med. Biol. 11:143-151; 1971.

34. Huston, R.L.; Weiser, P.C.; Dohm, G.L.; Askew, E.W.; Boyd, J.B. Effects of training, exercise and diet on muscle glycolysis and liver gluconeogenesis. Life Sci. 17:369-376; 1975.

35. Issekutz, B. The role of hypoinsulinemia in exercise metabolism. Diabetes 29:629-635; 1980.

36. Issekutz, B.; Vranic, M. Role of glucagon in regulation of glucose production in exercising dogs. Am. J. Physiol. 238:E13-E20; 1980.

37. Issekutz, B. Effects of glucose infusion on hepatic and muscle glycogenolysis in exercising dogs. Am. J. Physiol. 240:E451-E457; 1981.

38. Jenkins, A.B.; Chisholm, D.J.; James, D.E.; Ho, K.Y.; Kraegen, E.W. Exercise-induced hepatic glucose output is precisely sensitive to the rate of systemic glucose supply. Metabolism 34:431-441; 1985.

39. Jenkins, A.B.; Furler, S.M.; Chisholm, D.J.; Kraegen, E.W. Regulation of hepatic glucose output during exercise by circulating glucose and insulin in humans. Am. J. Physiol. 250:R411-R417; 1986.

40. John-Adler, H.B.; McAllister, R.M.; Terjung, R.L. Reduced running endurance in gluconeogenesis-inhibited rats. Am. J. Physiol. 251:R137-R142; 1986.

41. Juhlin-Dannfelt, A.; Ahlborg, G.; Hagenfeldt, L.; Jorfeldt, L.; Felig, P. Influence of ethanol on splanchnic and skeletal muscle substrate turnover during prolonged exercise in man. Am. J. Physiol. 233:E195-E202; 1977.

42. Kasperek, G.J.; Dohm, G.L.; Barakat, H.A.; Straus-Bauch, P.H.; Barnes, D.W.; Snider, R.D. The role of lysosomes in exercise-induced protein loss. Biochem. J. 202:281-288; 1982.

43. Katz, A.; Broberg, S.; Sahlin, K.; Wahren, J. Leg glucose uptake during maximal dynamic exercise in humans. Am. J. Physiol. 251:E65-E70; 1986.

44. Kjær, M.; Farrell, P.A.; Christensen, N.J.; Galbo, H. Increased epinephrine response and inaccurate glucoregulation in exercising athletes. J. Appl. Physiol. 61:1693-1700; 1986.

45. Kjær, M.; Secher, N.H.; Bach, F.W.; Galbo, H. Role of motor center activity for hormonal changes and substrate mobilization in humans. Am. J. Physiol. 253:R687-R695; 1987.

46. Kjær, M.; Secher, N.H.; Bach, F.W.; Sheikh, S.; Galbo, H. Hormonal and metabolic responses to exercise in humans: effect of sensory nervous blockade. Am. J. Physiol. 257:E95-E101; 1989.

47. Kjær, M.; Kiens, B.; Hargreaves, M.; Richter, E.A. Influence of active muscle mass on glucose homeostasis during exercise in humans. J. Appl. Physiol. 71:552-557; 1991.

48. Kjær, M.; Engfred, K.; Fernandes, A.; Secher, N.H.; Galbo, H. Regulation of hepatic glucose production during exercise in humans: role of sympatho-adrenergic activity. Am. J. Physiol. 265:E275-E283; 1993.

49. Kjær, M.; Engfred, K.; Galbo, H.; Sonne, B.; Rasmussen, K.; Keiding, S. Glucose homeostasis during exercise in humans with a liver or kidney transplant. Am. J. Physiol. In press.

50. Kjær, M.; Jurlander, J.; Galbo, H.; Kirkegaard, P.; Keiding, S.; Hage, E. No reinnervation of hepatic sympathetic nerves after liver transplantation in human subjects. J. Hepatol. 20:97-100; 1994.

51. Kjær, M.; Perko, G.; Secher, N.H.; Boushel, R.; Beyer, N.; Pollack, S.; Horn, A.; Fernandes, A.; Mohr, T.; Lewis, S.F.; Galbo, H. Cardiovascular and ventilatory responses to electrically induced cycling with complete epidural anaesthesia in humans. Acta Physiol. Scand. 151:199-207; 1994.

52. Kjær, M.; Pollack, S.F.; Mohr, T.; Weiss, H.; Gleim, G.W.; Bach, F.W.; Nico-laisen, T.; Galbo, H.; Ragnarsson, K.T. Regulation of glucose turnover and hormonal responses during exercise: Electrically induced cycling in tetraplegic humans. Am. J. Physiol. In press.

53. Knapik, J.J.; Meredith, C.N.; Jones, B.H.; Suek, L.; Young, V.R.; Evans, W.J. Influence of fasting on carbohydrate and fat metabolism during rest and exercise in men. J. Appl. Physiol. 64:1923-1929; 1988.

54. Lavoie, J.M.; Cardin, S.; Doiron, B. Influence of hepatic vagus nerve on pancreatic hormone secretion during exercise. Am. J. Physiol. 257:E855-E859; 1989.

55. Marker, J.C.; Arnall, D.A.; Conlee, R.K.; Winder, W.W. Effect of adreno-demedullation on metabolic responses to high-intensity exercise. Am. J. Physiol. 251:R552-R559; 1986.

56. Marker, J.C.; Hirsch, I.B.; Smith, L.J.; Parvin, C.A.; Holloszy, J.O.; Cryer, P.E. Catecholamines in prevention of hypoglycemia during exercise in humans. Am. J. Physiol. 260:E705-E712; 1991.

57. Marliss, E.B.; Simantirakis, E.; Miles, P.D.G.; Purdon, C.; Gougeon, R.; Field, C.J.; Halter, J.B.; Vranic, M. Glucoregulatory and hormonal responses to repeated bouts of intense exercise in normal male subjects. J. Appl. Physiol. 71:924-933; 1991.

58. Moates, J.M.; Lacy, D.B.; Cherrington, A.D.; Goldstein, R.E.; Wasserman, D.H. The metabolic role of the exercise-induced increment in epinephrine. Am. J. Physiol. 255:E428-E436; 1988.

59. Nobin, A.; Falck, B.; Ingemansson, S.; Järhult, J.; Rosengren, E. Organization and function of the sympathetic innervation of human liver. Acta Physiol. Scand. 452(Suppl): 103-106; 1977.

60. Rakestraw, N.W. Chemical factors in fatigue. J. Biol. Chem. 46:565-590; 1921.

61. Reichard, G.A.; Issekutz, B., Jr.; Kimbel, P.; Putnam, R.C.; Hochella, N.J.; Weinhouse, S. Blood glucose metabolism in man during muscular work. J. Appl. Physiol. 16:1001-1005; 1961.

62. Refsum, H.E.; Gjessing, R.; Strömme, S.B. Changes in plasma amino acid distribution and urine amino acids excretion during prolonged heavy exercise. Scand. J. Clin. Lab. Invest. 39:407-413; 1979.

63. Richter, E.A.; Galbo, H.; Sonne, B.; Holst, J.J.; Christensen, N.J. Adrenal medullary control of muscular and hepatic glycogenolysis and of pancreatic hormonal secretion in exercising rats. Acta Physiol. Scand. 108:235-242; 1980.

64. Richter, E.A.; Galbo, H.; Christensen, N.J. Control of exercise-induced muscular glycogenolysis by adrenal medullary hormones in rats. J. Appl. Physiol. 50:21-26; 1981.

65. Richter, E.A.; Galbo, H.; Holst, J.J.; Sonne, B. Significance of glucagon for insulin secretion and hepatic glycogenolysis during exercise in rats. Hormone Metab. Res. 13:323-326; 1981.

66. Rosell, S.; Ballard, K. Adrenergic neuro-humoral control of lipolysis in adipose tissue. In: Pernow, B.; Saltin, B., eds. Muscle metabolism during exercise. New York-London: Plenum Press; 1971: 111-117.

67. Rowell, L.B.; Masoro, E.J.; Spencer, M.J. Splanchnic metabolism in exercising man. J. Appl. Physiol. 20:1032-1037; 1965.

68. Rowell, L.B. Human circulation—regulation during physical stress. New York: Oxford University Press; 1986: 416.

69. Scheurink, A.J.W.; Steffens, A.B.; Benthem, L. Central and peripheral adrenoreceptors affect glucose, FFA and insulin in exercising rats. Am. J. Physiol. 255:R547-R556; 1988.

70. Sellers, T.L.; Jaussi, A.W.; Yang, H.T.; Heninger, R.W.; Winder, W.W. Effect of the exercise-induced increase in glucocorticoids on endurance in the rat. J. Appl. Physiol. 65:173-178; 1988.

71. Sestoft, L.; Trap-Jensen, J.; Lyngsøe, J.; Clausen, J.P.; Holst, J.J.; Nielsen, S.L.; Rehfeld, J.F.; Shaffalitsky de Muckadell, O. Regulation of gluconeogenesis and ketogenesis during rest and exercise in diabetic subjects and normal men. Clin. Sci. Mol. Med. 53:411-418; 1977.

72. Simonson, D.C.; Koivisto, V.; Sherwin, R.S.; Ferrannini, E.; Hendler, R.; De-Fronzo, R.A. Adrenergic blockade alters glucose kinetics during exercise in insulin-dependent diabetics. J. Clin. Invest. 73:1648-1658; 1984.

73. Sonne, B.; Galbo, H. Carbohydrate metabolism during and after exercise in rats: studies with radioglucose. J. Appl. Physiol. 59:1627-1639; 1985.

74. Sonne, B.; Mikines, K.J.; Richter, E.A.; Christensen, N.J.; Galbo, H. Role of liver nerves and adrenal medulla in glucose turnover of running rats. J. Appl. Physiol. 59:1640-1646; 1985.

75. Sonne, B.; Galbo, H. Carbohydrate metabolism in fructose-fed and food-restricted running rats. J. Appl. Physiol. 61:1457-1466; 1986.

76. Sonne, B.; Mikines, K.J.; Galbo, H. Glucose turnover in 48-hour-fasted running rats. Am. J. Physiol. 252:R587-R593; 1987.

77. Turcotte, L.P.; Rovner, A.S.; Roark, R.R.; Brooks, G.A. Glucose kinetics in gluconeogenesis-inhibited rats during rest and exercise. Am. J. Physiol. 258:E203-E211; 1990.

78. Tuttle, K.R.; Marker, J.C.; Dalsky, G.P.; Schwartz, N.S.; Shah, S.D.; Clutter, W.E.; Holloszy, J.O.; Cryer, P.E. Glucagon, not insulin, may play a secondary role in defense against hypoglycemia during exercise. Am. J. Physiol. 254:E713-E719; 1988.

79. Vissing, J.; Sonne, B.; Galbo, H. Role of metabolic feedback regulation in glucose production of running rats. Am. J. Physiol. 255:R400-R406; 1988.

80. Vissing, J.; Sonne, B.; Galbo, H. Regulation of hepatic glucose production in running rats studies by glucose infusion. J. Appl. Physiol. 65:2552-2557; 1988.

81. Vissing, J.; Iwamoto, G.A.; Rybicki, K.J.; Galbo, H.; Mitchell, J.H. Mobilization of glucoregulatory hormones and glucose by hypothalamic locomotor centers. Am. J. Physiol. 257:E722-E728; 1989.

82. Vissing, J.; Wallace, J.L.; Galbo, H. Effect of liver glycogen content on glucose production in running rats. J. Appl. Physiol. 66:318-322; 1989.

83. Vissing, J.; Wallace, J.L.; Scheurink, A.J.W.; Galbo, H.; Steffens, A.B. Ventromedial hypothalamic regulation of hormonal and metabolic responses to exercise. Am. J. Physiol. 256:R1019-R1026; 1989.

84. Vissing, J.; Lewis, S.F.; Galbo, H.; Haller, R.G. Effect of deficient muscular glycogenolysis on extramuscular fuel production in exercise. J. Appl. Physiol. 72:1773-1779; 1992.

84a. Vissing, J.; Iwamoto, G.A.; Fuchs, I.E.; Galbo, H.; Mitchell, J.H. Reflex control of glucoregulatory exercise responses by group III and IV muscle afferents. Am. J. Physiol. 266:R824-R830; 1994.

85. Vranic, M.; Kawamori, R.; Pek, S.; Kovacevic, N.; Wrenshall, G. The essentiality of insulin and the role of glucagon in regulating glucose utilization and production during strenuous exercise in dogs. J. Clin. Invest. 57:245-256; 1976.

86. Vranic, M.; Gauthier, C.; Bilinski, D.; Wasserman, D.; El Tayeb, K.; Hetenyi, G.; Lickley, H.L.A. Catecholamine responses and their interaction with other glucoregulatory hormones. Am. J. Physiol. 247:E145-E156; 1984.

87. Wahren, J.; Felig, P.; Ahlborg, G.; Jorfeldt, L. Glucose metabolism during leg exercise in man. J. Clin. Invest. 50:2715-2725; 1971.

88. Wahren, J.; Hagenfeldt, L.; Felig, P. Splanchnic and leg exchange of glucose, amino acids, and free fatty acids during exercise in diabetes mellitus. J. Clin. Invest. 55:1303-1314; 1975.

89. Wahren, J.; Sato, Y.; Östman, J.; Hagenfeldt, L.; Felig, P. Turnover and splanchnic metabolism of free fatty acids and ketones in insulin-dependent diabetics at rest and in response to exercise. J. Clin. Invest. 73:1367-1376; 1984.

90. Wasserman, D.H.; Lickley, H.L.A.; Vranic, M. Interactions between glucagon and other counterregulatory hormones during normoglycemic and hypoglycemic exercise in dogs. J. Clin. Invest. 74:1404-1413; 1984.

91. Wasserman, D.H.; Lacy, D.B.; Green, D.R.; Williams, P.E.; Cherrington, A.D. Dynamics of hepatic lactate and glucose balances during prolonged exercise and recovery in the dog. J. Appl. Physiol. 63:2411-2417; 1987.

92. Wasserman, D.H.; Williams, P.E.; Lacy, D.B.; Green, D.R.; Cherrington, A.D. Importance of intrahepatic mechanisms to gluconeogenesis from alanine during exercise and recovery. Am. J. Physiol. 254:E518-E525; 1988.

93. Wasserman, D.H.; Spalding, J.A.; Lacy, D.B.; Colburn, C.A.; Goldstein, R.E.; Cherrington, A.D. Glucagon is a primary controller of hepatic glycogenolysis and gluconeogenesis during muscular work. Am. J. Physiol. 257:E108-E117; 1989.

94. Wasserman, D.H.; Williams, P.E.; Lacy, D.B.; Goldstein, R.E.; Cherrington, A.D. Exercise-induced fall in insulin and hepatic carbohydrate metabolism during muscular work. Am. J. Physiol. 256:E500-E509; 1989.

95. Wasserman, D.H.; Lacy, D.B.; Goldstein, R.E.; Williams, P.E.; Cherrington, A.D. Exercise-induced fall in insulin and the increase in fat metabolism during prolonged muscular work. Diabetes 38:484-490; 1989.

96. Wasserman, D.H.; Spalding, J.A.; Bracy, D.; Lacy, D.B.; Cherrington, A.D. Exercise-induced rise in glucagon and ketogenesis during prolonged muscular work. Diabetes 38:799-807; 1989.

97. Wasserman, D.H.; Williams, P.E.; Lacy, D.B.; Bracy, D.; Cherrington, A.D. Hepatic nerves are not essential to the increase in hepatic glucose production during muscular work. Am. J. Physiol. 259:E195-E203; 1990.

98. Wasserman, D.H.; Geer, R.J.; Williams, P.E.; Becker, T.; Lacy, D.B.; Abumrad, N.N. Interaction of gut and liver in nitrogen metabolism during exercise. Metabolism 40:307-314; 1991.

99. Wasserman, D.H.; Lacy, D.B.; Colburn, C.A.; Bracy, D.; Cherrington, A.D. Efficiency of compensation for absence of fall in insulin during exercise. Am. J. Physiol. 261:E587-E597; 1991.

100. Winder, W.W.; Terry, M.L.; Mitchell, V.M. Role of plasma epinephrine in fasted exercising rats. Am. J. Physiol. 248:R302-R307; 1985.

101. Winder, W.W.; Yang, H.T.; Jaussi, A.W.; Hopkins, C.R. Epinephrine, glucose, and lactate infusion in exercising adrenodemedullated rats. J. Appl. Physiol. 62:1442-1447; 1987.

102. Wolfe, R.R.; Goodenough, R.D.; Wolfe, M.H.; Royle, G.T.; Nadel, E.R. Isotopic analysis of leucine and urea metabolism in exercising humans. J. Appl. Physiol. 52:458-466; 1982.

103. Wolfe, R.R.; Nadel, E.R.; Shaw, J.H.F.; Stephenson, L.A.; Wolfe, M.H. Role of changes in insulin and glucagon in glucose homeostasis in exercise. J. Clin. Invest. 77:900-907; 1986.

Chapter 4

Lipid Metabolism During Exercise

LORRAINE P. TURCOTTE, ERIK A. RICHTER, AND BENTE KIENS

Lipid fuel sources are important energy substrates for skeletal muscle metabolism during endurance exercise. Their contribution to total oxidative metabolism is dependent on a variety of factors, including exercise intensity and duration, as well as dietary and training status. Oxidizable lipid fuels include circulating plasma triacylglycerols (TG) and free fatty acids (FFA), as well as intramuscular TG. Whereas circulating albumin-bound FFA mobilized from adipose tissue contribute in significant proportion to lipid metabolism in skeletal muscle during exercise, the conditions during which FFA hydrolyzed from intramuscular TG and plasma TG-derived FFA contribute to lipid metabolism during exercise have not been clearly defined. This chapter will examine the contribution made by each of these lipid fuels to skeletal muscle metabolism during exercise and the regulatory mechanisms that control variations in their contributions.

Plasma Free Fatty Acid Metabolism

FFA derived from adipose tissue lipolysis constitute a major fuel oxidized by working muscles, especially when exercise duration is prolonged and intensity is low to moderate (33). The metabolism of albumin-bound long-chain FFA is a complex process that involves many steps: namely, FFA mobilization from adipose tissue, transport in plasma, permeation across cell membranes and interstitium, cytoplasmic transport, and intracellular metabolism.

Free Fatty Acid Mobilization

As the first committed step in the metabolism of FFA, the mobilization of lipids plays a key role in the regulation of FFA utilization during rest and exercise. Adipose tissue is quantitatively the most important store of energy in mammals. In humans, adipose tissue makes up between 10 and 25% of total body weight. For the most part, adipose tissue is located subcutaneously and around the abdominal organs, but smaller depots are located between skeletal muscles (19). The rate of mobilization of FFA from adipose tissue is dependent not only on the rate of lipolysis, but also on the plasma transport capacity for FFA and on the rate of reesterification of FFA by the adipocyte.

Adipose Tissue Lipolysis.   The rate of lipolysis is best estimated by measuring the release of glycerol. Glycerol appears in the blood only as a product of lipolysis, and once released it cannot be re-utilized by the adipocyte because adipose tissue lacks glycerol kinase (16). It is now possible to measure adipose tissue lipolysis *in situ* by using a microdialysis probe, which can measure glycerol release in the extracellular space of adipose tissue and deliver drugs or hormones locally (11). The rate of appearance of FFA can also be measured to estimate the rate of lipolysis, but it represents the net balance between adipose tissue lipolysis and intra-adipocyte FFA reesterification and, as such, it can only be used as an index of the rate of net FFA mobilization (21).

Effects of Acute Exercise.   Results from a number of studies show that the rate of adipose tissue lipolysis increases with exercise (97, 123, 126). In human gluteal fat cells isolated before and after 30 min of bicycle exercise, catecholamine-stimulated glycerol release was increased 35-50% after exercise (122, 123). Microdialysis of the extracellular space of abdominal subcutaneous adipose tissue showed that 30 min of moderate-intensity bicycle exercise increased glycerol concentration in adipose tissue (12). In dogs, the rate of appearance of glycerol was increased 4-4.5 times during 3 hr of submaximal exercise (97). In man, the rate of FFA uptake was increased threefold after 40 min of bicycle exercise at 60% of maximal oxygen uptake ($\dot{V}O_2$ max) (120), and the rate of appearance of glycerol and FFA were increased by more than five- and sixfold after 4 hr of submaximal treadmill exercise (126).

Hormonal Regulation of Lipolysis.   Adipose tissue lipolysis is under hormonal regulation. In isolated rat adipocytes, catecholamines, glucagon, growth hormone, adrenocorticotropic hormone, and various pituitary and intestinal hormones increase the lipolytic rate (56). In isolated human adipocytes only catecholamines, thyroid-stimulating hormone, and parathyroid hormone have consistently been shown to be good stimulators of lipolysis (56). Because only catecholamines can effectively stimulate lipolysis at physiological concentrations, they appear to be the most important stimulators of lipolysis in human adipose tissue *in vivo*. In human adipose tissue, catecholamines have both α_2-adrenergic inhibitory and β_1-adrenergic stimulatory effects on the rate of lipolysis via corresponding changes in the activity of adenylate cyclase and in the intracellular production of cAMP (32). In both rats and humans, insulin is the most potent hormone inhibiting lipolysis (56) (Figure 4.1).

The essential hormonal changes promoting increased lipolysis during whole-body exercise are increased sympathoadrenal β-adrenergic stimulation and decreased circulating insulin levels (47). In man, α_2-adrenergic inhibitory mechanisms modulate lipolysis at rest, whereas β_1-adrenergic stimulatory mechanisms are predominant during exercise. Thus, addition of the nonselective α-adrenergic blocker, phentolamine, to the ingoing solution perfusing subcutaneous adipose tissue more than doubled the glycerol concentration in the dialysate of resting subjects, whereas the addition of the nonselective β-adrenergic blocker, propranolol, did not alter glycerol concentration (12). On the other hand, the addition of propranolol to the ingoing perfusate diminished the exercise-induced increase

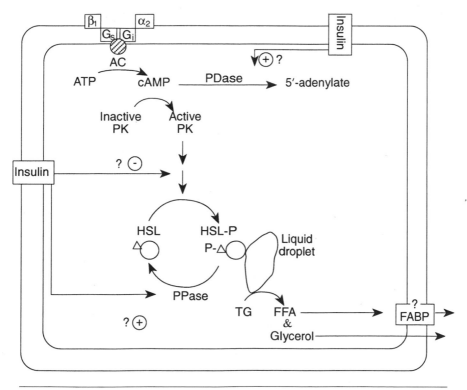

Figure 4.1 Schematic representation of the hormone-sensitive lipase system in rat adipocyte and its regulation by hormones. β_1 = adrenoceptor; α_2 = adrenoceptor; G_s: stimulatory G protein; G_i: inhibitory G protein; AC: adenylate cyclase; PDase: phosphodiesterase; PK: protein kinase; HSL: hormone-sensitive lipase; PPase: protein phosphatase; TG: triacylglycerol; FFA: free fatty acids; FABP: fatty acid binding protein.

in dialysate glycerol concentration by 65%, whereas the addition of phentolamine had no effect (12) (Figure 4.2). Furthermore, in exercising dogs, infusion of propranolol almost abolished the exercise-induced increase in the rate of appearance of FFA (70). In exercising man, acute β-adrenergic blockade with propranolol resulted in a significant reduction in exercise-induced increments in glycerol and FFA concentrations and was associated with an impairment of endurance performance (44). It has also been shown that exercise does not affect α- and β-adrenergic receptor binding to adipose tissue (122). Furthermore, the exercise-induced increase in lipolysis has been mimicked by agents acting at the levels of adenylate cyclase, coupling proteins, phosphodiesterase, and protein kinase (123). Thus, acute exercise appears to increase adipose tissue lipolysis through β-adrenergic enhancement of lipase activity (122).

The exercise-induced decrease in insulin concentration is directly related to work intensity (43) and is elicited by an α-adrenergic inhibition of insulin secretion (45). Thus, in man exercising during α-blockade with phentolamine, insulin concentrations were significantly higher than during exercise without drug administration (45). Compared with exercising

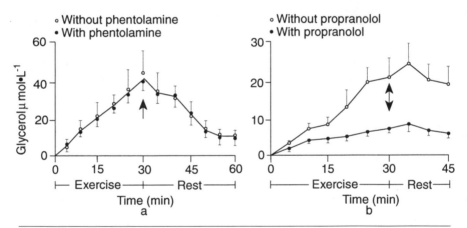

Figure 4.2 Effect of adrenoceptor blockade on exercise-induced glycerol levels in dialysates of abdominal subcutaneous adipose tissue. Two dialysis probes were inserted in the abdominal area of the same subject and perfused with Ringer's solution either in the absence (open circles) or presence (filled circles) of either 10^{-4} mol/liter of phentolamine (*a*) or 10^{-4} mol/liter of propranolol (*b*). The subjects rested for 35 min. Then, they exercised for 30 min at two-thirds of their maximum working capacity. Thereafter, they rested for a further 15-30 min. The mean glycerol levels in the first four fractions preceding exercise were determined. This baseline glycerol value was substracted from the subsequent exercise and postexercise values. Time 0 indicates the start of exercise. The arrow indicates the end of exercise. Values are means ± SE. *a* depicts experiments with and without phentolamine performed on two men and six women. *b* depicts experiments with and without propranolol performed on four men and two women. Reprinted with permission from Arner et al. (1990).

normal subjects, adipose tissue lipolysis is higher in exercising subjects who are in a hypoinsulinemic state (46, 120, 125). Thus, fasting (125) and fat-feeding (46) in normal subjects as well as insulin deprivation in diabetic subjects (12) have been shown to increase plasma concentrations of FFA and glycerol (46, 120) and the rate of appearance of FFA and glycerol (125). In exercising pancreatectomized dogs, it was shown that the larger exercise-induced rise in plasma FFA levels associated with hypoinsulinemia was due to an increased rate of release of FFA from adipose tissue and not to a decreased rate of uptake by skeletal muscle (67). In contrast, in exercising man, mild hyperinsulinemia induced by insulin infusion prevented the exercise-induced increase in plasma FFA concentration, suggesting an inhibition of lipolysis (22).

The Hormone-Sensitive Lipase System.   The rate of adipose tissue lipolysis is controlled by the hormone-sensitive triacylglycerol lipase (HSL) system, which hydrolyzes the glycerol-ester bonds of triacylglycerols into FFA and glycerol (127). HSL is an 84 kDa polypeptide, which *in vitro* is capable of completely hydrolyzing triacylglycerols to FFA and glycerol, even though the enzyme has a marked specificity for the ester bonds located at positions 1 and 3 (38). Monoacylglycerol lipase is responsible mainly for the hydrolysis of the ester bond in position 2 (39). *In vivo*, the action of both enzymes is required for complete hydrolysis of triacylglycerols (39). A diacylglycerol lipase also exists, but its action is not necessary for complete hydrolysis of triacylglycerols (127). In most instances, hydrolysis by HSL of the primary ester bonds of its acylglycerol substrates leads to an accumulation of monoacylglycerol and is the rate-limiting step in triacylglycerol hydrolysis (39).

Hormonal regulation of adipose tissue lipolysis occurs via regulation of the activity of HSL by a modification of its phosphorylation state (37). In isolated rat adipocytes, stimulation with lipolytic agents increases the phosphorylation state of HSL, whereas treatment with the antilipolytic hormone insulin decreases the phosphorylation state of the enzyme (84). Peptide mapping studies of intact rat adipocytes have identified two phosphorylation sites on serine residues of HSL, and these sites have been named the *regulatory* and *basal* sites (106). Stimulation of lipolysis by lipolytic agents increases phosphorylation on the regulatory site, and a close association exists between the activity of HSL and the phosphorylation state of the site (107). HSL is an excellent substrate of cAMP-dependent protein kinase *in vitro*, and peptide mapping studies indicate that the kinase phosphorylates the regulatory site (105, 106). Thus, the changes in the activity of adenylate cyclase and the intracellular production of cAMP, brought about by the interaction of catecholamines with α- and β-adrenergic receptors, regulate the phosphorylation state of the regulatory site.

It also has recently been proposed that the increased phosphorylation of HSL by cAMP-dependent protein kinase following lipolytic stimulation of rat adipocytes is associated not only with an increased activity of HSL, but also with a translocation of HSL from the cytosol to its substrate at the surface of lipid storage droplets (28). This translocation would explain the discrepancy existing between the fiftyfold increase in lipolytic rate of lipolytically-induced rat adipocytes and the twofold increase in catalytic HSL activity upon lipolytic stimulation.

Insulin can reverse the effects of lipolytic hormones on both the lipolytic rate and the phosphorylation state of the regulatory site (107). The mechanisms underlying the antilipolytic action of insulin remain uncertain. Whether insulin acts via a decrease in intracellular cAMP concentration by activating a low K_m cAMP phosphodiesterase (128) or by inhibiting cAMP-dependent protein kinase (42) or, alternatively, via a cAMP-independent pathway by activating a protein phosphatase that dephosphorylates both sites of HSL (86, 107), is still unclear (Figure 4.1).

Effects of Glucose Concentration.   Although the major regulatory factors controlling adipose tissue lipolysis are hormonal, glucose concentration can also influence lipolysis independently of changes in plasma hormones. Supporting evidence for this regulatory role of glucose on lipolysis has come from *in vitro* (10) and *in vivo* (125) studies. In isolated human adipocytes incubated with increasing concentrations of glucose, the antilipolytic effect of insulin was markedly increased (10). In healthy human subjects, glucose infusion suppressed the rate of appearance of glycerol (125). However, in this *in vivo* study it was difficult to separate the effects of glucose per se from the glucose-induced rise in insulin concentration on the suppression of lipolysis. With the use of a pancreatic-pituitary clamp to maintain basal insulin concentration, Carlson et al. (21) found that hyperglycemia (10 mM) equally suppressed the rate of appearance of FFA and glycerol by ~32% in healthy subjects. These results indicate that, independently of hormonal changes, glucose regulates FFA mobilization by suppressing lipolysis and not by stimulating FFA reesterification (21).

Plasma FFA Transport Capacity.   Although the major regulatory factors controlling adipose tissue mobilization are neuroendocrine, both the capacity to carry FFA away from adipose tissue and the rate of intra-adipocyte reesterification of FFA may influence net mobilization independently of changes in hormone concentrations. The capacity to carry FFA away from adipose tissue is determined by the blood albumin concentration, the arterial FFA/albumin molar ratio, and the perfusion rate through adipose tissue (19). Whereas albumin concentration is fairly constant in exercising humans and animals, arterial plasma FFA concentration can increase up to twentyfold during prolonged submaximal exercise, resulting in an increase in the FFA/albumin molar ratio from a resting value of less than 0.2 to an exercise value of 3 to 4. Because albumin binds

FFA with decreasing affinity (100), an increase in the FFA/albumin ratio is accompanied by an increase in the concentration of unbound FFA, and this increase favors the reesterification of FFA by adipose tissue at the expense of net mobilization. In contrast, the transport capacity of plasma for FFA is increased by an increase in adipose tissue blood flow (19). (In perfused adipose tissue, either an increase in the FFA/albumin molar ratio or a decrease in the perfusion flow decreases the net output of FFA by decreasing the plasma FFA transport capacity or by increasing the rate of reesterification (77). However, during prolonged submaximal exercise in humans and dogs, adipose tissue blood flow can increase up to three-fold, and this increase favors FFA mobilization and compensates, at least in part, for the simultaneously occurring increase in the FFA/albumin molar ratio (17, 18).

Rate of FFA Reesterification.   There exists a dynamic state between the rates of lipolysis and reesterification, and the net result of this triglyceride-fatty acid cycle determines the rate of FFA mobilization. The two metabolic pathways are not reversible. Whereas FFA released from adipose tissue can be reesterified to triacylglycerols after activation to acyl-CoA derivatives either in the adipocyte (intracellular recycling) or elsewhere (extracellular recycling), glycerol released cannot be reincorporated because the activity of glycerol kinase is extremely low (16, 126). Triglyceride-fatty acid cycling is under hormonal regulation, and it has been shown that changes in the rate of intracellular and extracellular recycling amplify the response of FFA flux to changes in substrate demand (81). During prolonged submaximal exercise when the rate of FFA oxidation increases by as much as tenfold, the percentage of FFA mobilized that were reesterified decreased from a resting value of 70% to an exercise value of 25%, and most of the change in the rate of reesterification was due to a decrease in the rate of extracellular recycling (126) (Figure 4.3).

Finally, it has been shown that lactate decreases FFA mobilization by increasing FFA reesterification without affecting lipolysis. Thus, in exercising dogs increased lactate concentration decreased the rate of appearance of FFA (66), and in isolated perfused adipose tissue from dogs lactate increased FFA reesterification without affecting lipolysis as measured by glycerol release (36). It is doubtful, however, that the presence of lactate would play a primary role in the regulation of FFA mobilization during prolonged submaximal exercise because blood lactate levels remain low in these conditions.

FFA Transport in Blood Plasma

Following their mobilization from adipose tissue, long-chain FFA need to be transported to other tissues. Due to their poor solubility in the aqueous media that prevails in most biological systems, 99.9% of FFA

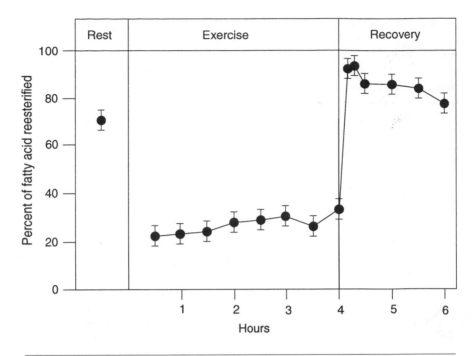

Figure 4.3   Percent reesterification of fatty acids made available via triglyceride hydrolysis during rest, 4 hr of treadmill exercise at 40% $\dot{V}O_2$ max and 2 hr of recovery (n=5). The total rate of reesterification was calculated as the difference between three times the rate of appearance of glycerol (total fatty acids released) and the rate of total fatty acid oxidation (determined by indirect calorimetry) and corrected for any increase in plasma free fatty acid concentration. Reprinted with permission from Wolfe et al. (1990).

circulate in plasma bound to albumin, a soluble protein that binds FFA with high affinity and allows total plasma FFA concentration to reach values as high as 2 mM. While there exist approximately 10 binding sites for FFA on each albumin molecule, only three of these sites have a high affinity for FFA (100). Thus, when total plasma FFA concentration increases, these sites fill up and the concentration of FFA not bound to albumin increases exponentially (100). Despite this, only a very small fraction of FFA (~0.1%) is actually dissolved in the plasmatic water, and this unbound fraction is assumed to be in equilibrium with the albumin-bound fraction (90).

FFA Permeation Across Plasma Membranes

Following dissociation from albumin, FFA cross the plasma membranes of skeletal muscle cells to be either stored as triacylglycerols or oxidized for ATP production. According to the conventional theory of cellular uptake for protein-bound ligand, only unbound ligand participates in the uptake process (15), and because of their lipid nature, FFA flux across plasma membranes has long been considered a passive diffusional process. This notion was reinforced by the existence of a linear relationship between total plasma FFA concentration and FFA utilization in humans and dogs at rest and during exercise (9, 54, 55, 58, 69). Arguing against the hypothesis of simple diffusion of FFA across cell membranes are several structural and physiological considerations (90). One argument is that the unbound FFA concentration is far too low to explain the high cellular influx rates observed *in vivo*. Another consideration relates to the tight structure of the phospholipid bilayer of plasma membranes, whose polar groups facing the extra- and intracellular space may hinder FFA permeation. Moreover, at physiologic pH, FFA exist in plasma as anions and thus have to be taken up against an unfavorable electrical gradient due to the negative charge on the cytosolic side of the plasma membrane. These theoretical considerations raise the possibility that transport mechanisms more efficient than simple diffusion exist for FFA.

Within the past decade, experimental evidence has emerged to suggest that FFA permeation across plasma membranes is indeed carrier-mediated and is dependent on the concentration of unbound FFA, as stated by the conventional theory of cellular uptake (15). In hepatocytes, adipocytes, and cardiac myocytes, evidence shows

- that cellular uptake of long-chain FFA is not limited by the dissociation of FFA from albumin and demonstrates saturation kinetics when plotted against the unbound plasma FFA concentration (3, 99, 108) (Figure 4.4);
- that long-chain FFA bind in a saturable fashion to freshly isolated plasma membranes (90, 108); and
- that such binding is attributable to a specific plasma membrane fatty acid binding protein (FABP$_{PM}$) (90, 108).

FABP$_{PM}$ have a molecular weight between 40 and 43 kDa, possess a high affinity for long-chain FFA, and are structurally and immunologically distinct from the 12-14 kDa cytosolic FABP described in many tissues (90). In each cell type studied to date, antibodies raised against the rat hepatic FABP$_{PM}$ inhibit both FFA binding to plasma membranes and cellular flux of FFA in a dose-dependent fashion, suggesting that FABP$_{PM}$ may constitute functional FFA transporters (90).

Evidence is also accumulating to suggest that permeation of FFA into skeletal muscle is carrier-mediated (73, 115-118). In untrained human subjects performing 2 or 3 hr of one-legged dynamic knee-extension exercise, FFA uptake into the exercising skeletal muscles determined either as net uptake (73) or with a tracer technique (116) was found to saturate with an increase in plasma unbound FFA concentration (Figure 4.5). Similarly, in isolated perfused rat skeletal muscle, palmitate uptake displayed

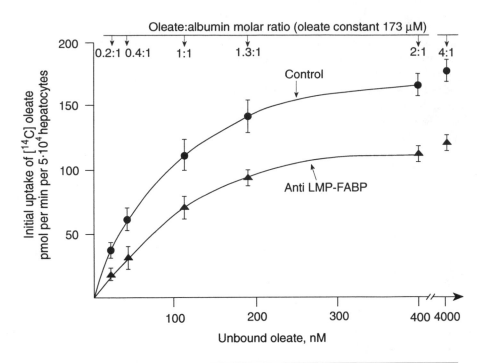

Figure 4.4 Inhibition of [^{14}C]oleate uptake into isolated hepatocytes by the anti-LPM-FABP IgG. Cells pretreated with 400 µg of the IgG fraction of the immune serum were compared to a control preparation pretreated with the preimmune serum. 250 µL of the cell suspensions, containing 2 · 10^6 cells/mL were incubated with 173 µM [^{14}C]oleate bound to albumin in various molar ratios at 37°C in 1 ml of PBS. The initial uptake rates as a function of the calculated unbound oleate concentrations in the incubation media are shown. [^{14}C]oleate influx is significantly reduced by the anti-LPM-FABP IgG. Values are means ± SD of three replicate experiments. LPM = liver plasma membranes; FABP = fatty acid binding protein. Reprinted with permission from Stremmel et al. (1986).

saturation kinetics when plotted against the unbound perfusate palmitate concentration (115) (Figure 4.6). The maximal velocity of the uptake of palmitate increased with acute muscle contractions induced by electrical stimulation (117) and decreased with low carbohydrate availability (94, 119), suggesting that physiological stimuli may alter membrane transport of FFA. Finally, immunoblotting of plasma membrane fractions of rat skeletal muscles with a polyclonal antibody against the rat hepatic FABP$_{PM}$ detected a single protein band with an apparent molecular weight of 42 kDa (118). Put together these results suggest that, as in other cell types, FFA permeation into skeletal muscle is mediated, at least in part, by a carrier-mediated process, which may play an important function in regulating the utilization of FFA by skeletal muscle.

Data collected in isolated adipocytes have suggested that epinephrine and insulin control FFA mobilization from adipose tissue by regulating the membrane transport system of fatty acids (3, 4), in addition to modulating the activity of HSL. Abumrad et al. (5) have shown that epinephrine stimulates the transport process by five- to tenfold and that the stimulation process is mediated by β-receptor interaction and cAMP accumulation (6). Furthermore, insulin at physiological concentrations has been shown to suppress epinephrine-stimulated membrane transport of long-chain FFA in isolated adipocytes by lowering cAMP level via an activation of phosphodiesterase (7). The molecular mechanism behind this phenomenon remains to be elucidated. Whether the plasma membrane transport

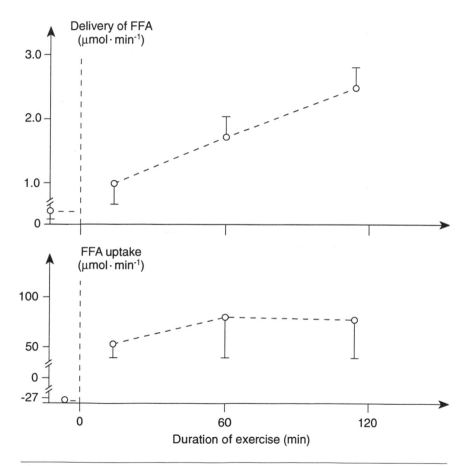

Figure 4.5 Net uptake of free fatty acids and plasma free fatty acid delivery at rest and during 2 hr of dynamic one-legged knee-extension exercise at 68% of maximum working capacity. Values are means ± SE of 8 observations. Adapted with permission from Kiens et al. (1993).

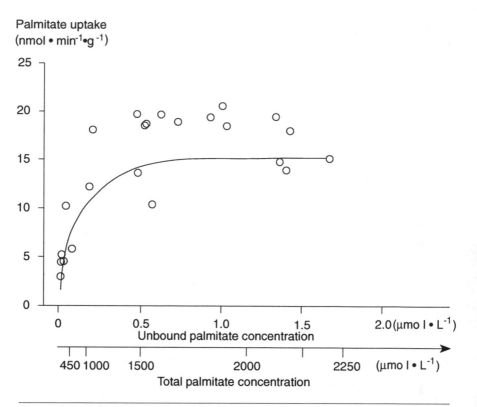

Figure 4.6   Palmitate uptake of perfused rat hindquarters as a function of unbound palmitate concentration. Abscissa also indicates the corresponding total
palmitate concentrations from which the unbound fraction was calculated by
the stepwise equilibrium method (albumin concentration = 510 µM). Each point
represents the average uptake value of one rat (n=23). Reprinted with permission
from Turcotte et al. (1991).

system for FFA in skeletal muscle is hormonally regulated also remains
to be elucidated.

Cytoplasmic Transport of FFA

Translocation of lipophilic substances across the aqueous environment
prevalent in the cytosol of cells is facilitated by several families of cellular
transport proteins. At least two different types of proteins implicated in
the intracellular transport of FFA and their fatty acyl-CoA and acyl-L-
carnitine esters have been identified in most tissues (50). Structurally
distinct cytoplasmic fatty acid binding proteins (FABP$_C$) with a molecular
weight between 12 and 14 kDa have been isolated from different tissues,
including liver, adipose tissue, heart, and intestine, and some isoforms

of these proteins have been characterized (50). Fatty acyl-CoA and acyl-L-carnitine esters bind to $FABP_C$ with an affinity comparable to that of their corresponding FFA (49). In rat skeletal muscle cytosols, the level of heart $FABP_C$ has been shown to be fiber type specific with high levels in slow-twitch oxidative (SO) fibers, intermediate levels in fast-twitch oxidative glycolytic (FOG) fibers, and low levels in fast-twitch glycolytic (FG) fibers (80). An acyl-CoA binding protein (ACBP) with a molecular weight of 10 kDa has also been identified in various tissues (82). So far, heterogeneity between tissues has not been observed, and only fatty acyl-CoA esters bind to ACBP (50).

The existence of distinct $FABP_C$ types and isoforms, the presence and separate regulation of two $FABP_C$ types in the same cell, and the existence of phosphorylated forms of these proteins have challenged the notion that $FABP_C$ are merely the cytoplasmic equivalent of serum albumin. The physiological functions attributed to $FABP_C$ are still largely speculative, but they include promoting cellular uptake of FFA and transport of FFA across the cytoplasm, protecting enzymes and cellular structures against the toxic effects of FFA, modulating enzyme activities, and targeting of FFA to specific metabolic pathways (101). In the heart, it has been shown that $FABP_C$ can transfer fatty acids to the mitochondria *in vitro*, suggesting that heart $FABP_C$ are a key factor in the utilization of FFA for energy production (35). The possible roles of $FABP_C$ in skeletal muscle have not yet been elucidated.

Intracellular Metabolism

Once inside the muscle cell, FFA are directed either to mitochondrial oxidation or to esterification in the intramuscular TG pool. Even in conditions of increased metabolic rate, the percentage of plasma FFA taken up that is directly oxidized never reaches a value of 100%, suggesting that a certain portion of plasma FFA are available for other metabolic pathways.

The rate of FFA oxidation is, to a large extent, dependent on exercise intensity and duration. As indicated by the observed increase in respiratory exchange ratio (RER), the relative contribution of lipids to total oxidative metabolism decreases as the intensity of exercise increases (23). However, during light- to moderate-intensity exercise, when lactate accumulation is minimal, the decrease in the relative contribution of lipids to oxidative metabolism is minimal compared with the increase in oxygen consumption, resulting in an increase in total lipid utilization until the intensity of exercise reaches a value equal to approximately 60-70% of $\dot{V}O_2$ max (48). Furthermore, as light- to moderate-intensity exercise progresses, the contribution of lipids to oxidative metabolism increases, as evidenced by a progressive decrease in RER during 4 hr of light-intensity exercise (8). Whereas factors such as the availability of FFA and other substrates and the oxidative capacity of skeletal muscle play a role in the regulation of FFA utilization, no convincing evidence has emerged to suggest that the process is under direct hormonal regulation.

The rate of FFA oxidation is, in part, a function of the plasma FFA concentration, and at a given FFA concentration it is also dependent on the metabolic rate (69, 89). In dogs (9) and humans (52, 69) plasma FFA turnover and oxidation have been shown to correlate with plasma FFA concentration, and during light- to moderate-intensity exercise FFA concentration increases with exercise intensity and duration (89, 91). In studies of men exercising at 30% of $\dot{V}O_2$ max, Ahlborg et al. (8) have shown that the gradual increase in plasma FFA level was accompanied by a progressive rise in the turnover rate of labeled oleate. The onset of exercise is usually accompanied by an immediate increase in the rate of FFA uptake and oxidation by the active muscles. Initially, this enhanced utilization of plasma FFA is not completely matched by an increased mobilization of FFA from adipose tissue, resulting in a small transient decrease in plasma FFA concentration (57, 59). As exercise continues, the rate of FFA mobilization increases and eventually exceeds the rate of FFA utilization, resulting in a gradual increase in plasma FFA concentration (89, 91); and the higher the work intensity, as long as it remains below the level at which lactate accumulates, the greater is the increase in FFA concentration. Thus, during prolonged mild- to moderate-intensity exercise in humans and dogs, the gradual increase in plasma FFA level is associated with an increase in the rate of FFA turnover and oxidation. At high FFA concentration, however, FFA uptake and oxidation plateau (73, 115, 116). It is interesting that this relationship between FFA concentration and FFA uptake is altered by endurance training, such that leveling off is not seen after training (73).

Although the capacity to oxidize FFA at a given FFA concentration has been shown to be dependent, in part, on the activity of β-oxidative and Krebs cycle enzymes such as β-hydroxyacyl-CoA dehydrogenase (HAD) and citrate synthase (CS), respectively (31, 51, 60), the oxidative potential of skeletal muscle certainly does not completely dictate the rate of lipid utilization during exercise (26, 73, 116). For example, in runners with similar rates of lipid oxidation during a 1-hr run at 70% $\dot{V}O_2$ max, significant differences were found in skeletal muscle carnitine palmitoyltransferase I (CPT-I) and succinate dehydrogenase (SDH) activities as well as in the capacity of skeletal muscle homogenates to oxidize palmitoyl CoA (26). These results suggest that other cellular factors may be implicated in the regulation of lipid oxidation by working skeletal muscles.

CPT-I, which is located on the outer surface of the inner mitochondrial membrane, has been proposed as an important site of regulation for hepatic FFA oxidation (104). The proposed regulator of CPT-I activity, malonyl-CoA, is formed by acetyl-CoA carboxylase in the rate-limiting reaction of fatty acid synthesis. *In vitro* studies have shown that, like hepatic CPT-I, skeletal muscle CPT-I is sensitive to regulation by fluctuations in malonyl-CoA concentration (79). In liver tissue, glucose abundance increases the rate of fatty acid synthesis, and the associated increase in the concentration of malonyl-CoA inhibits CPT-I and thereby β-oxidation. In conditions of glucose paucity such as fasting, acetyl-CoA carboxylase is inactivated, and the resulting decrease in malonyl-CoA concentration releases the inhibition on CPT-I and increases the rate of β-oxidation. Rat skeletal muscle malonyl-CoA levels have been shown to decrease in response to fasting and to 30 min of treadmill running, suggesting that malonyl-CoA levels may be a contributing factor in the regulation of FFA oxidation (79, 124) (Figure 4.7).

Evidence collected in isolated and perfused skeletal muscle suggests that the availability of carbohydrates may be an important factor determining the utilization of FFA (64, 94, 119). Hopp and Palmer (64) have shown in the isolated contracting rat flexor digitorum brevis (FDB) muscle that the oxidation of exogenous palmitate was lower in muscles incubated without glucose and insulin than in muscles incubated with both. These results suggest that the availability of exogenous glucose affected the utilization of exogenous FFA. In perfused contracting rat skeletal muscle, extreme carbohydrate deficiency, characterized by low muscle glycogen levels and by the absence of glucose in the perfusate, decreased total palmitate oxidation at high perfusate palmitate concentration (94, 119). Taken together these results suggest that with a decrease in the availability of total carbohydrate sources, FFA oxidation is decreased at high palmitate concentration. It has been suggested that low carbohydrate availability impairs high rates of aerobic energy production because the shift to fats as the predominant fuel leads to either a reduction in the production rate of acetyl-CoA units or an inability to maintain an adequate level of Krebs cycle intermediates (KCI) (83). Extreme carbohydrate deficiency in the perfused contracting skeletal muscle, however, was not associated with a decrease in muscle malate or citrate, two KCI that contribute 70-80% of the increase in the total level of KCI following skeletal muscle stimulation (34). These results suggest that KCI depletion was not the cause of the decreased palmitate oxidation at high palmitate concentration. Recent evidence collected in exercising humans suggests, however, that production of acetyl-CoA units is not limiting the function of the Krebs cycle in a state of glycogen depletion because the ratio of acetylcarnitine to carnitine, which is thought to reflect the availability of acetyl-CoA units, was maintained in exercising muscles at fatigue (95). Thus, the mechanisms linking carbohydrate depletion to impaired performance are still unclear.

It is difficult from the available evidence to accurately quantitate the percentage of plasma FFA uptake by muscle that is directed to metabolic pathways other than oxidation. Dagenais et al. (27) hypothesized that the immediate fate of all plasma FFA taken up by muscle was esterification in a large intramuscular TG pool. Using resting forearm skeletal muscle, the authors showed that the infusion of [1-^{14}C]oleic acid did not result in appreciable venous appearance of $^{14}CO_2$ for about 30 min, despite the fact

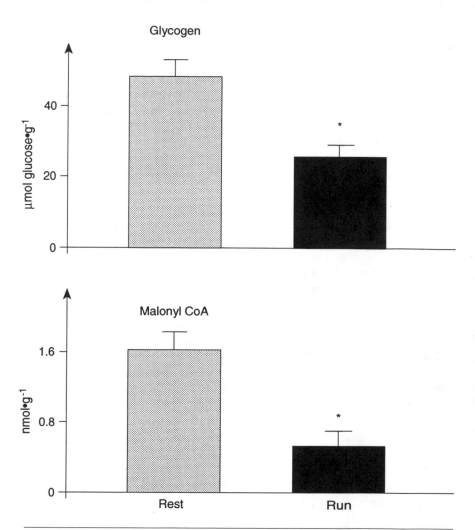

Figure 4.7 Effect of 30 min of treadmill exercise (21 m/min, 15% grade) on muscle glycogen and malonyl CoA in the gastrocnemius/plantaris muscles of rats. Values are means ± SE. * significantly different from the corresponding resting value, P<0.001. Adapted with permission from Winder et al. (1989).

that a significant oleate uptake occurred within 10 min, and they concluded that FFA taken up by muscle were first incorporated into intramuscular TG granules and subsequently underwent lipolysis at random. Thus, when muscle TG turnover is high, as it is during prolonged exercise, then FFA flux through the muscle pool would be high and plasma FFA taken up would be rapidly oxidized. During rest, the oxidation would lag markedly behind the uptake. This model thus argues against a direct pathway for plasma FFA oxidation. That a direct pathway may exist is evidenced by the findings of Hagenfeldt et al. (52). In exercising human forearm muscle, the percentage of radioactivity from plasma FFA recovered as $^{14}CO_2$ was on the average 60%, with the remaining radioactivity leaving the muscle as water soluble metabolites. Although no radioactivity was recovered in muscle lipids after 60 min of exercise, these results do not exclude the possibility that a small percentage of the FFA oxidized first passed through a small esterified pool of fatty acids with a rapid turnover.

Intramuscular Triacylglycerol Metabolism

It has been suggested that intramuscular TG is an important energy source for skeletal muscle metabolism, especially during prolonged exercise. These suggestions are based on the fact that isotopically determined plasma FFA oxidation does not match estimates of total lipid oxidation as calculated from RER measurements during prolonged exercise (58, 68). Thus, in postabsorptive exercising men and dogs, the oxidation of circulating plasma FFA can account for little more than half of the total lipid oxidation (58, 68). These results have led researchers to suggest that FFA released either from intramuscular TG pools or from adipose tissue located between muscle fibers are utilized for oxidative metabolism in working muscles (52, 58, 73).

Effects of Acute Exercise

Direct evidence for the utilization of intramuscular TG during exercise is available from some studies, but the exact quantitative contribution of this substrate is difficult to ascertain because of methodological limitations. To accurately quantify intramuscular TG content, it is imperative that all surrounding fat be dissected out before the muscle sample is analyzed; otherwise the contribution of adipocytes located between muscle fibers will be included in the measurement. In humans, the problem is compounded by the fact that the pre- and postexercise muscle biopsy samples usually do not have exactly the same fiber type composition. Because type I fibers have been shown to have a higher TG content than type II fibers (29), fiber type differences in muscle biopsy samples induce variation in biopsy TG concentrations.

Although the evidence collected from animal studies appears to be somewhat contradictory, the differences in results may reflect differences in the protocols and methods used to measure changes in TG concentration. The type and frequency of electrical stimulation employed to create muscle contractions appear to be two important factors that determine total intramuscular TG utilization. Intramuscular TG utilization has been measured in *in situ* mixed muscle (14) following prolonged stimulation at a twitch frequency of 5/sec but not at lower twitch frequencies (14,

78), suggesting that a minimal increase in metabolic rate is needed before intramuscular TG utilization can be measured during prolonged electrical stimulation. Similarly, intermittent stimulation of incubated FDB muscle resulted in a 39% decrease in TG content at a frequency of 5 Hz but not at lower frequencies (63, 64). The type of stimulation protocol may also affect total intramuscular TG utilization. Whereas continuous stimulation of incubated FDB muscle at 0.2 Hz for 30 min decreased TG content by 37%, there was no change in intramuscular TG concentration after intermittent stimulation at 0.2, 0.4, or 0.8 Hz (64). This suggests that a portion of intramuscular TG is constantly being synthesized and hydrolyzed and that the type and frequency of stimulation influence the relative rates of TG synthesis and hydrolysis and thus net intramuscular TG utilization. Similar considerations appear to affect intramuscular TG utilization during tetanic contractions. Whereas Barclay and Stainsby (14) found no change in mixed intramuscular TG content after stimulation at 40 tetani/min, Spriet et al. (102) found a 15-32% decrease in TG content of red muscle fibers after stimulation at 60 tetani/min.

Results collected from whole-body animal studies suggest that intramuscular TG utilization during exercise is dependent, at least in part, on exercise intensity and duration. Thus, a decrease in intramuscular TG content has been measured in red skeletal muscle after either exhaustive running (20, 114) or swimming (92, 103). When the intensity of exercise is mild to moderate, however, a net decrease in intramuscular TG has been difficult to demonstrate (40, 93), even after prolonged exercise.

In rats, intramuscular TG utilization is also dependent on the fiber type population sampled and is highest in FOG fibers, intermediate in SO fibers, and practically nonexistent in FG fibers (92). Differences in intramuscular TG utilization between fiber type populations follow the well-characterized differences in the capacity of muscle homogenates to oxidize FFA and in the activity of oxidative enzymes that exist between muscle fiber types (13).

Taking into consideration that skeletal muscle fiber recruitment is not the same between bicycle exercise, cross-country skiing, and running, researchers collected evidence from a number of studies in men that suggests TG content in vastus lateralis muscle decreases 25-50% during prolonged exercise at an exercise intensity of 55-75% of $\dot{V}O_2$ max (25, 29, 41). High-intensity exercise of short duration, however, may also result in significant intramuscular TG depletion. Thus, 5 min of intense bicycling exercise decreased intramuscular TG concentration by 29% (30).

Intramuscular TG utilization may also be influenced by the mode of exercise employed. Hurley et al. (65) observed a 20% decrease in intramuscular TG after 2 hr of bicycle exercise at 65% of $\dot{V}O_2$ max in untrained subjects. After 12 weeks of endurance training the decrease was twice as great. Thirty min of intermittent heavy resistance exercise activating the quadriceps femoris muscle has also been shown to decrease TG content by 30% (31). In contrast, Kiens et al. (73) found no change in intramuscular TG content following 2 hr of dynamic knee-extension exercise at 65% W_{max}. Although different, these results do not necessarily contradict each other but may, in fact, be a reflection of the different exercise modes employed. Bicycle and heavy-resistance exercise are associated with marked increases in plasma catecholamine levels, whereas one-legged knee-extension exercise is associated with catecholamine levels that are about one-third as high (47, 73, 113). This lower catecholamine response could affect the utilization of intramuscular TG because it has been shown in exercising humans that nonselective β-adrenergic blockade prevented muscle lipolysis (24). On the other hand, we have repeatedly been unable to obtain decreases in intramuscular TG concentration after prolonged exhaustive bicycle exercise (Kiens and Richter, unpublished observations). Thus, in 7 endurance-trained subjects with an average $\dot{V}O_2$ max of 4.5±0.1 L/min, 110 min of ergometer bicycling at 70% of $\dot{V}O_2$ max to exhaustion, at which point muscle glycogen stores were very low, did not decrease intramuscular TG concentrations (Table 4.1). Furthermore, in 10 untrained subjects with a mean $\dot{V}O_2$ max of 3.7 L/min, exhaustive ergometer bicycling at 77% of untrained $\dot{V}O_2$ max lasted on average 35 min before and 102 min after 8 weeks of endurance training. However, neither before nor after the training period did exercise cause a measurable decrease in intramuscular TG (Table 4.1).

It is thus apparent that the utilization of intramuscular TG is regulated by a number of factors that remain to be elucidated before a better understanding of the process can emerge. It is also important to keep in mind that the inability to measure an exercise-induced change in intramuscular TG content does not exclude the possibility that while FFA are being hydrolyzed from the intramuscular TG pool, TG is also being synthesized so that no net change in concentration is observed. As previously discussed, Dagenais et al. (27) have suggested that the intramuscular TG

Table 4.1   Muscle Triacylglycerol Concentrations Before and After Exercise

	Before	After
Endurance-trained ($n=7$)	48.9 ± 5.1	49.3 ± 7.6
Sedentary:		
Before training ($n=10$)	47.8 ± 3.2	43.4 ± 5.4
After 8 weeks of training ($n=10$)	47.5 ± 5.8	44.8 ± 4.2

Values are means ± SE. Muscle biopsies were obtained from the vastus lateralis before and after exhausting bicycle exercise. Triacylglycerol concentration was measured in freeze-dried muscle dissected free of visible fat, blood, and connective tissue, and is expressed as $mmol \cdot kg^{-1} d.w.$

pool is in constant turnover, and thus a net decrease in intramuscular TG would only be measured when the rate of utilization of intramuscular TG exceeds the rate of TG synthesis. In keeping with this notion, plasma-derived ^{14}C-FFA has been measured in the intramuscular TG pool during exercise conditions associated with no change in TG content (76). Finally, it is difficult to envision a role for intramuscular TG other than as a source of fuel.

Regulation of Intramuscular TG Utilization

Over the past decade, many attempts have been made to identify an enzyme responsible for the hydrolysis of intramuscular TG. In the early 1980s, Oscai et al. (88) proposed that the intracellular fraction of lipoprotein lipase (LPL) functioned as a TG lipase in skeletal muscle and heart. Evidence for this hypothesis included the fact that the activity of the intracellular fraction of LPL was increased in red skeletal muscle of exercising rats and that the increase was dependent on the intensity of the exercise bout (88). Perfusion of the rat hindquarter preparation with epinephrine increased intracellular LPL activity in SO, FOG, and FG fibers, indicating that the enzyme was sensitive to hormone stimulation (88). Furthermore, there was an inverse relationship between intracellular LPL activity and TG levels in skeletal muscle during exercise (87). One drawback of this hypothesis, however, was that LPL activity is negligible at neutral pH. Because the pH inside skeletal muscle cells is about 7 at rest and decreases during exercise, the role of intracellular LPL activity in intramuscular TG hydrolysis was challenged (96). Other investigators proposed that an HSL enzyme similar to the neutral pH optimum adipose tissue HSL could regulate intramuscular TG hydrolysis (96). Following the production of an antibody raised against the purified rat adipose tissue HSL, immunological evidence was presented to support this hypothesis. In rat skeletal muscle extracts, immunoblotting with this antibody revealed the presence of an antigenic protein with a molecular mass similar to the adipose tissue HSL (61). The use of a cDNA clone to perform Northern blotting showed that HSL mRNA in heart and skeletal muscle were also similar in size to that found in adipose tissue (62). Furthermore, cAMP-dependent protein kinase was able to phosphorylate HSL in rat cardiac myocyte preparations (98).

There is some evidence that, in skeletal muscle as in adipose tissue, the adrenergic system and insulin may play stimulatory and inhibitory roles in the activation of lipolysis (1, 2). In incubated diaphragm, stimulation of β-adrenergic receptors with isoproterenol increased both the intracellular cAMP level and the rate of appearance of glycerol into the incubation medium, suggesting the involvement of the cAMP cascade in the activation of intramuscular TG lipolysis. This hypothesis was supported by the activation of skeletal muscle lipolysis by dibutyryl cyclic-AMP and by the partial inhibition of isoproterenol-stimulated lipolysis by insulin (1, 2). In a study performed in swimming rats, Stankiewicz-Choroszucha and Gorski (103) showed that β-blockade with propranolol prevented the decrease in TG concentration in red skeletal muscle, emphasizing the importance of adrenergic stimulation in the regulation of intramuscular TG hydrolysis. In exercising humans, intramuscular lipolysis was inhibited by nonselective β-blockade (24). However, the decrease in intramuscular TG concentration measured after direct stimulation of a muscle with electrodes (63, 64) clearly suggests that lipolysis in contracting skeletal muscle may be activated by local nonadrenergic mechanisms.

Plasma Triacylglycerol Metabolism

Like long-chain FFA, plasma triacylglycerols (TG) are not soluble in water and thus are transported between tissues bound to lipoprotein complexes. Chylomicrons and very low density lipoproteins (VLDL) are TG-rich lipoproteins produced respectively by the intestinal tract (following the ingestion of a lipid-containing meal) and by the liver. Because the turnover rate of chylomicron-TG is as high as that of plasma FFA, the uptake of chylomicron TG-derived FFA during exercise in a fed condition could represent a potential source of fatty acids for β-oxidation or for the maintenance of the intramuscular TG pool in working muscles (111). For practical reasons, however, the contribution of chylomicron TG-derived FFA to skeletal muscle metabolism is usually minimal because exercise is usually not conducted in close proximity to a fatty meal.

Effects of Acute Exercise

Evidence collected from animal and human studies suggests that the contribution of TG-derived FFA to total oxidative metabolism does not exceed 10% during exercise in a postprandial state (71, 76, 85, 112). In rat skeletal muscle, the uptake of ^{14}C-TG was found to be higher in oxidative SO and FOG fibers than in FG fibers, and muscle stimulation increased the fractional uptake in all three fiber types (76).

In humans fasted overnight, no significant extraction of plasma TG was measured after 15 min of forearm exercise, even when plasma TG levels were increased by infusion of Intralipid (71, 85). Similarly, during prolonged bicycle exercise and one-legged knee-extension exercise the net extraction of plasma TG across the working muscles was found to be minimal (58, 116). When isolating VLDL-TG from total serum TG, however, Kiens et al. (73) found a net uptake of circulating VLDL-TG across the thigh during 2 hr of knee-extension exercise. These latter findings suggest that the VLDL-fraction of serum TG could serve, to some extent, as an available source of lipid for skeletal muscle during submaximal endurance exercise.

Regulation of Plasma TG Utilization

Lipoprotein lipase (LPL) is a tissue-bound triacylglycerol hydrolase located at the luminal surface of the endothelial cells of capillaries. The function of LPL is to hydrolyze the TG core of circulating chylomicrons and VLDL to release FFA prior to their uptake by extrahepatic tissues such as adipose tissue and skeletal muscle. In rat skeletal muscle LPL activity is correlated with the fiber's capacity for oxidative metabolism. Thus, LPL activity is highest in red oxidative fibers and lowest in white glycolytic fibers (109). There exists a high correlation between skeletal muscle LPL activity and the uptake of circulating TG. Thus, in rat skeletal muscle the fractional uptake of ^{14}C-labeled plasma TG was highest in SO fibers, intermediate in FOG fibers, and lowest in FG fibers, and the uptake varied with LPL activity, suggesting that the uptake is dependent on the hydrolic action of LPL on serum lipids (76).

Studies have suggested that skeletal muscle LPL activity may be elevated following prolonged exercise. Thus in overnight-fasted, well-trained men, prolonged running (20 km) or cross-country skiing (> 8 hr) was associated with a twofold increase in skeletal muscle LPL activity (75, 110). However, 1 hr of bicycle exercise was not associated with an increase in the skeletal muscle LPL activity of healthy young subjects (74). In knee extensors, LPL activity was not changed immediately following 1 hr of dynamic knee-extension exercise in healthy young men but was increased 4 hr later (72). Taken together these data suggest that the increase in skeletal muscle LPL activity may develop slowly and may not be evident until several hours after the onset of exercise.

Ketone Bodies Metabolism

Acetoacetate and β-hydroxybutyrate are the only freely soluble circulating lipid fuels and are known as *ketone bodies*. Although ketone bodies do not adhere to the strict biochemical definition of a lipid, they are generally classified as "water-soluble oxidizable lipid-fuel" (83). They arise from the partial oxidation of FFA in the liver and can be used by most aerobic tissues, including skeletal muscle, heart, and brain tissues, especially during conditions of carbohydrate starvation. The concentration of ketone bodies in the blood of fed, healthy humans is very low, but it can reach values of 2-3 mM after 3 days of fasting, 7-8 mM after 3 weeks of fasting, and as high as 25-30 mM in severely ketotic diabetic patients.

Effects of Acute Exercise

The rate of ketone bodies utilization by various tissues is dependent, in part, on their blood concentration. During exercise, blood ketone bodies levels vary with exercise duration. During 3 hr of knee-extension exercise, blood β-hydroxybutyrate concentration gradually increased from a basal value of 40 µM to 335 µM (116). However, the contribution of ketone bodies oxidation to total oxidative metabolism is usually minimal. In healthy postabsorptive men with low ketone bodies levels, the contribution of ketone bodies to basal skeletal muscle oxidative metabolism, as estimated from the arterial-venous concentration differences across the resting forearm muscle, was found to be less than 2% (53). Although bicycle and knee-extension exercise have been shown to increase the uptake of β-hydroxybutyrate by working muscles, the calculated percent contribution of ketone bodies oxidation to total energy expenditure does not exceed 1-2% (73, 116, 121). In ketotic diabetic patients with basal blood ketone bodies levels above 3 mM, although the leg uptake of ketone bodies was markedly increased by bicycle exercise, the calculated contribution of ketone bodies to leg oxidative metabolism still remained below 5% (120).

Summary

Plasma triacylglycerols (TG) and free fatty acids (FFA), as well as intramuscular TG, are oxidizable lipid fuel sources for skeletal muscle metabolism during endurance exercise.

Plasma FFA are a major fuel oxidized by skeletal muscle, and the mobilization of FFA from adipose tissue is the first committed step in their metabolism. The rate of FFA mobilization is dependent on the rate of adipose tissue lipolysis, the plasma transport capacity for FFA, and the rate of FFA reesterification. The rate of adipose tissue lipolysis increases during prolonged submaximal exercise. The essential hormonal changes promoting increased lipolysis during whole-body exercise are an increase in catecholamine levels and a decrease in insulin concentration, both of which facilitate the activation of the hormone-sensitive lipase system through changes in its phosphorylation state. Independently of the exercise-induced hormonal changes, glucose concentration also regulates FFA mobilization by suppressing lipolysis. The plasma transport capacity for FFA is dependent on blood flow and on the FFA/albumin molar ratio. During prolonged submaximal exercise the increase in adipose tissue blood flow compensates for the increase in the FFA/albumin molar ratio to favor an increase in FFA mobilization. As part of the triglyceride-fatty acid cycle, the exercise-induced decrease in the rate of FFA reesterification acts in concert with the exercise-induced increase in lipolysis to amplify the response and favor a net increase in FFA mobilization.

Following the transport of FFA in plasma, FFA permeation across the plasma membranes is the next step in the metabolism of FFA. In all cell types studied to date, evidence shows that at least part of the permeation of FFA across the plasma membranes is carrier-mediated and that a plasma membrane fatty acid binding protein may be the functional transporter. Possible regulation of FFA metabolism through changes in the rate of permeation remain to be elucidated. Cytoplasmic transport of FFA is facilitated by another family of fatty acid binding proteins whose level in skeletal muscle is correlated with the oxidative capacity of the muscle fiber types.

Intracellular metabolism of FFA is regulated by a number of factors. In skeletal muscle, the rate of FFA oxidation increases with an increase in the plasma FFA concentration. At a given FFA concentration, it increases with an increase in the metabolic rate. At high FFA concentration, the rate of FFA oxidation tends to plateau. The rate of FFA oxidation is also regulated in part by the oxidative capacity of the recruited fibers, the intramuscular concentration of malonyl-CoA, and the availability of carbohydrate sources.

Results from muscle biopsy and tracer studies indicate that intramuscular TG contribute to skeletal muscle oxidative metabolism during exercise. However, accurate quantitative assessment of their contribution is still lacking because of methodological considerations. Evidence shows that intramuscular TG utilization is dependent on exercise intensity, exercise duration, and exercise mode as well as fiber type recruitment. The exercise-induced increase in catecholamine levels and decrease in insulin concentration play stimulatory and inhibitory roles in the activation of intramuscular lipolysis through changes in the activity of intramuscular HSL.

During prolonged submaximal exercise, the contribution of plasma TG and ketone bodies to skeletal muscle oxidative metabolism is small. The rate of utilization of plasma TG is dependent on lipoprotein lipase (LPL) activity which is correlated with the fiber's capacity for oxidative metabolism. The rate of utilization of ketone bodies is dependent in part on their blood concentration. During prolonged exercise, blood ketone bodies' concentration increases slightly but their total contribution to skeletal muscle oxidative metabolism remains minimal.

Acknowledgments

The authors wish to thank Betina Bolmgreen for her expert technical assistance during all research projects conducted at the August Krogh Institute. The authors received support from the Danish Medical Research Council (12-9535), the Danish Natural Sciences Research Council (11-0082), Novo Research Foundation, and Nordisk Insulin Research Foundation. Lorraine P. Turcotte was supported by a postdoctoral fellowship from the Fonds de la Recherche en Santé du Québec.

References

1. Abumrad, N.A.; Stearns, S.B.; Tepperman, H.M.; Tepperman, J. Studies on serum lipids, insulin, and glucagon and on muscle triglyceride in rats adapted to high-fat and high-carbohydrate diets. J. Lipid Res. 19:423-432; 1978.

2. Abumrad, N.A.; Tepperman, H.M.; Tepperman, J. Control of endogenous triglyceride breakdown in the mouse diaphragm. J. Lipid Res. 21:149-155; 1980.

3. Abumrad, N.A.; Perkins, R.C.; Park, J.H.; Park, C.R. Mechanisms of long chain fatty acid permeation in the isolated adipocyte. J. Biol. Chem. 256(17):9183-9191; 1981.

4. Abumrad, N.A.; Park, J.H.; Park, C.R. Permeation of long-chain fatty acid into adipocytes. Kinetics, specificity, and evidence for involvement of a membrane protein. J. Biol. Chem. 259(14):8945-8953; 1984.

5. Abumrad, N.A.; Perry, P.R.; Whitesell, R.R. Stimulation by epinephrine of the membrane transport of long chain fatty acid in the adipocyte. J. Biol. Chem. 260(18):9969-9971; 1985.

6. Abumrad, N.A.; Park, C.R.; Whitesell, R.R. Catecholamine activation of the membrane transport of long chain fatty acids in adipocytes is mediated by cyclic AMP and protein kinase. J. Biol. Chem. 261(28):13082-13086; 1986.

7. Abumrad, N.A.; Harmon, C.M.; Barnela, U.S.; Whitesell, R.R. Insulin antagonism of catecholamine stimulation of fatty acid transport in the adipocyte. Studies on its mechanism of action. J. Biol. Chem. 263(29):14678-14683; 1988.

8. Ahlborg, G.; Felig, P.; Hagenfeldt, L.; Hendler, R.; Wahren, J. Substrate turnover during prolonged exercise in man. Splanchnic and leg metabolism of glucose, free fatty acids, and amino acids. J. Clin. Invest. 53:1080-1090; 1974.

9. Armstrong, D.T.; Steele, R.; Altszuler, N.; Dunn, A.; Bishop, J.S.; DeBodo, R.C. Regulation of plasma free fatty acid turnover. Am. J. Physiol. 201:9-15; 1961.

10. Arner, P.; Bolinder, J.; Ostman, J. Glucose stimulation of the antilipolytic effect of insulin in humans. Science 220:1057-1059; 1983.

11. Arner, P.; Bolinder, J.; Eliasson, A.; Lundin, A.; Ungerstedt, U. Microdialysis of adipose tissue and blood for *in vivo* lipolysis studies. Am. J. Physiol. 255:E737-E742; 1988.

12. Arner, P.; Kriegholm, E.; Engfeldt, P.; Bolinder, J. Adrenergic regulation of lipolysis *in situ* at rest and during exercise. J. Clin. Invest. 85:893-898; 1990.

13. Baldwin, K.M.; Reitman, J.S.; Terjung, R.L.; Winder, W.W.; Holloszy, J.O. Substrate depletion in different fiber types of muscles and liver during prolonged running. Am. J. Physiol. 225:1045-1050; 1973.

14. Barclay, J.K.; Stainsby, W.N. Intramuscular lipid store utilization by contracting dog skeletal muscle *in situ*. Am. J. Physiol. 223(1):115-119; 1972.

15. Brauer, R.W.; Pessotti, R.L. The removal of bromosulphthalein from blood plasma by the liver of the rat. J. Pharmacol. Exp. Ther. 97:358-370; 1949.

16. Brooks, B.; Arch, J.R.S.; Newsholme, E.A. Effects of hormones on the rate of the triacylglycerol/fatty acid substrate cycle in adipocytes and epididymal fat pads. FEBS Lett. 146:327-330; 1982.

17. Bulow, J.; Madsen, J. Adipose tissue blood flow during prolonged, heavy exercise. Pflugers Arch. 363:231-234; 1976.

18. Bulow, J.; Madsen, J. Human adipose tissue blood flow during prolonged exercise II. Pflugers Arch. 376:41-45; 1978.

19. Bulow, J. Regulation of lipid mobilization in exercise. Can. J. Spt. Sci. 12(Suppl):117S-119S; 1987.

20. Carlson, L.A. Lipid metabolism and muscular work. Fed. Proc. 26:1755-1758; 1967.

21. Carlson, M.G.; Snead, W.L.; Hill, J.O.; Nurjahan, N.; Campbell, P.J. Glucose regulation of lipid metabolism in humans. Am. J. Physiol. 261:E815-E820; 1991.

22. Chisholm, D.J.; Jenkins, A.B.; James, D.E.; Kraegen, E.W. The effect of hyperinsulinemia on glucose homeostasis during moderate exercise in man. Diabetes 31:603-608; 1982.

23. Christensen, E.H.; Hansen, O. Respiratorischer quotient und O_2-aufnahme. Scand. Arch. Physiol. 81:180-189; 1939.

24. Cleroux, J.; Van Nguyen, P.; Taylor, A.W.; Leenen, F.H.H. Effects of β_1- vs. $\beta_1+\beta_2$-blockade on exercise endurance and muscle metabolism in humans. J. Appl. Physiol. 66(2):548-554; 1989.

25. Costill, D.L.; Gollnick, P.D.; Jansson, E.; Saltin, B.; Stein, E.M. Glycogen depletion pattern in human muscle fibres during distance running. Acta Physiol. Scand. 89:374-383; 1973.

26. Costill, D.L.; Fink, W.J.; Getchell, L.H.; Ivy, J.L.; Witzmann, F.A. Lipid metabolism in skeletal muscle of endurance-trained males and females. J. Appl. Physiol. 47(4):787-791; 1979.

27. Dagenais, G.R.; Tancredi, R.G.; Zierler, K.L. Free fatty acid oxidation by forearm muscle at rest, and evidence for an intramuscular lipid pool in the human forearm. J. Clin. Invest. 58:421-431; 1976.

28. Egan, J.J.; Greenberg, A.S.; Chang, M.-K.; Wek, S.A.; Moos, M.C., Jr.; Londos, C. Mechanism of hormone-stimulated lipolysis in adipocytes: translocation of hormone-sensitive lipase to the lipid storage droplet. Proc. Natl. Acad. Sci. USA 89:8537-8541; 1992.

29. Essen, B. Intramuscular substrate utilization during prolonged exercise. Ann. N.Y. Acad. Sci. 301:30-44; 1977.

30. Essen, B. Studies on the regulation of metabolism in human skeletal muscle using intermittent exercise as an experimental model. Acta Physiol. Scand. 454(Suppl):1-32; 1978.

31. Essen-Gustavsson, B.; Tesch, P. Glycogen and triglyceride utilization in relation to muscle metabolic characteristics in men performing heavy-resistance exercise. Eur. J. Appl. Physiol. 61:5-10; 1990.

32. Fain, J.N.; Garcia-Sainz, J.A. Adrenergic regulation of adipocyte metabolism. J. Lipid. Res. 24:945-966; 1983.

33. Felig, P.; Wahren, J. Fuel homeostasis in exercise. N. Engl. J. Med. 293:1078-1084; 1975.

34. Flanagan, W.F.; Holmes, E.W.; Sabina, R.L.; Swain, J.L. Importance of purine nucleotide cycle to energy production in skeletal muscle. Am. J. Physiol. 251:C795-C802; 1986.

35. Fournier, N.C.; Rahim, M.H. Self-aggregation, a new property of cardiac fatty acid-binding protein. Predictable influence on energy production in the heart. J. Biol. Chem. 258(5):2929-2933; 1983.

36. Fredholm, B.B. The effect of lactate in canine subcutaneous adipose tissue *in situ*. Acta Physiol. Scand. 81:110-123; 1971.

37. Fredrikson, G.; Stralfors, P.; Nilsson, N.O.; Belfrage, P. Hormone-sensitive lipase of rat adipose tissue. Purification and some properties. J. Biol. Chem. 256(12):6311-6320; 1981.

38. Fredrikson, G.; Belfrage, P. Positional specificity of hormone-sensitive lipase from rat adipose tissue. J. Biol. Chem. 258(23):14253-14256; 1983.

39. Fredrikson, G.; Tornqvist, H.; Belfrage, P. Hormone-sensitive lipase and monoacylglycerol lipase are both required for complete degradation of adipocyte triacylglycerol. Biochim. Biophys. Acta 876:288-293; 1986.

40. Froberg, S.O. Effect of acute exercise on tissue lipids in rats. Metabolism 20(7):714-720; 1971.

41. Froberg, S.O.; Carlson, L.A.; Ekelund, L.-G. Local lipid stores and exercise. In: Pernow, B.; Saltin, B., eds. Muscle metabolism during exercise. New York: Plenum Press; 1971: 307-313.

42. Gabbay, R.A.; Lardy, H.A. Site of insulin inhibition of cAMP-stimulated glycogenolysis. cAMP-dependent protein kinase is affected independent of cAMP changes. J. Biol. Chem. 259(10):6052-6055; 1984.

43. Galbo, H.; Holst, J.J.; Christensen, N.J. Glucagon and plasma catecholamine responses to graded and prolonged exercise in man. J. Appl. Physiol. 38(1):70-76; 1975.

44. Galbo, H.; Holst, J.J.; Christensen, N.J.; Hilsted, J. Glucagon and plasma catecholamines during beta-receptor blockade in exercising man. J. Appl. Physiol. 40(6):855-863; 1976.

45. Galbo, H.; Christensen, N.J.; Holst, J.J. Catecholamines and pancreatic hormones during autonomic blockade in exercising man. Acta Physiol. Scand. 101:428-437; 1977.

46. Galbo, H.; Holst, J.J.; Christensen, N.J. The effect of different diets and of insulin on the hormonal response to prolonged exercise. Acta Physiol. Scand. 107:19-32; 1979.

47. Galbo, H. Hormonal and metabolic adaptation to exercise. Stuttgart, Germany: Beorg Thieme Verlag; 1983: 64-69.

48. Galbo, H. Exercise physiology: humoral function. Sport Sci. Rev. 1:65-93; 1992.

49. Glatz, J.F.C.; Veerkamp, J.H. Intracellular fatty acid-binding proteins. Int. J. Biochem. 17:13-22; 1985.

50. Glatz, J.F.C.; van der Vusse, G.J. Cellular fatty acid-binding proteins: current concepts and future directions. Mol. Cell. Biochem. 98:237-251; 1990.

51. Gollnick, P.D.; Saltin, B. Significance of skeletal muscle oxidative enzyme enhancement with endurance training: hypothesis. Clin. Physiol. 2:1-12; 1982.

52. Hagenfeldt, L.; Wahren, J. Human forearm muscle metabolism during exercise. II. Uptake, release and oxidation of individual FFA and glycerol. Scand. J. Clin. Lab. Invest. 21:263-276; 1968.

53. Hagenfeldt, L.; Wahren, J. Metabolism of free fatty acids and ketone bodies in skeletal muscle. In: Pernow, B.; Saltin, B., eds. Muscle metabolism during exercise. New York: Plenum Press; 1971: 153-163.

54. Hagenfeldt, L.; Wahren, J.; Pernow, B.; Raf, L. Uptake of individual free fatty acids by skeletal muscle and liver in man. J. Clin. Invest. 51:2324-2330; 1972.

55. Hagenfeldt, L. Turnover of individual free fatty acids in man. Fed. Proc. 34(13):2246-2249; 1975.

56. Hales, C.N.; Luzio, J.P.; Liddle, K. Hormonal control of adipose tissue lipolysis. Biochem. Soc. Symp. 43:97-135; 1978.

57. Havel, R.J.; Naimark, A.; Borchgrevink, C.F. Turnover rate and oxidation of free fatty acids of blood plasma in man during exercise: studies during continuous infusion of palmitate-1-C^{14}. J. Clin. Invest. 42(7):1054-1063; 1963.

58. Havel, R.J.; Pernow, B.; Jones, N.L. Uptake and release of free fatty acids and other metabolites in the legs of exercising men. J. Appl. Physiol. 23(1):90-99; 1967.

59. Henriksson, J. Training induced adaptations of skeletal muscle and metabolism during submaximal exercise. J. Physiol. 270:661-675; 1977.

60. Holloszy, J.O.; Coyle, E.F. Adaptations of skeletal muscle to endurance exercise and their metabolic consequences. J. Appl. Physiol. 56(4):831-838; 1984.

61. Holm, C.; Belfrage, P.; Fredrikson, G. Immunological evidence for the presence of hormone-sensitive lipase in rat tissue other than adipose tissue. Biochem. Biophys. Res. Commun. 148:99-105; 1987.

62. Holm, C.; Kirchgessner, T.G.; Svenson, K.L.; Fredrikson, G.; Nilsson, S.; Miller, C.G.; Shively, J.E.; Heinzmann, C.; Sparkes, R.S.; Mohandas, T.; Lusis, A.J.; Belfrage, P.; Schotz, M.C. Hormone-sensitive lipase: Sequence, expression, and chromosomal localization to 19 cent-q13.3. Science 241:1503-1506; 1988.

63. Hopp, J.F.; Palmer, W.K. Effect of electrical stimulation on intracellular triacylglycerol in isolated skeletal muscle. J. Appl. Physiol. 68(1):348-354; 1990.

64. Hopp, J.F.; Palmer, W.K. Electrical stimulation alters fatty acid metabolism in isolated skeletal muscle. J. Appl. Physiol. 68(6):2473-2481; 1990.

65. Hurley, B.F.; Nemeth, P.M.; Martin, W.H., III; Hagberg, J.M.; Dalsky, G.P.; Holloszy, J.O. Muscle triglyceride utilization during exercise: effect of training. J. Appl. Physiol. 60(2):562-567; 1986.

66. Issekutz, B., Jr.; Miller, H. Plasma free fatty acids during exercise and the effect of lactic acid. Proc. Soc. Exp. Biol. Med. 110:237-239; 1962.

67. Issekutz, B., Jr.; Miller, H.I.; Rodahl, K. Effect of exercise on FFA metabolism of pancreatectomized dogs. Am. J. Physiol. 205(4):645-650; 1963.

68. Issekutz, B., Jr.; Miller, H.I.; Paul, P.; Rodahl, K. Source of fat oxidation in exercising dogs. Am. J. Physiol. 207:583-589; 1964.

69. Issekutz, B., Jr.; Bortz, W.M.; Miller, H.I.; Paul, P. Turnover rate of plasma FFA in humans and in dogs. Metabolism 16:1001-1009; 1967.

70. Issekutz, B., Jr. Role of beta-adrenergic receptors in mobilization of energy sources in exercising dogs. J. Appl. Physiol. 44:869-876; 1978.

71. Kaijser, L.; Rossner, S. Removal of exogenous triglycerides in human forearm muscle and subcutaneous tissue. Acta Med. Scand. 197:289-294; 1975.

72. Kiens, B.; Lithell, H.; Mikines, K.J.; Richter, E.A. Effects of insulin and exercise on muscle lipoprotein lipase activity in man and its relation to insulin action. J. Clin. Invest. 84:1124-1129; 1989.

73. Kiens, B.; Essen-Gustavsson, B.; Christensen, N.J.; Saltin, B. Skeletal muscle substrate utilization during submaximal exercise in man: effect of endurance training. J. Physiol. (London) 469:459-478; 1993.

74. Lithell, H.; Hellsing, K.; Lundqvist, G.; Malmberg, P. Lipoprotein-lipase activity of human skeletal-muscle and adipose tissue after intensive physical exercise. Acta Physiol. Scand. 105:312-315; 1979.

75. Lithell, H.; Orlander, J.; Schele, R.; Sjodin, B.; Karlsson, J. Changes in lipoprotein-lipase activity and lipid stores in human skeletal muscle with prolonged heavy exercise. Acta Physiol. Scand. 107:257-261; 1979.

76. Mackie, B.G.; Dudley, G.A.; Kaciuba-Uscilko, H.; Terjung, R.L. Uptake of chylomicron triglycerides by contracting skeletal muscle in rats. J. Appl. Physiol. 49(5):851-855; 1980.

77. Madsen, J.; Bulow, J.; Nielsen, N.E. Inhibition of fatty acid mobilization by arterial free fatty acid concentration. Acta Physiol. Scand. 127:161-166; 1986.

78. Masoro, E.J.; Rowell, L.B.; McDonald, R.M.; Steiert, B. Skeletal muscle lipids: II. Nonutilization of intracellular lipid esters as an energy source for contractile activity. J. Biol. Chem. 244:2626-2634; 1966.

79. McGarry, J.D.; Mills, S.E.; Long, C.S.; Foster, D.W. Observations on the affinity for carnitine, and malonyl-CoA sensitivity, of carnitine palmitoyltransferase I in animal and human tissues. Biochem. J. 214:21-28; 1983.

80. Miller, W.C.; Hickson, R.C.; Bass, N.M. Fatty acid binding proteins in the three types of rat skeletal muscle. Proc. Soc. Exp. Biol. Med. 189:183-188; 1988.

81. Miyoshi, H.; Shulman, G.I.; Peters, E.J.; Wolfe, M.H.; Elahi, D.; Wolfe, R.R. Hormonal control of substrate cycling in humans. J. Clin. Invest. 81:1545-1555; 1988.

82. Mogensen, I.B.; Schulenberg, H.; Hansen, H.O.; Spener, F.; Knudsen, J. A novel acyl-CoA-binding protein from bovine liver: effect on fatty acid synthesis. Biochem. J. 241:189-192; 1987.

83. Newsholme, E.A.; Leech, A.R. Biochemistry for the medical sciences. New York: John Wiley and Sons; 1983: 246-300.

84. Nilsson, N.O.; Stralfors, P.; Fredrikson, G.; Belfrage, P. Regulation of adipose tissue lipolysis: effects of noradrenaline and insulin on phosphorylation of hormone-sensitive lipase and on lipolysis in intact rat adipocytes. FEBS Lett. 111(1):125-130; 1980.

85. Olsson, A.G.; Eklund, B.; Kaijser, L.; Carlson, L.A. Extraction of endogenous plasma triglycerides by the working human forearm muscle in the fasting state. Scand. J. Clin. Lab. Invest. 35:231-236; 1975.

86. Olsson, H.; Belfrage, P. The regulatory and basal phosphorylation sites of hormone-sensitive lipase are dephosphorylated by protein phosphatase-1, 2A and 2C but not by protein phosphatase-2B. Eur. J. Biochem. 168:399-405; 1987.

87. Oscai, L.B.; Caruso, R.A.; Wergeles, A.C. Lipoprotein lipase hydrolyzes endogenous triacylglycerols in muscles of exercised rats. J. Appl. Physiol. 52:1059-1063; 1982.

88. Oscai, L.B. Type L hormone-sensitive lipase hydrolyzes endogenous triacylglycerols in muscle in exercised rats. Med. Sci. Sports Exerc. 15(4):336-339; 1983.

89. Paul, P. FFA metabolism of normal dogs during steady-state exercise at different work loads. J. Appl. Physiol. 28(2):127-132; 1970.

90. Potter, B.J.; Sorrentino, D.; Berk, P.D. Mechanisms of cellular uptake of free fatty acids. Ann. Rev. Nutr. 9:253-270; 1989.

91. Pruett, E.D.R. FFA mobilization during and after prolonged severe muscular work in men. J. Appl. Physiol. 29(6):809-815; 1970.

92. Reitman, J.; Baldwin, K.M.; Holloszy, J.O. Intramuscular triglyceride utilization by red, white, and intermediate skeletal muscle and heart during exhausting exercise. Proc. Soc. Exp. Biol. Med. 142(2):628-631; 1973.

93. Richter, E.A.; Sonne, B.; Mikines, K.J.; Ploug, T.; Galbo, H. Muscle and liver glycogen, protein, and triglyceride in the rat. Effect of exercise and of the sympatho-adrenal system. Eur. J. Appl. Physiol. 52:346-350; 1984.

94. Richter, E.A.; Turcotte, L.P.; Hespel, P.; Graham, T.; Kiens, B. Regional substrate metabolism during exercise in humans. In: Devlin, J.; Horton, E.S.; Vranic, M., eds. Diabetes mellitus and exercise. London: Smith-Gordon and Company Limited; 1992: 129-138.

95. Sahlin, K.; Katz, A.; Broberg, S. Tricarboxylic acid cycle intermediates in human muscle during prolonged exercise. Am. J. Physiol. 259:C834-C841; 1990.

96. Severson, D.L. Regulation of lipid metabolism in adipose tissue and heart. Can. J. Physiol. Pharmacol. 57:923-937; 1979.

97. Shaw, W.A.S.; Issekutz, T.B.; Issekutz, B., Jr. Interrelationship of FFA and glycerol turnovers in resting and exercising dogs. J. Appl. Physiol. 39:30-36; 1975.

98. Small, C.A.; Garton, A.J.; Yeaman, S.J. The presence and role of hormone-sensitive lipase in heart muscle. Biochem. J. 258:67-72; 1989.

99. Sorrentino, D.; Robinson, R.B.; Kiang, C.-L.; Berk, P.D. At physiologic albumin/oleate concentrations oleate uptake by isolated hepatocytes, cardiac myocytes, and adipocytes is a saturable function of the unbound oleate concentration. Uptake kinetics are consistent with the conventional theory. J. Clin. Invest. 84:1325-1333; 1989.

100. Spector, A.A.; Fletcher, J.E.; Ashbrook, J.D. Analysis of long-chain free fatty acid binding to bovine serum albumin by determination of stepwise equilibrium constants. Biochem. 10:3229-3232; 1971.

101. Spener, F.; Borchers, T.; Mukherjea, M. On the role of fatty acid binding proteins in fatty acid transport and metabolism. FEBS Lett. 244(1):1-5; 1989.

102. Spriet, L.L.; Heigenhauser, G.J.F.; Jones, N.L. Endogenous triacylglycerol utilization by rat skeletal muscle during tetanic stimulation. J. Appl. Physiol. 60(2):410-415; 1986.

103. Stankiewicz-Choroszucha, B.; Gorski, J. Effect of decreased availability of substrates on intramuscular triglyceride utilization during exercise. Eur. J. Appl. Physiol. 40(1):27-35; 1978.

104. Stewart, H.B.; Tubbs, P.K.; Stanley, K.K. Intermediates in fatty acid oxidation. Biochem. J. 132:61-76; 1973.

105. Stralfors, P.; Belfrage, P. Phosphorylation of hormone-sensitive lipase by cyclic AMP-dependent protein kinase. J. Biol. Chem. 258(24):15146-15152; 1983.

106. Stralfors, P.; Bjorgell, P.; Belfrage, P. Hormonal regulation of hormone-sensitive lipase in intact adipocytes: identification of phosphorylated sites and effects on the phosphorylation by lipolytic hormones and insulin. Proc. Natl. Acad. Sci. USA 81:3317-3321; 1984.

107. Stralfors, P.; Honnor, R.C. Insulin-induced dephosphorylation of hormone-sensitive lipase. Correlation with lipolysis and cAMP-dependent protein kinase activity. Eur. J. Biochem. 182:379-385; 1989.

108. Stremmel, W.; Strohmeyer, G.; Berk, P.D. Hepatocellular uptake of oleate is energy dependent, sodium linked, and inhibited by an antibody to a hepatocyte plasma membrane fatty acid binding protein. Proc. Natl. Acad. Sci. USA 83:3584-3588; 1986.

109. Tan, M.H.; Sata, T.; Havel, R.J. The significance of lipoprotein lipase in rat skeletal muscles. J. Lipid Res. 18:363-370; 1977.

110. Taskinen, M.-R.; Nikkila, E.A.; Rehunen, S.; Gordin, A. Effect of acute vigorous exercise on lipoprotein lipase activity of adipose tissue and skeletal muscle in physically active men. Artery 6(6):471-483; 1980.

111. Terjung, R.L.; Budohoski, L.; Nazar, K.; Kobryn, A.; Kaciuba-Uscilko, H. Chylomicron triglyceride metabolism in resting and exercising fed dogs. J. Appl. Physiol. 52:815-820; 1982.

112. Terjung, R.L.; Kaciuba-Uscilko, H. Lipid metabolism during exercise: influence of training. Diabetes/Metabolism Rev. 2:35-51; 1986.

113. Tesch, P.A. Acute and long-term metabolic changes consequent to heavy-resistance exercise. Med. Sport. Sci. 26:67-89; 1987.

114. Therriault, D.G.; Beller, G.A.; Smoake, J.A.; Hartley, L.H. Intramuscular energy sources in dogs during physical work. J. Lipid Res. 14:54-60; 1973.

115. Turcotte, L.P.; Kiens, B.; Richter, E.A. Saturation kinetics of palmitate uptake in perfused skeletal muscle. FEBS Lett. 279(2):327-329; 1991.

116. Turcotte, L.P.; Richter, E.A.; Kiens, B. Increased plasma FFA uptake and oxidation during prolonged exercise in trained vs. untrained humans. Am. J. Physiol. 262:E791-E799; 1992.

117. Turcotte, L.P.; Petry, C.; Kiens, B.; Richter, E.A. Electrical stimulation increases the V_{max} for the uptake and oxidation of palmitate in perfused skeletal muscle. Med. Sci. Sports Exerc. 24(5):S178; 1992.

118. Turcotte, L.P.; Richter, E.A.; Srivastava, A.K.; Chiasson, J.-L. First evidence for the existence of a fatty acid binding protein in the plasma membrane of skeletal muscle. Diabetes 41(Suppl. 1):172A; 1992.

119. Turcotte, L.P.; Hespel, P.J.L.; Graham, T.E.; Richter, E.A. Impaired plasma FFA oxidation imposed by extreme CHO deficiency in contracting rat skeletal muscle. J. Appl. Physiol. 77:517-525; 1994.

120. Wahren, J.; Hagenfeldt, L.; Felig, P. Splanchnic and leg exchange of glucose, amino acids, and free fatty acids during exercise in diabetes mellitus. J. Clin. Invest. 55:1303-1314; 1975.

121. Wahren, J.; Sato, Y.; Ostman, J.; Hagenfeldt, L.; Felig, P. Turnover and splanchnic metabolism of free fatty acids and ketones in insulin-dependent diabetics at rest and in response to exercise. J. Clin. Invest. 73:1367-1376; 1984.

122. Wahrenberg, H.; Engfeldt, P.; Bolinder, J.; Arner, P. Acute adaptation in adrenergic control of lipolysis during physical exercise in humans. Am. J. Physiol. 253:E383-E390; 1987.

123. Wahrenberg, H.; Bolinder, J.; Arner, P. Adrenergic regulation of lipolysis in human fat cells during exercise. Eur. J. Clin. Invest. 21:534-541; 1991.

124. Winder, W.W.; Arogyasami, J.; Barton, R.J.; Elayan, I.M.; Vehrs, P.R. Muscle malonyl-CoA decreases during exercise. J. Appl. Physiol. 67(6):2230-2233; 1989.

125. Wolfe, R.R.; Peters, E.J.; Klein, S.; Holland, O.B.; Rosenblatt, J.; Gary, H., Jr. Effect of short-term fasting on lipolytic responsiveness in normal and obese human subjects. Am. J. Physiol. 252:E189-E196; 1987.

126. Wolfe, R.R.; Klein, S.; Carraro, F.; Weber, J.-M. Role of triglyceride-fatty acid cycle in controlling fat metabolism in humans during and after exercise. Am. J. Physiol. 258:E382-E389; 1990.

127. Yeaman, S.J. Hormone-sensitive lipase—a multipurpose enzyme in lipid metabolism. Biochim. Biophys. Acta 1052:128-132; 1990.

128. Zinman, B.; Hollenberg, C.H. Effect of insulin and lipolytic agents on rat adipocyte low K_m cyclic adenosine 3':5'-monophosphate phosphodiesterase. J. Biol. Chem. 249(7):2182-2187; 1974.

Chapter 5

Skeletal Muscle Amino Acid Metabolism and Ammonia Production During Exercise

TERRY E. GRAHAM, JAMES W.E. RUSH,
AND DAVE A. MacLEAN

The area of amino acid metabolism is an enormous topic and involves every tissue of the body. In this chapter we will focus on human skeletal muscle; nonhuman animal studies will be referred to only when comparable information is not available because large species differences exist. In addition, tissues other than skeletal muscle will be referred to only within the context of their roles in providing substrate to and clearing metabolic products from skeletal muscle.

Protein and amino acids are often ignored in discussions of metabolism during exercise probably for two reasons: firstly, amino acids contribute only a minor portion (perhaps 5-15%) of the energy consumed during exercise and secondly, little is known about this complex aspect of metabolism. On the other hand, one must recognize that even a minor contribution to the energy consumption is important in conditions of high energy demands over a prolonged period of time. In addition, the protein composition of skeletal muscle is critical to the specific character of the tissue, and exercise puts considerable stress on the integrity and turnover of the muscle's protein pool. Furthermore, the metabolism of the amino groups (both as ammonia and as glutamine and alanine) is very dynamic and may be critical to the overall regulation of metabolism. For example, amino group metabolism plays a key role in hepatic gluconeogenesis, and it has even been suggested that it contributes to peripheral and/or central fatigue. Numerous amino acid pathways directly involve glycolytic or TCA intermediates as either substrates or products. Thus, by investigating amino acid metabolism one not only learns more about amino acids but, more importantly, also begins to explore the integration of fat and carbohydrate metabolism. By studying such processes, we finally begin to appreciate the complexity of skeletal muscle metabolism.

It is well established that skeletal muscle produces ammonia during both short-term, intense exercise and prolonged, submaximal exercise. (In physiological conditions, both ammonia and the ion, ammonium, exist. In this review, NH_3 will represent the sum of both forms.) It has been suggested that the NH_3 produced during both types of exercise comes from the same source, namely the AMP deaminase reaction of the purine nucleotide cycle (PNC). Amino acid catabolism can produce NH_3, and the oxidation of the branched chain amino acids (BCAA) isoleucine, leucine, and valine increases in skeletal muscle during exercise, but this has seldom been considered a source of NH_3. Recent studies have reevaluated this possibility, and evidence suggests that the BCAA may be a source of considerable NH_3 production during prolonged, submaximal exercise.

This review will focus on amino acid and NH_3 metabolism in skeletal muscle during exercise. We will discuss the role of amino acids as energy substrates and the primary source of these amino acids during exercise. We will also discuss NH_3 metabolism and evaluate both of the potential sources of NH_3. Similarly, we will consider the interaction of other energy substrates on amino acid and NH_3 metabolism in muscle. Lastly, we will address the effects of training and the possible role that NH_3 has on fatigue.

Protein Synthesis and Degradation During Exercise

Skeletal muscle constitutes approximately 40% of the body weight and is the second largest store of potential energy in the body after fat. Because the free amino acid pool is small and constant, the amino acids catabolized for energy or converted to glucose during exercise must come predominantly from endogenous liver and skeletal muscle protein. The amount of amino acids available from endogenous protein depends upon the balance between the rates of protein synthesis and protein degradation. It is generally accepted that during endurance exercise there is a net breakdown of body protein, predominantly in liver and muscle. This is accomplished by a decrease in the rate of protein synthesis and an increase· in the rate of protein degradation in these tissues. In muscle, however, the increase in the rate of degradation seems to be isolated to the noncontractile proteins, whereas the rate of contractile protein degradation appears to be suppressed.

Some of the early investigations into protein degradation during exercise measured the levels of protein in different tissues of rodents exercised to exhaustion (31). Researchers observed that following exhaustive exercise there was significantly less protein in both liver and skeletal muscle, indicating that net protein breakdown had occurred (31). A complementary approach is to measure the concentrations of the essential amino acids (EAA) because the body cannot synthesize them, and any change in tissue EAA concentrations must come only from exchange with the plasma or endogenous protein breakdown. Because diet is not a significant source of amino acids during exercise, increases in the tissue EAA concentration or efflux would reflect an increase in net tissue protein breakdown.

Dohm and coworkers (33, 34) demonstrated a significant increase in tyrosine (an EAA) and leucine (another EAA) concentrations in muscle, liver, and plasma of rodents exercised to exhaustion. Similarly, Haralambie and Berg (54) found that the free plasma concentrations of tyrosine increased progressively with exercise duration in humans. It has also been shown (3) in humans that the splanchnic bed releases the three branched-chain amino acids (BCAA), leucine, isoleucine, and valine (which are also EAA), whereas the exercising leg has a large net EAA release (49) and the intramuscular EAA pool also rises (89) during prolonged exercise.

It has been estimated that the amount of leucine oxidized during endurance exercise is greater than the total leucine pool in the body. Leucine concentration in plasma and muscle, however, does not change, suggesting that protein catabolism is the source of leucine (89). It is evident that exercise causes a net breakdown of both liver and muscle protein; however, these studies cannot determine whether this is a result of decreased protein synthesis, increased protein degradation, or both.

Protein Synthesis During Exercise

A considerable number of studies have reported that protein synthesis is decreased as the result of an exercise bout (14, 19, 29, 30, 35, 112). Several researchers utilizing a constant infusion, labeled amino acid approach have examined *in vivo* whole-body protein synthesis rates in humans, and all have reported that exercise decreased protein synthesis (53, 112, 146). Other researchers have focused on muscle protein synthesis using a variety of other approaches, such as isolated or perfused muscle preparations, *in vitro* perfusion following exercise, or the *in vivo* administration of radioactive label, and they have consistently found that protein synthesis is depressed as a result of exercise.

The effect of exercise on liver protein synthesis has also been investigated. In a study of subjects who performed 1 hr of treadmill running, Dohm et al. (33) found that liver protein synthesis was depressed by 20%, and exercise to exhaustion resulted in a 65% decrease in protein synthesis. In another study Dohm found that muscle protein synthesis was reduced to a greater extent (35-55%) following progressively longer work bouts than in work bouts of lighter intensities (34). Therefore, the degree to which protein synthesis is reduced in liver and muscle is influenced by both exercise intensity and duration.

It should be noted that these tracer studies involve the labeling of one or more amino acids, the introduction of this label into the whole-body or muscle preparation, and the measurement of this label in tissues, fluids, and/or gases. Although this technique is extremely useful and direct, some methodological problems have led researchers to question the accuracy of this approach in obtaining precise quantitative information. The problems arise from the assumptions surrounding the type of tracer used, the mode of injection, the precursor labeling, and then the measurement of the various enriched products (for complete review consult reference 125). In fact, these problems have led some researchers to report erroneous estimates and directions of protein turnover. Despite some drawbacks, advances in techniques have allowed this approach to produce very informative qualitative data.

Protein Degradation During Exercise

Investigators have reported an increase, no change, and a decrease in protein degradation (34, 35, 53, 68, 70, 112, 146) in response to exercise. The explanation for the differing results has been attributed to the different experimental methods used and the difficulty in measuring protein degradation. It is also possible that protein degradation may be increased, decreased, or unchanged under various exercise conditions, such as different exercise durations and intensities. However, the literature generally supports the contention that exercise results in an increase in the rate of protein degradation in liver and noncontractile muscle protein. In contrast, there is a suppression in the rate of contractile protein degradation in muscle.

There are two classes of protein in skeletal muscle: contractile and noncontractile. In humans contractile and noncontractile proteins comprise 66% and 34% of the total muscle protein, respectively (20). Tyrosine and phenylalanine have been used as indicators of noncontractile protein degradation because they are not subject to intermediary metabolism in muscle (125). Furthermore, 3-methylhistidine (3-MH) has been used as a specific index of contractile protein degradation because it is a direct by-product of actin and myosin degradation, and there are no enzymatic pathways for its degradation or other metabolic fates for 3-MH in the body.

Several studies with both rodents and humans have shown that muscle releases tyrosine and phenylalanine to a greater extent during exercise than during rest (30, 39). Furthermore, the magnitude of efflux, and thus degradation, is proportional to the intensity and duration of the exercise bout. Kasperek et al. (68) have demonstrated in rodents that after 2 to 3 hr of treadmill running, the livers had lost up to 25% of their protein. This loss was greater than that which could be accounted for by a decrease in protein synthesis alone, and thus protein degradation must also have been elevated. These findings have been supported by reports of increased lysosomal activity in muscle and liver, which would promote an increase in protein degradation (68).

The most common index of contractile protein degradation has been 3-MH, and it has been measured in plasma and urine in both *in vivo* and *in vitro* studies. The measurement of 3-MH in the urine has been the most widely used approach, and it has yielded conflicting results. Some studies have observed either an increase (32), a decrease (112), or no change (27, 106) in 3-MH excretion after exercise. Most of these studies have measured the excretion of 3-MH after an exercise bout, and this would reflect the behavior of the contractile proteins during both the exercise period and the recovery period. Furthermore, these studies usually calculate the excretion as a total for a given time period (i.e., 24 hr), so the changes may be considerably different during the early, middle, and late stages of exercise and recovery. Thus, when summed, the overall effects may be masked or misleading. With these points in mind Dohm et al. (35) have reassessed most of the data available in the literature and have demonstrated a biphasic response of 3-MH excretion to exercise. When the time course of change in 3-MH was considered, most studies showed a decrease in 3-MH excretion during exercise and an increase in excretion during recovery.

It also seems likely that the degree of contractile protein breakdown depends on the intensity and duration of the exercise bout, as well as the type of exercise (concentric vs. eccentric). It has been shown that 3-MH excretion is not elevated during recovery from light exercise (21) but is elevated to a greater extent following exercise of greater duration and intensity (35). Similarly, 3-MH excretion has been shown to be increased in rodents exercised eccentrically (70); however, this has not yet been substantiated in humans (106). There seems to be general agreement that during an endurance exercise bout, the rate of 3-MH excretion is decreased, whereas the rate of excretion during recovery depends on when the sample is taken and the duration and intensity of the exercise bout.

It is true that 3-MH production provides some index of contractile protein degradation, but there are a number of limitations to this approach and there are doubts about the usefulness of this method (125). There are small pools of contractile proteins in the gut and skin that turn over rapidly enough to contribute significantly to 3-MH excretion. Although muscle constitutes the bulk of the depot, it has been estimated in humans that these peripheral sources can contribute up to 25% of the total 3-MH excretion (2), and this may be even greater in rodents (35). It has been argued that during an exercise bout it is unlikely that these other sources are significantly affected, and if the extent of contractile protein degradation is of interest, regardless of its source, then 3-MH excretion is a valuable measure. Caution should be used, however, when interpreting 3-MH data from whole-body *in vivo* studies.

This approach is much more useful when applied directly to muscle fluxes and biopsies where the influences from gut and skin are eliminated.

It has been shown that 3-MH release is significantly decreased during contraction in the perfused rodent hindlimb (19). Similarly, Rennie et al. (112) demonstrated a 30% decrease in muscle 3-MH concentration in subjects performing 40 min of exercise. These data support the finding from urinary 3-MH studies and strongly suggest that contractile protein degradation in muscle is decreased during exercise.

Neither the effects of exercise intensity nor the effects of exercise duration on protein synthesis and degradation are completely clear. At the present time much of the data suggests that there is an increase in the net protein degradation of both muscle and liver, accomplished in part by a decrease in the rate of protein synthesis in both these tissues. Protein degradation is stimulated in the liver and can account for a significant portion of the amino acids released by the liver during exercise. In skeletal muscle there is a decrease in the degradation of contractile proteins and an increase in the degradation of noncontractile proteins.

Regulation of Protein Synthesis and Degradation During Exercise

Many recent investigations into protein turnover have focused on the potential regulators of protein synthesis and degradation. It has been shown that protein synthesis is increased in response to insulin (93), growth hormone (43), leucine, and other amino acids (138), but it is decreased by exercise (35), reduced intake of dietary protein (129), and a decreased energy state of the cell (19). On the other hand, protein degradation was increased in response to fasting (42), exercise (6), and glucocorticoids (9), and decreased by infusion of leucine (98), decreases in dietary protein (129), and the infusion of medium chain triglycerides (9). There are many different potential regulators of both protein synthesis and degradation, and the net change in protein turnover is most likely a reflection of the summation of these regulators. However, during prolonged exercise there is an increase in glucagon and glucocorticoids, which could promote a decrease in protein synthesis and an increase in protein degradation. Thus, the endocrine signals, considered to be the most potent regulators, support the findings of net protein breakdown as discussed here.

Amino Acid Metabolism in Muscle

There are three principal sources of amino acids for energy metabolism:

- dietary protein,
- tissue free amino acid pools, and
- endogenous tissue protein.

Under normal conditions during exercise, dietary protein is a relatively minor source of amino acids because few people would consume a large protein meal prior to an extensive exercise bout. The free amino acid pool of human skeletal muscle is greater than that of plasma; due to its mass (40% of body weight), muscle contains approximately 75% of the whole-body, free amino acids (125). However, this is considerably smaller than the amount of amino acids available from endogenous protein breakdown. In fact, it has been estimated that the intramuscular amino acid pool contains less that 1% of the metabolically active amino acids (125). It has also been estimated that the amount of leucine oxidized during a prolonged exercise bout is approximately 25 times greater than the free leucine concentration in muscle, liver, and plasma (33). Therefore, the free amino acid pool is only a minor source of amino acids during exercise, whereas the most important source is endogenous protein breakdown (34).

Pathways of Amino Acid Metabolism in Muscle

There are at least six amino acids that can be oxidized by skeletal muscle: alanine, aspartate, glutamate, and the three BCAA. Not all of these amino acids, however, have the same metabolic potential in muscle. It appears that the BCAA are the dominant amino acids oxidized by skeletal muscle (22, 44, 46, 85). The catabolism of amino acids involves the removal of the alpha-amino group by transamination or oxidative deamination, followed by conversion of the carbon skeleton to metabolites that are common to the pathways of carbohydrate and fat metabolism. It should be noted that the avenues available for amino acid catabolism and conversion are extensive, and the final products, their fates, and the pathways available to them are all quite complex.

Transamination and Transdeamination of BCAA

The first step in BCAA metabolism is the reversible removal of the NH_3 group. Figure 5.1 demonstrates that the NH_3 group from a BCAA is donated to 2-oxoglutarate to form glutamate and branched chain oxo acids (BCOA), catalyzed by BCAA aminotransferase (BCAAT). Glutamate can then combine with other oxo acids to reform amino acids, or it can combine with oxaloacetate to form aspartate and 2-oxoglutarate. Glutamate plays a central role in BCAA metabolism (Figure 5.2), and the amino group from BCAA can be used to form quite a wide variety of compounds.

Glutamate can also be oxidatively deaminated by glutamate dehydrogenase (GDH) to form NH_3 and 2-oxoglutarate. By coupling BCAAT and GDH, a transdeamination reaction is formed (99), with the net process being BCAA $\rightarrow NH_3$ + BCOA. This has been suggested to be the primary pathway for BCAA deamination in skeletal muscle. These two reactions are near equilibrium; therefore, for BCAA catabolism to proceed, both of these products must be either removed or further metabolized.

The BCAAT is a pyridoxal phosphate-dependent enzyme, which accepts all three BCAA as substrates. It is widely distributed among tissues with the highest activity in the heart and kidneys, intermediate activity in skeletal muscle, and the lowest activity in the liver (55). Furthermore, the

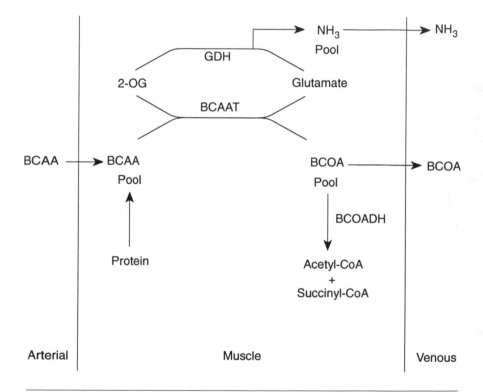

Figure 5.1   Branched chain amino acid (BCAA) transdeamination. The BCAA donate their NH_3 group to 2-oxoglutarate (2-OG) forming glutamate and branched chain oxo acid (BCOA), catalyzed by BCAA amino transferase (BCAAT). Glutamate is deaminated by glutamate dehydrogenase (GDH) and both 2-OG and NH_3 are formed. The BCOA can be effluxed from muscle for further metabolism in the liver or undergo decarboxylation in muscle via branched chain oxo acid dehydrogenase (BCOADH). This enzyme catalyzes the rate limiting step in BCAA oxidation and the products, acetyl-CoA and succinyl-CoA, are TCA cycle intermediates. Both liver and muscle protein breakdown are the predominant sources of BCAA for intramuscular metabolism during exercise.

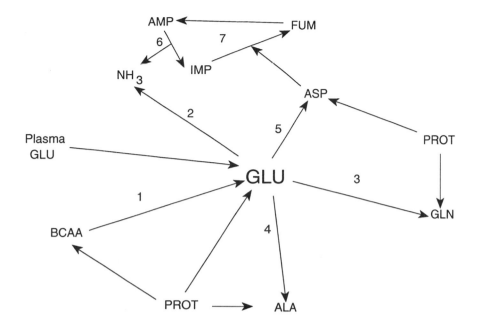

Figure 5.2   A schematic illustration of the potential sources of ammonia and of the interactions of various amino acids with the intramuscular free glutamate pool. Ammonia (NH₃) can be produced by the AMP deaminase (reaction 6) as it produces IMP from AMP. This is a portion of the purine nucleotide cycle (reaction 7). If this process cycles it requires aspartate (ASP) and produces fumarate (FUM). Intramuscular glutamate (GLU) is central in the transamination reactions. It can be derived from the plasma (plasma GLU), from intramuscular protein catabolism (PROT), and from the transamination (reaction 1) of the branched-chain amino acids (BCAA). GLU can be transaminated to ASP (reaction 5; ASP aminotransferase) and to alanine (ALA; reaction 4; ALA aminotransferase). It can also be used for glutamine (GLN) synthesis (reaction 3; GLN synthase) and can be a source of NH₃ via glutamate dehydrogenase (reaction 2).

BCAAT enzyme has been isolated in both the cytosolic and mitochondrial compartments. In rodents the distribution of activity in skeletal muscle was found to be dependent on fiber type, with the highest cytosolic activity occurring in white fibers and the highest mitochondrial activity occurring in red fibers (63). A specific regulatory mechanism for BCAAT has never been identified, but the K_ms for the major tissue BCAAT enzymes are two- to fourfold higher than tissue BCAA concentrations (55). As a result, the rate of BCAA transamination in muscle should be sensitive to changes in intramuscular BCAA levels.

GDH is located exclusively in the mitochondrial matrix (77), and there are very few reported values for GDH activity in the literature. It has been suggested that GDH activity in contracting human muscle is low or negligible (15), based solely on early reported values determined in rodent muscle. However, Wibom and Hultman (141, 142) have reported much higher levels for human GDH, and that the activity of GDH increases with training (142). Similarly, Henriksson et al. (57) demonstrated that following chronic stimulation, rabbit tibialis anterior muscle increased its GDH activity sixfold. These findings are not surprising, as one would expect GDH to follow changes in mitochondrial density. Furthermore, given the mitochondrial location of GDH, it would appear that BCAA transdeamination should be greatest in the most oxidative muscle fibers.

BCOA Decarboxylation and Its Regulation

The second and rate limiting step in BCAA oxidation is the nonreversible oxidative decarboxylation of the BCOA by branched-chain oxo acid dehydrogenase (BCOADH). The BCOADH is located on the inner surface of the inner mitochondrial membrane, giving further support to the speculation that mitochondrially rich oxidative fibers would have the greatest BCAA catabolism. BCOADH is a classic example of a multicomplex enzyme (147). The content of this enzyme is higher in the liver than in skeletal muscle, and under resting conditions only 4% of the enzyme is active in muscle versus 97% in liver (133, 134). The activity of the BCOADH is regulated by reversible phosphorylation, whereby the complex is inactivated by BCOADH kinase and activated by BCOADH phosphatase. The phosphorylation of the enzyme complex results in a dramatic reduction in V_{max} (as reviewed by Yeaman, 147). This enzyme complex is under strict regulation and many allosteric regulators have been identified; however, not all of these have been identified in skeletal muscle. The activity of the BCOADH complex has been shown to increase in response to elevated levels of leucine (121) and H^+ (62, 94), as well as to increases in mitochondrial ADP and possibly $NAD^+/NADH$ ratios (78, 105). Meanwhile, BCOADH activity has been shown to be inhibited by increases in ATP and acetyl-CoA (78), and by increases in other energy substrates such as pyruvate, free fatty acids, and ketone bodies (17). It is evident that the BCOADH complex is sensitive not only to changes in substrate and products, but also to the energy state of the cell. Despite a low activity in resting muscle, activation can result in a significant increase in BCAA oxidation. It has been demonstrated that the complex is stimulated by exercise, and the degree of activation is proportional to the intensity and duration of the exercise bout (69, 71, 134). It is not clear which factors are important to the *in vivo* regulation of BCOADH in skeletal muscle, and very little is known about the intramitochondrial concentrations of the putative regulators.

Metabolic Intermediates

The BCOA have many metabolic fates; some may be effluxed from the cell (111) and further oxidized in other tissues, particularly the liver.

Regardless of the tissue, the most important fate of BCOA is the degradation of the carbon skeleton to TCA cycle intermediates initiated by BCOADH (Figure 5.1). Both isoleucine and valine form succinyl-CoA, whereas leucine forms acetyl-CoA. Of these, only the carbons of acetyl-CoA from leucine can be oxidized directly in the TCA cycle (99); the other intermediates must first be converted to pyruvate via phosphoenolpyruvate before their carbons are available for oxidation in the TCA cycle as acetyl CoA.

Amino Acid Oxidation During Exercise

As mentioned previously, skeletal muscle can utilize alanine, aspartate, glutamate, and the BCAA. Alanine is the only amino acid consistently released from skeletal muscle at rest and during exercise (3, 39). Although muscle can oxidize this amino acid, its primary fate is as a gluconeogenic precursor for the liver, and its direct utilization by muscle is negligible. Glutamate plays a central role in amino acid metabolism as mentioned earlier (Figure 5.2). Aspartate is used as an NH_3 donor for the reamination of IMP to AMP and subsequently produces fumarate, which can be used to replenish the TCA cycle; however, the use of this mechanism during a submaximal exercise bout is not clear. Most research suggests that the BCAA are the major amino acids metabolized in skeletal muscle.

Wagenmakers et al. (134) demonstrated in humans that only 4% of the BCOADH enzyme was active in muscle at rest. Meanwhile, researchers have illustrated that liver BCOADH is almost completely active regardless of the energy demand (69, 133). Due to the extremely low BCAAT activity in liver and its high activity in muscle, it has been suggested that at rest the BCAA are deaminated in muscle and the BCOA transported to the liver for further oxidation (112). This is supported by the findings of Rennie et al. (112), who showed that at rest BCOA were effluxed from resting skeletal muscle to the liver for oxidation. However, with such a low resting muscle BCOADH activity, the potential for increase in muscle BCAA utilization during exercise is great.

The ability of skeletal muscle to utilize amino acids as an energy source has generally been regarded as limited, but not insignificant. The total oxidation of 1 mole of leucine, isoleucine, and valine yields 43, 42, and 32 moles of ATP, respectively. It has been estimated that amino acids may contribute anywhere from 3 to 18% of the total energy required for a prolonged exercise bout (16, 107). Despite the low basal BCOADH activity, skeletal muscle has 60% of the body's total specific enzymes for amino acid oxidation (74). It has been demonstrated in rodents that the proportion of the BCOADH complex in the active form is increased during exercise in proportion to intensity and duration. These findings have now been substantiated in human muscle (134). The amount of activation reported (13-66%) may be underestimated because the techniques used do not allow rapid sampling and processing of the tissue. Nevertheless, it is apparent that active skeletal muscle increases its capacity to oxidize BCAA.

Previous studies have shown that at rest there is a net efflux of amino acids from human leg muscle (3, 39). During exercise there is an uptake of several amino acids (predominantly the BCAA) by leg tissues, and if the exercise is prolonged there is a significant release of BCAA from the liver (3). Furthermore, MacLean et al. (89) demonstrated that during a prolonged exercise bout lasting 2 to 3 hr, there was no net accumulation of BCAA in the plasma or in contracting muscle. This suggests that active muscle was responsible for their removal and oxidation. This hypothesis is supported by Rennie et al. (112), who illustrated that, following the initiation of an exercise bout, there was a significant drop in the efflux of BCOA from muscle, suggesting that BCOA were oxidized in the muscle.

The use of tracers has also substantiated these findings. Most of these studies have assessed amino acid oxidation by monitoring the production of $^{13}CO_2$ or $^{14}CO_2$ from a labeled BCAA. The amino acid most often used is leucine, because it is purely ketogenic and has quantitatively the highest oxidation rate of all the BCAA. Leucine oxidation has been shown to increase during exercise in both rodents (56, 59, 60, 79) and humans (53, 75, 146). Henderson et al. (56) have further demonstrated that the degree of leucine oxidation is proportional to the metabolic rate. Therefore, it appears that as exercise intensity and duration increase so does leucine oxidation.

A limitation to most of the human studies is that the measurement of the CO_2 enrichment represents whole-body leucine metabolism, and the actual site of the increased leucine oxidation is not indicated. However, Hood and Terjung (59, 60) have examined leucine metabolism in the perfused rat hindlimb during electrical stimulation and have provided direct estimates of muscle leucine oxidation. They demonstrated a significant increase in muscle leucine oxidation, and their values could reasonably account for the rates of whole-body leucine oxidation observed in untrained subjects during steady state *in vivo* tracer studies. Since skeletal muscle accounts for more than 40% of the body mass and is the primary site of peripheral BCAA metabolism, it is generally accepted that the increase in BCAA oxidation observed during exercise is a direct result of elevated BCAA oxidation in active skeletal muscle.

Hood and Terjung (61) also noted that most estimates of leucine oxidation during exercise in human muscle were considerably higher than those in rodent muscle. This demonstrates a potential hazard in trying to extrapolate findings from rodents to humans. This is especially true for amino acid metabolism because the type (isozyme), distribution, and activity of some key enzymes in amino acid metabolism vary greatly between rodent and human, as reviewed by Lund (88). For example, the rat has an uneven distribution of the BCAAT and BCOADH between skeletal muscle and liver. This results in a significant release of BCOA from skeletal muscle and subsequent removal by the liver for further oxidation. In contrast, the human has a more even distribution of these enzymes, suggesting that a smaller release of BCOA from skeletal muscle and greater intramuscular oxidation should occur. The rodent liver has predominantly the low activity, high K_m isozyme II BCAAT so that BCAA are not metabolized by the liver. On the other hand, the human liver has a low K_m isozyme I BCAAT, and thus it is possible that the BCAA are metabolized to a greater extent in the human liver.

As compared with other tissues, human skeletal muscle has the enzyme distribution to uniquely promote BCAA utilization and is the primary site of peripheral BCAA metabolism. During exercise the BCAA are made available for oxidation by muscle from intramuscular free pools (minor) as well as from protein breakdown (major). Exercise stimulates the activation of the BCOADH complex, the rate limiting enzyme in BCAA metabolism, thus promoting BCAA oxidation. As exercise progresses, BCAA oxidation increases, and this together with the amino acids involved in gluconeogenesis may account for a significant portion (3-18%) of the energy required for sustained exercise.

Amino Metabolism in Muscle

Whereas the carbon skeletons of amino acids can be oxidized within contracting skeletal muscle, the amino groups are released. The major amino carriers are ammonia, alanine, and glutamine.

Ammonia Responses During Exercise

Many studies have measured plasma NH_3 levels during exercise, but very few have measured intramuscular NH_3 concentrations or muscle NH_3 flux. It has been demonstrated that during exercise of approximately 40% $\dot{V}O_2$ max and greater, NH_3 production was increased proportionally to intensity (50, 87). At lower exercise intensities, the muscle NH_3 release tends to balance the clearance and little change in plasma NH_3 is found. However, plasma and muscle NH_3 concentrations rise rapidly during more intense exercise because clearance cannot match the NH_3 release from active muscle. Although there have been a few isolated reports of plasma NH_3 of 200-250 μM in healthy subjects, values of 100-150 μM are more typically observed at exhaustion. When NH_3 flux is examined, the changes are qualitatively similar to concentration changes but quantitatively much more dramatic. Several studies during prolonged submaximal exercise have also demonstrated that NH_3 production increases as exercise progresses (15, 49). Although the production rate is greatest in intense exercise, total production is greatest in prolonged activity. Eriksson et al.

(38) further demonstrated that during moderate exercise liver NH_3 uptake is not altered. Therefore, the increases in plasma NH_3 levels during exercise are a direct reflection of increases in muscle NH_3 production and not decreases in NH_3 removal. Overall, the basic conclusion is that during exercise a rise in plasma NH_3 correlates with both muscle NH_3 concentrations and muscle NH_3 efflux.

Other Amino Carriers

As demonstrated in Figure 5.2, both glutamine and alanine (depending on whether or not the glutamate is synthesized within the muscle) are also amino carriers. During exercise their plasma concentrations generally rise (3, 38, 90, 91) due to large effluxes from the active muscle. Their release appears to increase with exercise intensity (38, 72) and duration (3, 39, 49), with fluxes as high as 100-150 µmol/min being reported (i.e., values similar to those of NH_3).

We have quantified release of NH_3, glutamine, and alanine from the human quadriceps during an hour of leg extensor work (80% $\dot{V}O_2$ max) (49). The net NH_3 efflux was 4.4 mmol, and the net glutamine and alanine effluxes were 3.4 and 2.5 mmol, respectively. Thus, NH_3 efflux alone drastically underestimated the total amino release.

In short-term, exhaustive exercise, NH_3 flux can reach 300 µmol/min (48). There are few data available addressing alanine and glutamine release under these conditions. We recently measured the amino acid exchange across the thigh of 3 males exercising to exhaustion in approximately 3 minutes (unpublished data). Although there was an NH_3 efflux of 0.5 mmol during the exercise and a further 1.7 mmol in recovery, the fluxes of glutamine and alanine were extremely variable and generally small. The reasons for this could lie in the intense competition that must exist for intramuscular glutamate and pyruvate by a variety of enzymes during such exercise, resulting in little alanine and glutamine synthesis. In addition, the synthesis of glutamine requires energy.

Transport of NH_3 From Muscle

It is frequently stated that ammonium, the common form of NH_3, cannot cross the cell membrane and that ammonia is the form that is permeable. Furthermore, it has been speculated that with the metabolic acidosis of exercise, more of the NH_3 would exist as ammonium and hence accumulate in the cell. We examined this hypothesis (48) and found exactly the opposite; during intense exercise intramuscular acidosis occurred, but there was a large NH_3 release (about 25% of the net NH_3 production was released during 3 min of exhaustive exercise). Furthermore, the muscle/plasma NH_3 ratio did not rise as the theory would predict, but fell, implying that NH_3 release was facilitated.

When one considers the pK_a of NH_3 and the small increase in hydrogen ion associated with exercise, it is obvious that the impact this has on the ammonia/ammonium distribution is negligible (less than 1%). Thus, hydrogen ion is unlikely to be an important inhibitory factor in NH_3 transport in physiological systems. In fact, one could speculate that if the proton gradient plays a role, it may facilitate NH_3 release. This is important not only for tissue release but also for intracellular movements. If mitochondrial GDH and BCOADH are important components of NH_3 production, then the flux of NH_3 out of the mitochondria must be considered, and according to the "hydrogen ion theory" this would be difficult. The specific processes by which NH_3 crosses the membranes are not known. Ammonia diffusion could be a major process, but there are also reports (76) that ammonium can compete with potassium ions for K^+ channels.

Wagenmakers et al. (135) noted that cultured endothelial cells contain a high concentration of glutaminase. This raises the possibility that some of the measured NH_3 efflux may have left the muscle cell as glutamine and entered the plasma as NH_3 only after being metabolized by the endothelial cells. Such a process would offer the advantage of conserving some of the rapidly declining muscle glutamate stores. Rapidly dividing cells, however, often have high glutaminase activity, and therefore this finding may reflect the fact that cultured cells were studied. Recently Willholf et al. (144), using immunocytochemical and enzymological techniques, found that glutaminase activity was relatively low in rat plantaris muscle compared with glutamine synthase. They concluded that the glutaminase was not quantitatively significant.

This latter study also reported that the slow oxidative fibers had the greatest glutamine synthase activity. This suggests that there may be differences in amino carriers with slow-twitch fibers favoring glutamine and fast-twitch fibers predominantly employing AMP deaminase and NH_3. However, this is speculation and more research is needed.

Plasma NH₃ Clearance

Active muscle can release several millimoles of NH_3 into the plasma. This represents a substantial NH_3 load, as arterial NH_3 at rest is 20-50 µM. Because the splanchnic bed metabolizes muscle-derived alanine and glutamine, it can be confronted with an even larger quantity of NH_3. Certainly the liver metabolizes NH_3 via the urea cycle; however, the sole investigation of splanchnic NH_3 uptake during exercise found no change from that at rest, despite an increased plasma NH_3 concentration (38). In this and other studies (34), the plasma urea levels were unchanged for at least an hour of exercise. Thus, the liver does not appear to be a major NH_3 clearance tissue during exercise. Lemon (80) points out that the vast majority (85%) of the nitrogen from protein is excreted in the urine as urea. However, this occurs predominantly after exercise and can continue for several days. Similarly, the decreased kidney blood flow and urine production during exercise make renal nitrogen clearance a minor route at that time. Rennie et al. (112) reported that urinary NH_3 represented 10-15% of total urinary nitrogen excretion at rest and that it did not increase until after 2.5 hr of exercise. Presumably this NH_3 is derived from glutamine that is taken up by the kidney because the kidney does not take up NH_3. Sweat is another possible NH_3 clearance mechanism. Lemon (80) has clearly demonstrated that sweat is a vehicle for urea excretion; however, the absolute amount is small. Recently, Czarnowski and Gorski (26) have reported that sweat may also contain significant amounts of NH_3. It is not clear, however, whether this is NH_3 cleared from the plasma or produced by the sweat glands.

Several investigators (38, 72) have speculated that uptake by resting muscle and general distribution into the body water is the major fate of NH_3. Resting muscle does take up NH_3, but at a very low rate. We (48) demonstrated that arterial NH_3 rose during the initial recovery phase of exercise, even though the flux from the previously active muscle declined rapidly (50% in 1-2 min). This signifies that NH_3 clearance decreased even more rapidly than muscle release. The clearance mechanisms such as the liver, kidney, resting muscle, and sweat glands would not be expected to decline this rapidly. We speculated that the lung was the major clearance organ during exercise, and with the rapid fall in ventilation during recovery this removal route decreased. Expired air has been shown to contain NH_3 (65), but no one has examined this during exercise.

Despite the large efflux of alanine and glutamine and smaller effluxes of many other amino acids, there is usually little or no change in arterial amino acids concentration during exercise (49). Many of these amino acids (particularly alanine) are gluconeogenic, and it is highly likely that the liver is clearing them from the circulation as rapidly as the muscle is releasing them.

There are two potential sources of NH_3 from skeletal muscle during exercise: 1) the deamination of BCAA and 2) the deamination of AMP as one of the steps in the purine nucleotide cycle (PNC). The increase in amino acid oxidation during exercise has already been discussed; however, several researchers have neglected to consider amino acids as a NH_3 source and have instead attributed all the NH_3 produced during any type of exercise bout to the reactions of the PNC. This pathway and its potential for NH_3 production will now be considered.

The Purine Nucleotide Cycle

The purine nucleotide cycle (PNC) consists of three reactions catalyzed by AMP deaminase (AMPD), adenylosuccinate synthetase (AS), and adenylosuccinate lyase (AL) (Figure 5.3), all of which occur in the cytosol.

The cycle is often functionally defined as having a deaminating (AMPD) and a reaminating (AS and AL) portion (Figure 5.3). This group of reactions is important to the present discussion of NH_3 and amino acid metabolism because AMPD is a potential source of NH_3 production, and AS consumes an NH_3 equivalent directly from aspartate. Because of the transamination reactions that can convert other amino acids to aspartate (Figure 5.2), the alpha amino group consumed in the AS reaction may originate from one of a number of amino acids.

The PNC is also involved in the regulation of adenine nucleotide status in muscle. Consumption of AMP by AMPD allows the near equilibrium enzyme adenylate kinase to continue functioning in the ATP production direction during severe energy demands (Figure 5.3).

Much of the experimental work investigating the regulation of the PNC has used rat hindlimb muscle. This model facilitates investigation of basic

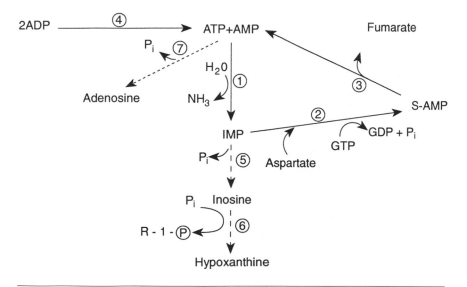

Figure 5.3   The purine nucleotide cycle and some aspects of adenine nucleotide management. In states of excessive energy demand adenylate kinase (reaction 4) catalyzes the formation of ATP and AMP from ADP. AMP deaminase (reaction 1) is the entry point to the PNC. IMP may be reaminated to AMP when adenylosuccinate synthetase (reaction 2) and adenylosuccinate lyase (reaction 3) are active. If excessive IMP accumulation occurs or if reaction 2 or 3 is inhibited, IMP may be converted to inosine by a cytoplasmic 5'-nucleotidase (reaction 5). Inosine may be further catabolized to hypoxanthine via purine nucleoside phosphorylase (reaction 6). Inosine and hypoxanthine readily leave the muscle and their formation thus represents potential net purine nucleotide loss. If AMP accumulates excessively or if AMP deaminase is inhibited, AMP may be converted to adenosine via a 5'-nucleotidase (reaction 7). Adenosine also readily leaves the muscle. Abbreviations: S-AMP = adenylosuccinate, R-1-P = ribose-1-phosphate.

metabolic regulation questions because different muscle fiber types can be studied, flow and delivery of metabolites and oxygen can be controlled if a perfusion system is used, and pharmacological manipulations can be performed. Thus, most of the data discussed in this section come from experiments with rodents. Whenever possible, human data are included to support the arguments. One should keep in mind that there are numerous inter-species differences. For example, the differences in metabolic capacity and in fatigue resistance between fast- and slow-twitch fibers are much more pronounced in the rodent.

Deamination and PNC Function

The deamination of AMP serves a number of important functions and is catalyzed by AMP deaminase.

Regulation of AMP Deaminase Activity.   AMPD catalyzes the irreversible deamination of free AMP (AMP_f) to IMP via hydrolytic liberation of NH_3 (Figure 5.3). This reaction is generally considered the entry point to the PNC. The regulation of AMPD activity is complex and occurs on several levels, including isoenzymes, allosteric modifiers, substrate driven catalysis, and binding of the enzyme to myosin.

Isozymes.   White muscles deaminate AMP several times more effectively than red muscles. This is apparent in the higher specific activities and K_m values for AMPD in white muscle as compared with red muscle and heart muscle (108). These differences in activity among fiber types are due to differences in isozyme distribution.

For the purposes of this discussion, attention will be given only to adult muscle AMPD, and the isozyme nomenclature of Raggi et al. (108) will be used. Two distinct isozymes of AMPD can be isolated from rabbit red muscle (forms A and B). Form A accounts for approximately 70% of the total AMPD activity in red muscle. In the heart, all of the activity of AMPD could be accounted for by form A, whereas rabbit white muscle contained exclusively form B, the second isoform from red muscle. The A form of AMPD extracted from heart muscle is not sensitive to varying energy charges (ATP/ADP ratios). AMPD activity from both red and white fibers, however, was increased as energy charge decreased. Thus, the isozyme distribution varies between fiber types due to differences in the aerobic capacity and stability of the energy charge of the fiber.

Substrate and Allosteric Effects.   At rest the physiological concentrations of orthophosphate (K_i = 1-2 mM) and GTP are probably the most important inhibitors of AMPD (8, 109). ATP increasingly inhibits rabbit skeletal muscle AMPD in the concentration range of 0.005-0.1 mM, but above 0.1 mM, ATP inhibition is reversed. This reversal of inhibition also occurs with GTP when the [GTP] is greater than 1 mM. Because the physiological concentrations of ATP and GTP are approximately 6-10 mM and 0.2-0.3 mM, respectively, GTP, but not ATP, is in the inhibitory range (87, 116).

Elevation in [AMP_f] is a major activator of AMPD during contraction (36, 72, 73, 139). The K_m for AMPD is well above the intracellular [AMP_f]. AMPD is in a relatively low activity state at rest, and therefore during contractions the deaminase is very sensitive to increases in [AMP_f] and should form IMP stoichiometrically.

Free ADP (ADP_f) is probably the most important allosteric activator of AMPD, because an increase in [ADP_f] associated with a declining ATP/ADP ratio decreases the apparent affinity of AMPD for inhibitors. Increasing H^+ decreases the K_m of AMPD for AMP (102). In combination with the ADP effect on inhibitor affinity, acidosis lessens the inhibition of AMPD by P_i, (139). Thus, H^+ may perform a secondary but not a primary role in the activation of AMPD.

Myosin Binding.   It has been demonstrated that purified AMPD will bind to myosin *in vitro* and that the activity of the deaminase is increased by binding (8, 123). At rest, most of the AMPD activity is in the free cytosolic fraction, and little is bound to myosin. When energy demanding contractions are initiated, however, a significant shift in distribution to the bound fraction occurs. It is proposed that myosin binding is important in AMPD activation.

Recently, the role of myosin binding in the activation of AMPD has been investigated in different rat hindlimb muscle sections during contractions (114, 115). The total activity of AMPD in the fast-twitch white gastrocnemius (WG) was highest and that in the slow-twitch red soleus (SOL) was lowest. The activity in the fast-twitch, red gastrocnemius (RG) was intermediate between the other two muscles.

Binding of AMPD to myosin precedes deamination of AMP, occurs in all fiber types when contraction conditions elicit high rates of AMP deamination, and can occur during contractions in the absence of cellular acidosis. Binding does not occur simply as a consequence of contractions; relatively mild contraction conditions of 0.5 Hz (for WG) or 5 Hz (for RG and SOL), which resulted in no IMP formation, did not trigger binding of AMPD to myosin. Thus, it seems that excessive energy demand and not simply contraction causes binding of AMPD to myosin, which is coincident with high AMPD activity.

Rundell et al. (115) evaluated the impact of binding on the kinetic behavior of AMPD in skeletal muscle of the rat. Free (unbound) AMPD extracted from resting muscle had a K_m of 1.71 mM and a V_{max} of 152 over 0.05-2.0 mM AMP. At AMP concentrations of 0.20-2.0 mM, the kinetics of the myosin bound AMPD were similar to those of the free enzyme, but at lower [AMP] (0.05-0.20 mM) a low K_m, low V_{max} kinetic profile was apparent. The low K_m, high affinity state of the bound enzyme could promote high rates of AMP deamination at physiological free AMP concentrations, even though V_{max} is lower.

The observation that elevated ADP (50 μM) decreases the inhibition of bound AMPD by orthophosphate but does not affect the activity of the free fraction of AMPD further confirms the primary importance of binding in AMPD activity.

Functions of AMP Deamination

Lowenstein (86) originally proposed several potential functions of the PNC. With a few additions, these putative functions have remained the subject of debate. The proposed functions related to the AMPD reaction only are

- maintenance of high ATP/ADP ratio (energy charge),
- prevention of adenine nucleotide degradation (net loss of nucleotides),
- production of ammonia to buffer H^+, and
- regulation of carbohydrate metabolism; NH_3 as an activator of phosphofructokinase (PFK) and IMP as an activator of phosphorylase b.

Maintenance of ATP/ADP Ratio During Contraction.   As previously mentioned, AMPD is the major removal pathway for AMP_f formed during situations of net ATP hydrolysis. Attenuating the rise in AMP_f promotes adenylate kinase activity in the ATP formation direction. This activity lessens the increase in ADP_f caused by excessive ATPase activity and attempts to maintain a high ATP/ADP_f ratio to facilitate further contraction.

It has been demonstrated that the ability of muscle to maintain cellular [ATP] during electrical stimulation-induced contractions is related to the inherent functional aerobic capacity of the fibers comprising the muscle (36). Thus, red fibers with higher mitochondrial contents and blood flow maintain [ATP] (energy balance) and have no rise in IMP during moderate contractions (36, 37). In contrast, white fibers do not maintain [ATP] as well as red fibers, and IMP content increases progressively throughout moderate contractions. The functional aerobic capacity of red fibers can be impaired by ischaemia, and that of white fibers can be increased by exercise training-induced increases in mitochondrial content. When these treatments are employed and the functional aerobic capacity is altered, the differences in [ATP] maintenance and IMP formation among fiber types can be diminished. Thus, it appears that excessive energy demand or limiting aerobic metabolism creates the cellular conditions necessary to activate AMPD, which attempts to maintain the ATP/ADP_f ratio necessary for continued contractile activity and high rates of ATP hydrolysis.

Prevention of Net Adenine Nucleotide Loss.   Purine salvage and *de novo* adenine nucleotide synthesis are time consuming and energetically costly processes. Thus, the prevention of adenine nucleotide degradation to purine nucleosides and bases, which readily leave the cell (66) and represent a potentially large net loss of adenine nucleotides, should be a cellular priority. The production of IMP via AMPD during intense contractions could function to conserve cellular nucleotides (116); IMP remains in the cell and can quickly and relatively nonenergetically be reaminated to replenish the adenine nucleotide pool, when cellular conditions favor this process.

In patients with AMPD deficiency, AMP is not deaminated, and IMP therefore is not formed to any considerable extent. These patients have lower increases in blood inosine and hypoxanthine (the two primary degradation products of IMP, Figure 5.3) than control subjects during exercise (124). In contrast, plasma and muscle concentrations of adenosine (the major degradation product of AMP if AMPD is inactive, Figure 5.3) rise several fold more in deficient patients (117, 124). This results in an increase in net adenine nucleotide loss due to the activity of 5'-nucleotidase when AMPD is not present to shunt adenine nucleotides to IMP to prevent excess degradation.

Ammonia as a Proton Buffer. NH_3 is present in muscle as both ammonia and ammonium:

$$NH_3 + H^+ \longleftrightarrow NH_4^+, pK_a = 9.3$$

The formation of ammonium consumes H^+ stoichiometrically, and this has led to the speculation by some investigators that ammonium formation may be important for buffering the increase in H^+ that occurs during exercise. In light of the large disparity between total net NH_3 and lactate production during short-term intense work (2 mmol NH_3 vs. 127 mmol lactate in single leg extensor work; 48), however, a role for NH_3 as a buffer for this large amount of lactate (H^+) seems unlikely and quantitatively unimportant. The potential buffering role of ammonia is further challenged by the occurrence of a large ratio of intramuscular lactate/NH_3 during prolonged moderate leg exercise (15, 47).

Regulation of Carbohydrate Metabolism.   The contraction conditions that cause activation of AMPD are usually fueled by anaerobic metabolism. Thus, the regulation of carbohydrate metabolism by products of AMPD will be most important during conditions of anaerobiosis. The regulation of carbohydrate metabolism under these conditions has been addressed in this volume by Spriet (see chapter 1). Here only some brief comments on the putative roles of NH_3 and IMP will be made.

Ammonium as an Activator of PFK.   Ammonium has been shown *in vitro* to activate PFK, one of the regulatory enzymes of glycolysis (1). Because of the coincidence of increased NH_3 and increased lactate (indicating increased glycolytic rate) in some exercise situations, many authors believe that ammonium produced when AMP is deaminated stimulates PFK activity *in vivo*, causing increased rates of glycolysis. It is likely that other factors that regulate glycolysis are more important than ammonium in activating PFK during contractions.

Several arguments can be made to divorce ammonium responses and PFK activity. There is a temporal mismatch in the ammonium/PFK argument in some exercise situations. Glycolytic rate is already high (and therefore lactate accumulation is already high) during intense human thigh exercise when NH_3 starts to accumulate (48). In prolonged moderate-intensity exercise situations, muscle and plasma NH_3 concentrations increase progressively, whereas lactate concentrations plateau or decrease (15, 47). Muscle and blood lactate concentrations are significantly lower in humans during prolonged submaximal exercise when they breathe hyperoxic gas as opposed to room air (47). In contrast, there is no difference in the muscle and blood NH_3 responses as a result of hyperoxic gas breathing.

These data imply that glycolysis can be influenced independently from NH_3 in intense and prolonged exercise. It is possible that ammonium has a sustaining influence on PFK activity in some situations, such as the later phase of sprint type exercise.

IMP as a Regulator of Phosphorylase b.   Because IMP may activate phosphorylase b (PHOS b) (4), it has been proposed to be a sustaining stimulus to glycogenolysis *in vivo*. This proposal can be refuted from several lines. Again there is a temporal mismatch of putative stimulus and response variables in some exercise situations. IMP and NH_3 increase stoichiometrically in intense exercise, so the same temporal mismatch argument used to divorce NH_3 production from stimulation of glycolysis can be applied to separate IMP from glycolytic stimulation, at least in the early phase of intense exercise.

Studies measuring IMP and calculating the degree of activation of PHOS b have demonstrated that the IMP increases cannot stimulate PHOS b activity enough to even approach the rates of glycogenolysis elicited by intense contractions (4, 110). It is doubtful that during contractions that produce very high IMP contents (i.e., 3 μmol/g wet wt), IMP activation of PHOS b to sustain a high rate of glycogenolysis is physiologically significant.

Under moderately intense contraction conditions, there is no IMP or NH_3 accumulation in slow twitch fibers of the rat hindlimb unless the muscle is made anoxic or ischaemic, yet glycogenolysis and presumably PHOS *b* are active to fuel contraction (37, 131, 140). In prolonged exercise situations it has been demonstrated that there is no increase in [IMP] in human type I or II muscle fibers until the fibers have a dramatic decrease in glycogen (101).

Based on the aforementioned results it is apparent that the regulation of glycogenolysis and PHOS *b* activity can occur independently of IMP accumulation. It seems more likely that the decreased glycogen content causes the elevated IMP than that the elevated IMP stimulates glycolysis. Other activators may be more important or act in concert with IMP in the regulation of PHOS *b*.

Reamination and PNC Function

The reamination arm of the PNC involves two steps catalyzed by adenylo-succinate synthetase and adenylosuccinate lyase.

Adenylosuccinate Synthetase.   Adenylosuccinate synthetase (Figure 5.3) catalyzes the rate limiting step in the PNC (the formation of adenylo-succinate, GDP, and P_i from IMP) at the expense of stoichiometric amounts of aspartate and GTP. AS binds to the thin filaments of myofibrils, and it has been calculated that over 99% of the AS content occurs in this bound form (92). Because AMPD can bind to myosin and AS can bind to actin, the potential proximity of the two enzymes has been argued to be an important coupling mechanism in the regulation of flux through these reactions. However, AS content is much lower than that of AMPD in the same muscle extracts, and the distribution of AS across fiber types does not coincide with that of AMPD; AS is highest in red muscle and lowest in white muscle.

IMP can cause significant inhibition of AS at concentrations greater than 260 μM *in vivo* (128), and [IMP] in contracting skeletal muscle can significantly exceed this value. P_i inhibits AS, and P_i is increased during contractions due to PCr hydrolysis (128). In addition, AS is subject to product inhibition by both adenylosuccinate (103) and AMP (128).

Adenylosuccinate Lyase.   Adenylosuccinate lyase (Figure 5.3) cata-lyzes the trans-elimination of fumarate from adenylosuccinate to form AMP. Purified rat leg muscle AL has a high K_m compared with the concen-tration of adenylosuccinate found in resting (undetectable) or exercising (4-5 nmol · g^{-1} wet in mild stimulation) muscle. This suggests that the activity of AL is very sensitive to changes in adenylosuccinate concentra-tion (5, 45). There is little information regarding the specific regulation of this enzyme.

Cycling of the Purine Nucleotide Cycle

The role that the reactions of the PNC perform in skeletal muscle may change under differing contraction protocols. In some situations including intense contractions, it is clear that the cycle is not functioning concomitantly, but is dominated by AMP deamination. In other situations such as low- to moderate-intensity contractions, some concomitant deamination and reamination may occur at the level of whole muscles.

The arguments opposing the concomitant cycling of the PNC usually focus on substrate and energy availability and the kinetic and allosteric limits of the PNC enzymes. If the PNC is cycling the net result is

$$\text{Aspartate} + \text{GTP} \rightarrow \text{Fumarate} + NH_3 + \text{GDP} = P_i$$

This means that there is no net formation of IMP or removal of AMP by this series of reactions (Figure 5.3) and that they cannot contribute in any way to nucleotide management. What is accomplished is the deamination of the amino acid aspartate and the formation of both NH_3 and the TCA cycle intermediate, fumarate. This anaplerotic action could contribute to the regulation of the TCA cycle (see Peripheral Fatigue, page 162, and PNC as a Source of TCA Cycle Intermediates, page 156).

The intramuscular aspartate concentration is small and tends to be constant during exercise (11, 89). Muscle generally does not take up plasma aspartate; thus for cycling to occur there must be a continuous supply of aspartate from endogenous sources. It may be derived from intramuscular protein catabolism or from transamination reactions. Glutamate can readily be transaminated to form aspartate (Figure 5.2); however, this would place an even greater demand on the glutamate pool. Glutamate is already heavily involved in the production of alanine and glutamine and possibly NH_3. Thus, while PNC cycling would serve an anaplerotic function for the TCA cycle, an even greater generation of glutamate would be essential.

The activities of the enzymes of the PNC cycle are all sensitive to increases in their substrates, but the activity of AMPD is several fold greater than those of AS and AL in all fiber types. AS is the rate limiting enzyme of the cycle, and its activity therefore dictates potential cycle flux. Ironically, IMP, the substrate for AS, inhibits AS at concentrations reached during moderate exercise. The inhibition of AS by both P_i and by the primary and secondary products adenylosuccinate and AMP (87) further questions a role for this enzyme and the cycle during contractions.

In contraction conditions causing AMP accumulation there is obviously an energy imbalance in the cell. Because the reamination of IMP is energetically costly, (1 GTP per IMP reaminated), it would seem difficult for the reamination portion of the PNC to function while excessive energy demands of contraction were occurring. In any situation in which there is a large decrement in TAN it seems reasonable that PNC cycling cannot be functioning to any consequential extent, because if significant cycling were occurring it would prevent large decreases in TAN due to stoichiometric reamination of IMP to AMP.

During high-intensity stimulation, when there can potentially be a large decrease in TAN, there is no proof that the PNC cycles. It appears that deamination of AMP to IMP is the function of the PNC under these conditions. In fact, blocking reamination with hadacidin, a specific inhibitor of AS, had no effect on IMP accumulation compared with controls in rat red muscle under low, moderate, or intense stimulation conditions (95). There was, however, an increase in IMP in white muscle under moderate- and high-intensity stimulation when hadacidin was used (95).

During moderate stimulation, it is clear that cycling of the PNC can occur at the level of active whole muscles (of variable fiber type composition) and muscle groups. Rats treated with hadacidin have a greater accumulation of intramuscular IMP in whole hindlimb homogenates within 1 min of moderate stimulation than that of control rats. The excess IMP accumulation represents the cycling that normally occurs under this stimulation protocol. These results could support the view that in less demanding contractions the PNC normally is cycling, and thus modifying the increases in IMP.

Fiber type analysis demonstrates that the IMP accumulation occurs in white muscle fibers only, and the time course of the IMP accumulation in rat white hindlimb muscle illustrates that even though stimulation to the nerve continued for 30 minutes, the IMP production occurred in the first 5 minutes of contractions (95). In the subsequent 25 minutes of stimulation there was a reamination of IMP to AMP in the absence, but not in the presence, of hadacidin. These data suggest that the deamination and reamination reactions of the PNC normally function out of phase and probably in different fibers. The white fibers probably produce large amounts of IMP and fatigue quickly after contractions are initiated. When they are in a state of minimal tension development (fatigue), there is the potential for some degree of metabolic recovery, including AMP and ATP resynthesis, to occur over the rest of the time course of stimulation, while these particular fibers are not contributing to tension development at the whole muscle level.

A pharmacological blocker of AL, 5-amino-4-imidazolecarboxamide riboside (AICAr) has also been used to study PNC cycling. AICAr-treated rats had impaired performance characteristics during electrical stimulation. ATP content decreased more and IMP content rose more in the muscles of animals with inhibited AL (40). These investigators concluded that the PNC cycles under normal conditions and that the fumarate produced acts anaplerotically to the TCA cycle, enhancing mitochondrial respiration and contributing to the maintenance of tension.

The utility of AICAr as a tool to study AL has been questioned, however, because of its systemic effects (41). AICAr-treated animals had persistently lower (20 Torr lower) mean arterial pressures than control animals. AICAr is a potent competitive inhibitor of adenosine deaminase. It is feasible that the lower tension in the AICAr-treated animals in Flanagan's work (40) is due to AICAr-induced increases in tissue adenosine concentrations, which caused vasodilation, decreased cardiovascular tone, decreased blood pressure, and finally decreased muscle tension, independently of the PNC.

In light of the disparity in activity of the enzymes of the PNC, the energy and substrate requirements of cycling, and the results obtained with pharmacological blockers of reamination, it is unlikely that the PNC is cycling or acting anaplerotically to the TCA cycle in active muscle fibers during electrical stimulation (see the next section).

In normal exercise situations there is not maximal stimulation of all motor units as there is in the hindlimb stimulation model. During human leg exercise there is an increase in IMP and NH_3 as fatigue ensues in certain fibers (15, 100, 118), at which point other motor units are probably recruited to maintain performance while reamination and adenine nucleotide recovery could occur in inactive, recovering fibers, to maintain an excellent energy balance at the level of the whole muscle.

During prolonged exercise situations in humans there is a moderate rate of NH_3 production and release from skeletal muscle early in the exercise and a progressively rising rate as exercise progresses. If the PNC is the source of the NH_3 during this type of exercise, then it must be functioning as a cycle because there is no accumulation of IMP nor decrease in TAN in muscle under these conditions until glycogen is low (100, 101). If PNC cycling is responsible for the NH_3 production in these situations, it would have to be moderately activated early in the exercise bout and then be progressively activated as exercise continues to account for the NH_3 production. This is unlikely because there is little or no change in the known modulators of AMPD, AS, and AL as prolonged submaximal exercise progresses. Thus, it appears that deamination and reamination do not concurrently occur in individual active exercising muscle fibers.

In addition to the proposed functions of AMPD, Lowenstein (86) proposed two functions for the entire PNC. These are deamination of amino acids (see Figure 5.3) and anaplerocity to the TCA cycle via fumarate produced by the AL reaction.

PNC as a Source of TCA Cycle Intermediates.   Aragon et al. (4) have enzymatically analyzed mixed rat hindlimb muscle for TCA cycle intermediates under conditions of 5 Hz stimulation for 15 minutes. These authors report decreased ATP and increased AMP, IMP, and adenylosuccinate as a result of stimulation. Total TCA cycle intermediates were elevated twofold, whereas fumarate and malate were increased fourfold in the first 10 min of exercise.

When AS was competitively inhibited by hadacidin, fumarate production and TCA cycle intermediate responses to exercise were decreased compared with controls. The authors argue that the principal source of the increased TCA cycle intermediates in the control condition is the PNC and that increased TCA cycle intermediates increase aerobic function of the muscle fibers.

Some methodological considerations in the Aragon et al. study, however, confound the data. The rat hindlimb is a mixture of low and high oxidative fibers, and the measurement of metabolite levels in homogenates of the entire hindlimb musculature therefore represents an average across fiber types and includes both active and fatigued fibers. It is apparent that reamination and concomitant fumarate production were occurring under the conditions of this protocol, but is is unclear if concurrent deamination/reamination to increase aerobic function is occurring in *active* muscle fibers or whether the reamination/fumarate production occurred strictly in *fatigued* noncontracting recovering fibers.

It is possible that the decreased muscle oxygen consumption associated with contraction failure in the low-oxidative, fast-twitch white fibers caused a decrease in flux through the TCA cycle, which resulted in a transient increase in TCA intermediates, obscuring the interpretation of this whole muscle group homogenate analysis. This argument is integrated and reviewed by Tullson and Terjung (132). There is no evidence for increased aerobic function (increased oxygen consumption) without hadacidin. It is clear that if increased aerobic capacity due to increased TCA intermediates is the argument of Aragon et al., the functional or physiological consequences must be demonstrable.

Deamination of AMP is clearly important in NH_3 and adenine nucleotide management. AMPD is subject to regulation on several levels, and this tight regulation ensures that the enzyme is active only when excessive energy demand is imposed on muscle fibers. During very high-intensity stimulation or exercise it appears that AMP deamination is the only reaction of the PNC that is functioning to any considerable extent. Some of the originally proposed functions of this enzyme have been adequately refuted. It is probable that maintenance of the cellular energy state (ATP/ADP) and the prevention of excess adenine nucleotide degradation are the most important functions of AMPD.

At the whole muscle level of analysis under some conditions cycling of the PNC can be demonstrated. At the individual muscle fiber level of analysis, however, it is clear that deamination and reamination do not concomitantly occur. Though some increases in TCA cycle intermediates can be demonstrated under certain contraction conditions, whether the source of the intermediates is the PNC and the functional consequences of this observation remains obscure because no enhancement of aerobic function has been demonstrated. Reamination probably occurs almost exclusively in recovering fibers to repay the adenine nucleotide pool debt that is created during contractions by AMPD.

Influence of Other Substrates

Investigators have tried to alter the degree of amino acid metabolism during long-term work by altering the availability of other energy substrates. The majority of these studies have focused on the effects of other energy substrates on the oxidation of just one amino acid, leucine. Furthermore, these studies have been conducted on a wide variety of different species and tissues and have employed preparations ranging from whole-body kinetics to incubated diaphragms. However, very few investigations have evaluated the effects of these other substrates on NH_3 metabolism. This section will focus primarily on the effects of altered carbohydrate, fat, and amino acid availability on muscle amino acid and NH_3 metabolism during exercise.

Carbohydrates

It is well established that fatigue from prolonged exercise correlates well with low levels of liver and muscle glycogen. To investigate this relationship, researchers have employed the method of either increasing or decreasing endogenous muscle glycogen, as well as offering athletes a carbohydrate based supplement during exercise. In light of the fact that amino acid oxidation in muscle increases as exercise progresses, researchers have speculated that by altering the availability of endogenous carbohydrates the muscle will be forced to increase or decrease BCAA metabolism, and this will be reflected in plasma NH_3 levels.

Several studies have demonstrated that by depleting initial muscle glycogen stores prior to exercise, plasma NH_3 levels are significantly increased during exercise as compared with when initial muscle glycogen stores are normal or abundant (15, 52, 90, 136). Broberg and Sahlin (15) have further illustrated that muscle NH_3 efflux was significantly increased during a prolonged exercise bout when initial muscle glycogen was depleted. Similarly, it has been demonstrated that plasma NH_3 levels were lower when subjects ingested a carbohydrate drink during exercise as compared with placebo (136). MacLean et al. (90) also found that manipulation of initial muscle glycogen by the traditional manner of exhaustive exercise and diet resulted in elevated plasma BCAA prior to exercise. These BCAA were significantly decreased during exercise, indicating removal, presumably by active muscle. Similar findings were reported for McArdle's disease patients (myophosphorylase deficiency), who demonstrated a much larger uptake of BCAA by exercising muscle than normal subjects demonstrated (135). These results were further supported by Wagenmakers et al. (136), who showed that the BCOADH complex was activated to a much greater extent during exercise when initial muscle glycogen was depleted, as compared with when it was abundant.

On the other hand, MacLean et al. (89, 90) found no significant differences in plasma NH_3 levels during prolonged exhaustive exercise when initial muscle glycogen was normal or supercompensated. The authors also found no significant differences in either the plasma or the muscle BCAA levels during exercise. Thus, it appears that muscle NH_3 production is affected to a greater extent when carbohydrates are limiting, as compared with when they are normal or increased.

It must be noted that some investigators (15) attribute this NH_3 response exclusively to the reactions of PNC. PNC cycling and AMP deaminase activity may be a major NH_3 producer early during glycogen depletion; however, the responses of BCOADH and BCAA to alterations in carbohydrate availability suggest that transdeamination may also be important.

Free Fatty Acids and Ketones

Much of the research into the effects of free fatty acids (FFA) and ketones on amino acid metabolism has focused on their effects on the rate of leucine oxidation and protein turnover. Furthermore, these effects are controversial because both an increase (18, 104) and a decrease (10, 130) in leucine oxidation have been reported. A critical review of the studies in this area suggests that the conflicting reports about the effectiveness of FFA to increase or decrease amino acid oxidation may be related to the different species (dog, human, rodent) and tissue types (fast, slow, diaphragm) coupled with the varying methodologies (incubation, infusion, perfusion) and fatty acid chain lengths used (short-, medium-, long-chain triglycerides). In contrast, ketone infusion has consistently caused a decrease in leucine oxidation (17, 120, 122). However, there is very little data available addressing the effects of these substrates on the entire spectrum of amino acids and on NH_3 metabolism in exercising human muscle.

To the authors' knowledge there is only one study that has examined the effects of FFA on NH_3 and amino acid metabolism during exercise in humans. Graham et al. (49) examined the effects of Intralipid infusion on muscle metabolism during prolonged, steady state, one-legged exercise at 80% of work max. Although there were no significant differences in total amino efflux from muscle, the arterial concentration of nine amino acids (alanine, methionine, lysine, hydroxyproline, serine, glycine, proline, asparagine, and ornithine) decreased when Intralipid was introduced, compared with control. Furthermore, the net release of NH_3 was approximately one-half that of the control trial. These data support the general contention that FFA and ketones decrease muscle amino acid metabolism and NH_3 production.

Amino Acids

Muscle readily removes amino acids, more specifically BCAA, from the circulation. In fact Gelfand et al. (44) infused amino acids in resting humans and observed that muscle was responsible for the removal of 65 to 70% of the total BCAA load. In a similar experiment, Louard et al. (85) infused BCAA and reported a significant increase in both oxidative and non-oxidative leucine disposal. Because skeletal muscle preferentially removes BCAA, any perturbation in their concentration may have a significant effect on muscle NH_3 production.

Human liver has a very low BCAAT activity and, therefore, ingested BCAA selectively escape uptake by the liver and can quickly affect circulating BCAA levels (137). MacLean et al. (91) used an oral supplement of BCAA to significantly elevate plasma BCAA levels prior to exercise in humans. During 1 hr of moderate-intensity exercise, plasma NH_3 and glutamine concentrations were significantly elevated as compared with placebo. Wagenmakers et al. (135) reported similar findings when BCAA were administered to a McArdle's disease patient prior to exercise. In contrast, when the BCOA were given to the patient, plasma NH_3 was less than during the placebo trial. These data clearly suggest that elevated BCAA levels prior to exercise result in significantly elevated NH_3 production, presumably by contracting muscle.

Overall, the literature supports the hypothesis that when other energy substrates are altered prior to exercise, amino acid metabolism is subsequently altered during exercise. It appears that the greatest effects on amino acid and NH_3 metabolism during exercise occur when muscle glycogen is limited and when FFA and BCAA are elevated. However, there does not appear to be an effect when carbohydrates are abundant.

Central and Peripheral Effects of NH_3

There has been interest in the physiological effects of NH_3 production during exercise. Most attention has focused on the potential link between ammonia and fatigue and the effect of ammonia on ventilation.

Ammonia and Ventilation

As discussed previously, ventilation during exercise may serve as a means of reducing the NH_3 load on the circulation. In addition, it has been suggested that the increase in plasma NH_3 may stimulate the ventilatory response during exercise. Certainly the temporal patterns in plasma NH_3 during exercise in which the power output rises rapidly (e.g., a standard, progressive $\dot{V}O_2$ max test) follow the curvilinear rise in ventilation. Similarly during prolonged, steady state exercise, the plasma NH_3 concentration tends to drift upward, as does ventilation. However, these correlations cannot be considered proof of a causal relationship.

In some pathological conditions associated with chronically high plasma NH_3, as well as when plasma NH_3 is massively elevated by infusion, ventilation may be stimulated. For example, Wichser and Kazemi (143) infused NH_3 in anesthetized dogs to a blood NH_3 concentration of 400 µM and observed a marked increase in ventilation. Similarly direct infusion of the ventriculocisternal system with a high glutamate concentration also stimulated ventilation (23). Obviously these are extreme treatments, and one must keep in mind that the plasma NH_3 concentrations very rarely exceed 150 µM during exercise and that such a high concentration only occurs transiently. The authors are unaware of any evidence that such increases will alter the amino acid metabolism of the central nervous system in any way or will stimulate ventilation.

Central Fatigue

There have been various theories that either plasma NH_3 or a shift in the plasma amino acid profile may cause the varied sensations of fatigue. Banister and Cameron (7) speculate that exhaustive exercise may result in a state of "acute NH_3 toxicity," which leads to an altered CNS function and impaired motor functioning. Iles and Jack (64) point out that a high NH_3 concentration can produce lethargy, convulsions, ataxia, and even coma. The mechanisms for these CNS effects may include changes in intracellular pH, changes in intra- and extracellular electrolyte concentrations, a hyperpolarizing shift of the IPSP-equilibrium potential toward the resting potential in both cortical and lower motor neurons, and changes in a variety of reactions in the CNS, causing altered levels of neurotransmitters such as glutamate, glutamine, and GABA.

There is no question that these responses can occur in metabolic encephalopathies and in experimental manipulations in which large, perhaps pharmacological, doses of NH_3 are introduced (25). But one should keep in mind that these levels are rarely seen *in vivo*. We are aware of no evidence in exercising humans or other animals that plasma NH_3 affects CNS function. Thus, NH_3 as a cause of central fatigue remains an interesting theory that will be very difficult to test accurately.

NH_3 does cross the blood brain barrier by diffusion (25), which is facilitated by a high blood pH (84). Thus the acidosis of strenuous exercise would not facilitate the CNS uptake of NH_3. While the brain readily takes up NH_3, the astrocytes act as an "enzymatic barrier." They have a high concentration of glutamine synthase, and the NH_3 is largely metabolized to glutamine and released back into the blood and CSF (25). The efflux of glutamine represents a carbon drain on the astrocytes. If this process continues for a prolonged time, it will tax the glutamate pool in the astrocytes, and this in turn could lead to disturbances in the concentrations of glutamine, glutamate, etc., within the neurons (7, 25). Cooper and Plum (25) state that the normal brain NH_3 concentration is 1.5-3.0 times that of the blood, and that brain and blood NH_3 do not mix freely. Rises in blood NH_3 must be sustained before the CNS concentration is affected.

The other theory for a central fatigue mechanism that pertains to this discussion focuses on the plasma amino acid profile during exercise. Blomstrand et al. (12, 13) have proposed that the ratio of plasma trypto-phan to branched-chain amino acids could affect CNS function. Trypto-phan is the precursor for the synthesis of the neurotransmitter serotonin (5-hydroxytryptamine). High concentrations of serotonin are known to cause impaired mental performance and to induce sleep. It is thought that the flux generating step for the synthesis of serotonin is the availability of tryptophan from the plasma. Tryptophan has a low concentration in the plasma and exists as both free and bound (to albumin) forms. The synthesis of serotonin can be increased through diet. For example, when carbohydrates are ingested, the high insulin concentration can cause an increase in the uptake of plasma BCAA by tissues, predominantly muscle. Tryptophan is present in low concentrations and competes with several amino acids, including the BCAA for a transport carrier at the blood brain barrier. Thus by lowering the BCAA level, insulin is increasing the opportunity for tryptophan uptake and serotonin synthesis.

Blomstrand et al. (12, 13) reported that during marathon runs and other forms of prolonged exercise, the plasma BCAA level fell (probably due to muscle metabolism) and free tryptophan rose (perhaps because the rise in free fatty acids displaces some of the bound tryptophan). They speculate that this impact on the CNS serotonin level resulted in the heightened perception of fatigue. We are aware of no direct evidence with which to evaluate this theory, and at present it remains an interesting hypothesis.

Peripheral Fatigue

It has also been proposed that NH_3 and/or the metabolic events associated with its production within active muscle could be linked to the processes of fatigue. Processes that could cause peripheral fatigue in relationship to NH_3 and amino acids include an increase in intramuscular NH_3 stimulating afferent neurons, a disturbance in the anapleorotic TCA-related reactions of amino acids, and a failure of the PNC to rephosphorylate ADP at an adequate rate to balance ATP dephosphorylation.

In addition to the Ia, Ib, and II afferents that originate from muscle spindles, Golgi tendon organs, and Pacinian corpuscles, skeletal muscle also has group III and IV afferents. Their receptors are "free" nerve terminals or unencapsulated nerve endings. These receptors are responsible for reflex cardiovascular responses that occur with static contractions (96), and some of the receptors are termed *nociceptors*. These are activated by noxious chemical stimuli and are responsible for the sensation of muscle pain. Rotto and Kaufman (113) demonstrated that lactate, adenosine, and inorganic phosphate were ineffective stimuli of the group III and IV afferents, but lactic acid and cyclo-oxygenase products (prostaglandins and thromboxanes) were potent stimuli.

Lewis and Haller (82) speculated that NH_3 would also be a stimulus for the group III and IV afferents because McArdle's disease patients have an exaggerated NH_3 production and pressor responses to dynamic exercise. However, they demonstrated that NH_3 had little or no effect on these afferents (81).

It is important to appreciate that the TCA cycle is not a closed system but a series of reactions that include a number of substances that also serve as substrates or products to other, non-TCA reactions. Thus, intermediates of the cycle can be consumed or produced even while the muscle is active. Little is known about the concentrations of the TCA intermediates or the *in vivo* regulation of the TCA reactions. However, investigators (119, 135) have suggested that the removal of intermediates and/or the failure to maintain high concentrations of the intermediates may lead to a slowing of the TCA cycle and ultimately ATP supply during prolonged exercise.

It has been clearly demonstrated that human skeletal muscle has a net NH_3 production during prolonged exercise (15, 49). The production begins early in the exercise and increases progressively. It has also been shown that the TCA intermediate, citrate, increases in the muscle early in the activity, and then the concentration decreases over time but remains several fold higher than the resting concentration even at the time of fatigue (119, 127). Sahlin's group (119) has also followed the time course of several intermediates (malate, citrate, fumarate, and oxaloacetate). All of these intermediates rise approximately tenfold within 5 minutes and then slowly decline to 5 to 6 times rest concentration at fatigue.

On the other hand, acetylcarnitine rises but does not show this decline over time during exercise. Sahlin et al. (119) suggest that glycogenolysis and glycolysis are reduced as the exercise progresses. This decrease in pyruvate formation would reduce its availability for anaplerotic reactions:

$$\text{glutamate} + \text{pyruvate} \xrightarrow{\text{AT}} \text{2-oxoglutarate} + \text{alanine}$$

$$\text{pyruvate} + CO_2 + \text{ATP} \xrightarrow{\text{PC}} \text{ADP} + \text{Pi} + \text{oxaloacetate}$$

$$\text{phosphoenolpyruvate} + CO_2 + \text{IDP} \xrightarrow{\text{PEPCK}} \text{oxaloacetate} + \text{ITP}$$

$$\text{pyruvate} + CO_2 + \text{NADH} \xrightarrow{\text{MDH}} \text{NAD} + \text{malate}$$

AT = alanine transaminase, PC = pyruvate carboxylase,
PEPCK = phosphoenolpyruvate carboxykinase,
and MDH = malate dehydrogenase.

Of these, there is at least indirect evidence that alanine transaminase is active. As Sahlin et al. (119) pointed out, active muscle experiences an initial rapid decline in glutamate and a rise in alanine, suggesting that the glutamate pyruvate transaminase reaction is involved in the initial increase in TCA intermediates.

However, little is known about the other reactions during exercise, and there is little evidence to suggest that the alanine transaminase reaction would be compromised during prolonged exercise. In fact, muscle glutamate uptake and alanine release continue to occur at the initial rate or even higher throughout exercise (49). Furthermore, alanine release in muscle working at 80% $\dot{V}O_2$ max represents only 1% of the net pyruvate formation. It is unlikely that changes in pyruvate availability will have a profound effect in limiting this process.

If the source of the increasing rate of NH_3 production during prolonged exercise is glutamate dehydrogenase, then this process would generate 2-oxoglutarate (Figure 5.2). Similarly, if the source is PNC cycling, then fumarate is supplied (Figures 5.2 and 5.3). In addition, if the aspartate for the PNC cycling is derived from BCAA (i.e., aspartate transaminase: BCAA + Glu → Asp + BCOA), then the BCAA are a source of TCA intermediates. Because AMP deamination (as reflected by IMP accumulation) cannot be the main source of NH_3 in prolonged exercise, the NH_3 formation should be associated with an anaplerotic function regardless of its origin in prolonged exercise, and obviously this association would not be directly linked with fatigue.

The final aspect to be considered in the area of peripheral fatigue is that of inadequate rephosphorylation of ADP. It is clear that during the main portion of prolonged exercise there is little or no change in the nucleotide pool or IMP (100, 101). At the point of fatigue, however, the muscle is characterized by a marked rise in AMP and IMP. At this time AMP deaminase is obviously quite active. Sahlin and coworkers (119) suggest that this is a reflection of the inability of the metabolic processes to rephosphorylate the ATP rapidly enough. They propose that the decrease in glycolysis, in association with a declining glycogen concentration, limits the amount of pyruvate and thus the various anaplerotic reactions associated with pyruvate and phosphoenolpyruvate. The resulting decrease in TCA intermediates would reduce TCA cycle flux and oxidative phosphorylation. As a consequence, ADP and AMP would increase in the cytosol, and phosphocreatine would decline. Although this seems logical, there are no data to suggest that mitochondrial $\dot{V}O_2$ declines, nor do their data show a decrease in NADH (in fact, it is 30% above rest concentration). If the TCA flux decreases, one would expect both to occur. As with many theories for fatigue, this one will be difficult to test, and one needs to know the free concentrations of the various metabolites as well as the concentrations in various metabolic compartments.

NH_3 and amino acids have been proposed to be associated with a variety of fatigue processes. None of these have been supported with direct evidence. We cannot come to definitive conclusions, but the bulk of the data do not support that either central or peripheral fatigue are directly related to the metabolism of NH_3 in healthy, active humans.

NH_3 and Amino Acid Metabolism in Trained Muscle

In 1984 Holloszy and Coyle (58) reviewed the area of NH_3 metabolism and endurance training. They hypothesized that trained muscle with a greater mitochondrial population would experience a smaller rise in ADP and thus have lower muscle AMP, IMP, and NH_3 concentrations. These adaptations would result in less glycolytic activation, glycogen degradation, and lactate production. Although we now know much more about NH_3 metabolism, and their hypothesis appears to be correct, we still must speculate a great deal about the responses of NH_3 to training by humans. As we learn more, the situation becomes more complicated. For example, Holloszy and Coyle (58) focused only on PNC related events, but we must also consider amino acid metabolism.

Despite our level of understanding of muscle NH_3 metabolism, the data available regarding humans and training are restricted almost exclusively to changes in plasma NH_3 concentration. Lo and Dudley (83) appear to have been the first to study NH_3 responses to training in humans. They reported that after training the subjects had less accumulation in plasma NH_3 for a given absolute workload during an incremental work test. Recently Snow et al. (126) demonstrated that "sprint" training resulted in subjects performing more total work during a 30-s maximal sprint test but having less increase in plasma NH_3. Under these circumstances AMP deaminase is likely to be the prime NH_3 source, but these studies are extremely restricted in that nothing is known about muscle NH_3 production or release or about plasma NH_3 clearance. Two other reports (28, 51) have found that training resulted in less plasma NH_3 increase during prolonged, steady state exercise. These findings cannot resolve which NH_3 processes (production, release, or clearance) are affected, but the long-term nature of the exercise suggests that amino acid metabolism could be involved.

Nothing is known about training and plasma NH_3 clearance, and in order to assess the possible impact of training on muscle NH_3 production we are restricted to animal models at present. Winder et al. (145) found that rats had no change in muscle adenylosuccinate lyase after 12 weeks of training, but AMP deaminase was decreased 29% in the fast-twitch red quadriceps and unchanged in other muscle groups. The data are compatible with studies reporting less plasma NH_3 in trained humans during exercise (83, 126). In a similar study, during intense electrical stimulation lasting a few minutes, trained rodent muscle had less muscle AMP, IMP, and NH_3 accumulation, even though force development was greater (24, 36). These studies support the theory that training reduces AMP deaminase. This, combined with the expanded mitochondrial pool giving a greater ability to maintain the ATP concentration and minimize the AMP_f level during intense work, could account for a lower NH_3 production in trained muscle during intense work.

In contrast, Ji et al. (67) found that training increased aspartate aminotransferase, suggesting that training could cause greater cycling of the PNC. This could explain low levels of AMP and IMP, but would result in a higher production of NH_3.

It is far more difficult to account for the lower plasma NH_3 in trained subjects during prolonged exercise because one must consider the PNC as well as amino acids as NH_3 sources, and also because nothing is known about training and alternative amine carriers such as glutamine. Leucine oxidation has been shown to be greater in trained rats (29, 56). In agreement with this, Dohm et al. (29) found that the mitochondrially based BCOADH was greater in trained rodent muscle. In a similar study, Ji et al. (67) found that trained, exercising rats had a markedly lower plasma BCAA/BCOA ratio, suggesting a greater intramuscular oxidation of the BCOA with training. In addition, Wibom et al. (142) found that glutamate dehydrogenase (another mitochondrial enzyme) increases with training in humans. These enzyme responses suggest that amino acid metabolism and NH_3 production would be greater in trained muscle during prolonged exercise, yet plasma NH_3 is lower. It is possible that other amino carriers become more important. Alanine aminotransferase increases with training (67, 97). It is unknown how glutamine synthase responds to training. It is an energy-requiring process, and thus the greater potential to generate high energy phosphates in trained muscle could make glutamine production more viable during exercise.

There have been few investigations into NH_3 metabolism and training. The training may not equally affect all muscle or involve all fiber types within a muscle. Therefore, it will be difficult to resolve the mechanisms involved in training that result in dampening the NH_3 response to exercise. In brief, intense exercise, the lower NH_3 response may be associated with a reduced AMP deaminase concentration or less rise in the positive modulators of the enzyme. In prolonged, steady state exercise the situation appears more complex; the increased concentration of mitochondrial enzymes would suggest that NH_3 production should be enhanced. However, it may be that either the activation is dampened or the amino group is transferred to another carrier.

Summary

Protein is a very dynamic component of skeletal muscle, and there is a net degradation of noncontractile proteins during exercise. The regulating events for these processes are not understood. The free amino acid pool does not change during exercise; the amino acids liberated from endogenous protein may be released into the circulation before or after transamination reactions, or they may be oxidized in the active muscle. The latter is a major fate of the BCAA. The amino acids released from the muscle do not accumulate in the circulation, but are rapidly cleared, predominantly by the liver, where many can be used for gluconeogenesis.

The metabolism of amino acids in skeletal muscle results in dynamic changes in glutamate, glutamine, and alanine. The latter are amino carriers and may act to minimize the net NH_3 accumulation. During most exercise conditions, the active muscle releases glutamine, alanine, and NH_3 in similar quantities. Glutamate is taken up by the muscle; however, glutamate is a central component of many reactions and the glutamate pool must be supplemented. This occurs by protein catabolism and by amino acid transaminations.

NH_3 can be produced by both amino acid metabolism and AMP deamination. The former appears to be important during prolonged exercise, and the latter is the main source of NH_3 in intense exercise. The degree to which the two processes act simultaneously is not known, and the regulation of NH_3 production from either source is poorly understood.

There is a great deal of speculation about the possible physiological roles played by NH_3 production and the reactions associated with its metabolism. Although there are numerous theories linking NH_3 to aspects of peripheral and central fatigue, there is little evidence to support these hypotheses in healthy humans.

It is evident that NH_3 and amino acid metabolism is a vast, complex area. There are numerous examples of interactions between these processes and fat and carbohydrate metabolism. While the metabolism of amino acids is not a major source of ATP during exercise, it is obvious that their metabolism is critical to metabolic homeostasis and is involved with such processes as maintaining the concentrations of the TCA intermediates.

Acknowledgments

The work of the authors has been supported by NSERC of Canada. D. MacLean has been supported by an Ontario graduate studentship, and J. Rush by an NSERC studentship. The authors gratefully acknowledge the outstanding technical support of P. Sathasivam in their research.

References

1. Abrahams, S.L.; Younathan, E.S. Modulation of the kinetic properties of phosphofructokinase by ammonium ions. J. Biol. Chem. 246:2464-2467; 1971.

2. Afting, E.G.; Bernhardt, W.; Janzen, R.W.C.; Rothig, H.J. Quantitative importance of non-skeletal muscle N-methylhistidine and creatinine in human urine. Biochem. J. 220:449-452; 1981.

3. Ahlborg, G.; Felig, P.; Hagenfeldt, L.; Hendler, R.; Wahren, J. Substrate turnover during prolonged exercise in man. J. Clin. Invest. 53:1080-1090; 1974.

4. Aragon, J.J.; Tornheim, K.; Lowenstein, J.M. On a possible role of IMP in the regulation of phosphorylase activity in skeletal muscle. FEBS Lett. 117(Suppl.):K56-K64; 1980.

5. Aragon, J.J.; Tornheim, K.; Goodman, M.N.; Lowenstein, J.M. Replenishment of citric acid cycle intermediates by the purine nucleotide cycle in rat skeletal muscle. Curr. Top. Cell. Regul. 18:131-149; 1981.

6. Balon, T.W.; Zorzano, A.; Treadway, J.L.; Goodman, M.N.; Ruderman, N.B. Effect of insulin on protein synthesis and degradation in skeletal muscle after exercise. Am. J. Physiol. 258:E92-E97; 1990.

7. Banister, E.W.; Cameron, B.J.C. Exercise-induced hyperammonemia: peripheral and central effects. Int. J. Sports Med. 11(Suppl. 2):S129-S142; 1990.

8. Barshop, B.A.; Frieden, C. Analysis of the interaction of rabbit skeletal muscle adenylate deaminase with myosin subfragments. J. Biol. Chem. 259:60-66; 1984.

9. Beaufrere, B.; Tessari, P.; Cattalini, M.; Miles, J.; Haymond, W. Apparent decreased oxidation and turnover of leucine during infusion of medium-chain triglycerides. Am. J. Physiol. 249:E175-E182; 1985.

10. Beaufrere, B.; Horber, F.F.; Schwenk, W.F.; Marsh, H.M.; Matthews, D.; Gerich, J.E.; Haymond, M.W. Glucocorticoids increase leucine oxidation and impair leucine balance in humans. Am. J. Physiol. 257:E712-E721; 1989.

11. Bergstrom, J.; Furst, P.; Hultman, E. Free amino acids in muscle tissue and plasma during exercise in man. Clin. Physiol. 5:155-160; 1985.

12. Blomstrand, E.; Celsing, F.; Newsholme, E.A. Changes in plasma concentrations of aromatic and branched-chain amino acids during sustained exercise in man and their possible role in fatigue. Acta Physiol. Scand. 133:115-121; 1988.

13. Blomstrand, E.; Hassmen, P.; Ekblom, B.; Newsholme, E.A. Administration of branched-chain amino acids during sustained exercise-effects on performance and on plasma concentration of some amino acids. Eur. J. Appl. Physiol. 63:83-88; 1991.

14. Booth, F.W.; Watson, P.A. Control of adaptations in protein levels in response to exercise. Fed. Proc. 44:2293-2300; 1985.

15. Broberg, S.; Sahlin, K. Adenine nucleotide degradation in human skeletal muscle during prolonged exercise. J. Appl. Physiol. 67:116-122; 1989.

16. Brooks, G.A. Amino acid and protein metabolism during exercise and recovery. Med. Sci. Sport Exerc. 19:S150-S156; 1987.

17. Buffington, C.K.; DeBuysere, M.S.; Olson, M.S. Studies on the regulation of the branched chain alpha-keto acid dehydrogenase in the perfused rat heart. J. Biol. Chem. 254:10453-10458; 1979.

18. Buse, M.G.; Biggers, F.; Friderici, K.G.; Buse, J.F. Oxidation of branched chain amino acids by isolated hearts and diaphragms of the rat. J. Biol. Chem. 247:8085-8096; 1972.

19. Bylund-Fellenius, A.C.; Ojamaa, K.M.; Flaim, K.E.; Li, J.B.; Wassner, S.J.; Jefferson, L.S. Protein synthesis versus energy state in contracting muscles of perfused rat hindlimb. Am. J. Physiol. 246:E297-E305; 1984.

20. Cahill, G.F. Metabolic role of muscle. In: Pernow, B.; Saltin, B., eds. Muscle metabolism during exercise. New York: Plenum Press; 1971: 103-109.

21. Calles-Escandon, J.; Cunningham, J.J.; Snyder, P.; Jacob, R.; Huszar, G.; Loke, J.; Felig, P. Influence of exercise on urea, creatinine, and 3-methylhistidine excretion in normal human subjects. Am. J. Physiol. 246:E334-E338; 1984.

22. Chang, T.W.; Goldberg, A.L. Leucine inhibits oxidation of glucose and pyruvate in skeletal muscles during fasting. J. Biol. Chem. 253:3696-3701; 1978.

23. Chiang, C-H.; Pappagianopoulos, P.; Hoop, B.; Kazemi, H. Central cardiorespiratory effects of glutamate in dogs. J. Appl. Physiol. 60:2056-2062; 1986.

24. Constable, S.H.; Favier, R.J.; McLane, J.A.; Fell, R.D.; Chen, M.; Holloszy, J.O. Energy metabolism in contracting rat skeletal muscle: adaptation to exercise training. Am. J. Physiol. 253:C316-C322; 1987.

25. Cooper, A.J.L.; Plum, F. Biochemistry and physiology of brain ammonia. Physiol. Rev. 67:440-519; 1987.

26. Czarnowski, D.; Gorski, J. Sweat ammonia excretion during submaximal cycling exercise. J. Appl. Physiol. 70:371-374; 1991.

27. Decombaz, J.; Reinhardt, P.; Anantharaman, K.; von Glutz, G.; Poortmans, J.R. Biochemical changes in a 100 km run: free amino acids, urea, and creatinine. Eur. J. Appl. Physiol. 41:61-72; 1979.

28. Denis, C.; Linossier, M.-T.; Dormois, D.; Cottier-Perrin, M.; Geyssant, A.; Lacour, J.-R. Effects of endurance training on hyperammonaemia during a 45-min constant exercise intensity. Eur. J. Appl. Physiol. 59:268-272; 1989.

29. Dohm, G.L.; Hecker, A.L.; Brown, W.E.; Klain, G.J.; Puente, F.R.; Askew, E.W.; Beecher, G.R. Adaptation of protein metabolism to endurance training. Biochem. J. 164:705-708; 1977.

30. Dohm, G.L.; Kasperek, G.J.; Tapscott, E.B.; Beecher, G.R. Effect of exercise on synthesis and degradation of muscle protein. Biochem. J. 188:255-262;1980.

31. Dohm, G.L.; Beecher, G.R.; Warren, R.Q.; Williams, R.T. The influence of exercise on amino acid concentrations in rat tissues. J. Appl. Physiol. 50:41-44; 1981.

32. Dohm, G.L.; Williams, R.T.; Kasperek, G.J.; van Rij, A.M. Increased excretion of urea and N-methylhistidine by rats and humans after a bout of exercise. J. Appl. Physiol. 52:27-33; 1982.

33. Dohm, G.L.; Kasperek, G.J.; Tapscott, E.B.; Barakat, H.A. Protein metabolism during endurance exercise. Fed. Proc. 44:348-352; 1985.

34. Dohm, G.L. Protein as a fuel for endurance exercise. Exerc. Sport Sci. Rev. 14:143-173; 1986.

35. Dohm, G.L.; Tapscott, E.B.; Kasperek, G.J. Protein degradation during endurance exercise and recovery. Med. Sci. Sports Exerc. 19:S166-S171; 1987.

36. Dudley, G.A.; Terjung, R.L. Influence of aerobic metabolism on IMP accumulation in fast-twitch muscle. Am. J. Physiol. 248:C37-C42; 1985.

37. Dudley, G.A.; Terjung, R.L. Influence of acidosis on AMP deaminase activity in contracting fast twitch muscle. Am. J. Physiol. 248:C43-C50; 1985.

38. Eriksson, L.S.; Broberg, S.; Bjorkman, O.; Wahren, J. Ammonia metabolism during exercise in man. Clin. Physiol. (Oxf) 5:325-336; 1985.

39. Felig, P.; Wahren, J. Amino acid metabolism in exercising man. J. Clin. Invest. 50:2703-2714; 1971.

40. Flanagan, W.F.; Holmes, E.W.; Sabina, R.L.; Swain, J.L. Importance of purine nucleotide cycle to energy production in skeletal muscle. Am. J. Physiol. 251:C795-C802; 1986.

41. Foley, J.M.; Adams, G.R.; Meyer, R.A. Utility of AICAr for metabolic studies is diminished by systemic effects in situ. Am. J. Physiol. 257:C488-C494; 1989.

42. Fryburg, D.A.; Barrett, E.J.; Louard, R.J.; Gelfand, R.A. Effect of starvation on human muscle protein metabolism and its response to insulin. Am. J. Physiol. 259:E477-E482; 1990.

43. Fryburg, D.A.; Gelfand, R.A.; Barrett, E.J. Growth hormone acutely stimulates forearm muscle protein synthesis in normal humans. Am. J. Physiol. 260:E499-E504; 1991.

44. Gelfand, R.A.; Glickman, M.G.; Jacob, R.; Sherwin, R.S.; DeFronzo, R.A. Removal of infused amino acids by splanchnic and leg tissues in humans. Am. J. Physiol. 250:E407-E413; 1986.

45. Goodman, M.N.; Lowenstein, J.M. The purine nucleotide cycle. Studies of ammonia production by skeletal muscle *in situ* and in perfused preparations. J. Biol. Chem. 252:5054-5060; 1977.

46. Goodman, M.N.; Ruderman, N.B. Influence of muscle use on amino acid metabolism. Exerc. Sport Sci. Rev. 10:1-26; 1982.

47. Graham, T.E.; Pedersen, P.K.; Saltin, B. Muscle and blood ammonia and lactate responses to prolonged exercise with hyperoxia. J. Appl. Physiol. 63:1457-1462; 1987.

48. Graham, T.E.; Bangsbo, J.; Gollnick, P.D.; Juel, C.; Saltin, B. Ammonia metabolism during intense dynamic exercise and recovery in humans. Am. J. Physiol. 259:E170-E176; 1990.

49. Graham, T.E.; Kiens, B.; Hargreaves, M.; Richter, E.A. Influence of fatty acids on ammonia and amino acid flux from active human muscle. Am. J. Physiol. 261:E168-E176; 1991.

50. Graham, T.E.; MacLean, D.A. Ammonia and amino acid metabolism in human skeletal muscle during exercise. Can. J. Physiol. Pharmacol. 70:132-141; 1992.

51. Green, H.J.; Jones, S.; Ball-Burnett, M.; Fraser, I. Early adaptations in blood substrates, metabolities, and hormones to prolonged exercise training in man. Can. J. Physiol. Pharmacol. 69:1222-1229; 1991.

52. Greenhaff, P.L.; Leiper, J.B.; Ball, D.; Maughan, R.J. The influence of dietary manipulation on plasma ammonia accumulation during incremental exercise in man. Eur. J. Appl. Physiol. 63:338-344; 1991.

53. Hagg, S.A.; Morse, E.L.; Adibi, S.A. Effect of exercise on rates of oxidation turnover, and plasma clearance of leucine in human subjects. Am. J. Physiol. 242:E407-E410; 1982.

54. Haralambie, G.; Berg, A. Serum urea and amino nitrogen changes with exercise duration. Eur. J. Appl. Physiol. 36:39-48; 1976.

55. Harper, A.E.; Miller, R.H.; Block, K.P. Branched-chain amino acid metabolism. Ann. Rev. Nutr. 4:409-454; 1984.

56. Henderson, S.A.; Black, A.L.; Brooks, G.A. Leucine turnover and oxidation in trained rats during exercise. Am. J. Physiol. 249:E137-E144; 1985.

57. Henriksson, J.; M.-Y. Chi, M.; Hintz, C.S.; Young, D.A.; Kaiser, K.K.; Salmons, S.; Lowry, O.H. Chronic stimulation of mammalian muscle: changes in enzymes of six metabolic pathways. Am. J. Physiol. 251:C614-C632; 1986.

58. Holloszy, J.O.; Coyle, E.F. Adapations of skeletal muscle to endurance exercise and their metabolic consequences. J. Appl. Physiol. 56:831-838; 1984.

59. Hood, D.A.; Terjung, R.L. Leucine metabolism in perfused rat skeletal muscle during contractions. Am. J. Physiol. 253:E636-E647; 1987.

60. Hood, D.A.; Terjung, R.L. Effect of endurance training on leucine metabolism in perfused rat skeletal muscle. Am. J. Physiol. 253:E648-E656; 1987.

61. Hood, D.A.; Terjung, R.L. Amino acid metabolism during exercise and following endurance training. Sports Med. 9:23-35; 1990.

62. Hutson, S.M. Branched chain alpha-keto acid oxidative decarboxylation in skeletal muscle mitochondria. J. Biol. Chem. 261:4420-4425; 1986.

63. Hutson, S.M. Subcellular distribution of branched-chain aminotransferase activity in rat tissues. J. Nutr. 118:1475-1481; 1988.

64. Iles, J.F.; Jack, J.J.B. Ammonia: assessment of its action on postsynaptic inhibition as a cause of convulsions. Brain 103:555-578; 1980.

65. Jacquez, J.A.; Popell, J.W.; Jeltsch, R. Partial pressure of ammonia in alveolar air. Science 129:269-270; 1959.

66. Jennings, R.B.; Steenbergen, C., Jr. Nucleotide metabolism and cellular damage in myocardial ischemia. Ann. Rev. Physiol. 47:727-749; 1985.

67. Ji, L.L.; Miller, R.H.; Nagle, F.J.; Lardy, H.A.; Stratman, F.W. Amino acid metabolism during exercise in trained rats: the potential role of carnitine in the metabolic fate of branched-chain amino acids. Metabolism 36:748-752; 1987.

68. Kasperek, G.J.; Dohm, G.L.; Barakat, H.A.; Strausbauch, P.H.; Barnes, D.W.; Snider, R.D. The role of lysosomes in exercise-induced hepatic protein loss. Biochem. J. 202:281-288; 1982.

69. Kasperek, G.J.; Dohm, G.L.; Snider, R.D. Activation of branched-chain keto acid dehydrogenase by exercise. Am. J. Physiol. 248:R166-R171; 1985.

70. Kasperek, G.J.; Snider, R.D. Increased protein degradation after eccentric exercise. Eur. J. Appl. Physiol. 54:30-34; 1985.

71. Kasperek, G.J.; Snider, R.D. Effect of exercise intensity and starvation on activation of branched-chain keto acid dehydrogenase by exercise. Am. J. Physiol. 252:E33-E37; 1987.

72. Katz, A.; Broberg, S.; Sahlin, K.; Wahren, J. Muscle ammonia and amino acid metabolism during dynamic exercise in man. Clin. Physiol. (Oxf) 6:365-379; 1986.

73. Katz, A.; Sahlin, K.; Henrikson, J. Muscle ammonia metabolism during isometric contraction in humans. Am. J. Physiol. 250:C834-C840; 1986.

74. Khatra, B.S.; Chawla, R.K.; Sewell, C.W.; Ruderman, D. Distribution of branched chain alpha-keto acid dehydrogenases in primate tissues. J. Clin. Invest. 59:558-564; 1977.

75. Knapik, J.; Meredith, C.; Jones, B.; Fielding, R.; Young, V.; Evans, W. Leucine metabolism during fasting and exercise. J. Appl. Physiol. 70:43-47; 1991.

76. Knepper, M.A.; Packer, R.; Good, D.W. Ammonium transport in the kidney. Physiol. Rev. 69:179-249; 1989.

77. Kovacevic, Z.; McGivin, J.D. Mitochondrial metabolism of glutamine and glutamate and its physiological significance. Physiol. Rev. 63:547-605; 1983.

78. Lau, K.S.; Fatania, H.R.; Randle, P.J. Regulation of the branched chain 2-oxoacid dehydrogenase kinase reaction. FEBS Lett. 144:57-62; 1982.

79. Lemon, P.W.R.; Nagle, F.J.; Mullin, J.P.; Benevenga, N.J. *In vivo* leucine oxidation at rest and during two intensities of exercise. J. Appl. Physiol. 53:947-954; 1982.

80. Lemon, P.W.R. Protein and exercise: update. Med. Sci. Sports 19:S179-S190; 1987.

81. Lewis, S.F.; Kaufman, M.P. Lack of pressor response to ammonium chloride injections in cat hindlimb. Physiologist 28:292; 1985.

82. Lewis, S.F.; Haller, R.G. The pathophysiology of McArdle's disease: clues to regulation in exercise and fatigue. J. Appl. Physiol. 61:391-401; 1986.

83. Lo, P.-Y; Dudley, G.A. Endurance training reduces the magnitude of exercise-induced hyperammonemia in humans. J. Appl. Physiol. 62:1227-1230; 1987.

84. Lockwood, A.H.; Finn, R.D.; Campbell, J.A.; Richman, T.B. Factors that affect the uptake of ammonia by the brain: the blood-brain pH gradient. Brain Res. 181:259-266; 1980.

85. Louard, R.J.; Barrett, E.J.; Gelfand, R.A. Effect of infused branched-chain amino acids on muscle and whole-body amino acid metabolism in man. Clin. Sci. 79:457-466; 1990.

86. Lowenstein, J.M. Ammonia production in muscle and other tissues: the purine nucleotide cycle. Physiol. Rev. 52:382-414; 1972.

87. Lowenstein, J.M. The purine nucleotide cycle revised. Int. J. Sports Med. 11:537-546; 1990.

88. Lund, P. Metabolism of glutamine, glutamate and aspartate. In: Waterlow, J.C.; Stephen, J.M.L., eds. Nitrogen metabolism in man. Essex, U.K.: Applied Science Publishers; 1980: 155-169.

89. MacLean, D.A.; Spriet, L.L.; Hultman, E.; Graham, T.E. Plasma and muscle amino acid and ammonia responses during prolonged exercise in humans J. Appl. Physiol. 70:2095-2103; 1991.

90. MacLean, D.A.; Spriet, L.L.; Graham, T.E. Plasma amino acid and ammonia responses to altered dietary intakes prior to prolonged exercise in humans. Can. J. Physiol. Pharmacol. 70:420-427; 1992.

91. MacLean, D.A.; Graham, T.E. Branched chain amino acid supplementation augments plasma ammonia responses during exercise in humans. J. Appl. Physiol. 74:2711-2717; 1993.

92. Manfredi, J.P.; Marquetent, R.; Magid, A.D.; Holmes, E.W. Binding of adenylosuccinate synthetase to contractile proteins of muscle. Am. J. Physiol. 257:C29-C35; 1989.

93. Marshal, S.; Monzon, R. Amino acid regulation of insulin action in isolated adipocytes. J. Biol. Chem. 264:2037-2042; 1989.

94. May, R.C.; Hara, Y.; Kelly, R.A.; Block, K.P.; Buse, M.G.; Mitch, W.E. Branched-chain amino acid metabolism in rat muscle: abnormal regulation in acidosis. Am. J. Physiol. 252:E712-E718; 1987.

95. Meyer, R.A.; Terjung, R.L. AMP deamination and IMP reamination in working skeletal muscle. Am. J. Physiol. 239:C32-C38; 1980.

96. Mitchell, J.H. Neural control of the circulation during exercise. Med. Sci. Sports Exerc. 22:141-154; 1990.

97. Molé, P.A.; Baldwin, K.M.; Terjung, R.L.; Holloszy, J.O. Enzymatic pathways of pyruvate metabolism in skeletal muscle: adaptations to exercise. Am. J. Physiol. 224:50-54; 1973.

98. Nair, K.S.; Schwartz, R.G.; Welle, S. Leucine as a regulator of whole body and skeletal muscle protein metabolism in humans. Am. J. Physiol. 263:E928-E934; 1992.

99. Newsholme, E.A.; Leech, A.R. Biochemistry for the medical sciences. New York: John Wiley and Sons; 1983.

100. Norman, B.; Sollevi, A.; Kaijser, L.; Jannson, E. ATP breakdown products in human skeletal muscle during prolonged exercise to exhaustion. Clin. Physiol. 7:503-509; 1987.

101. Norman, B.; Sollevi, A.; Jansson, E. Increased IMP content in glycogen-depleted muscle fibres during submaximal exercise in man. Acta Physiol. Scand. 133:97-100; 1988.

102. Odessey, R.; Goldberg, A.L. Oxidation of leucine by rat skeletal muscle. Am. J. Physiol. 223:1376-1383; 1972.

103. Ogawa, H.; Shiraki, H.; Matsuda, Y.; Kakiuchi, K.; Nakagawa, H. Purification, crystallization and properties of adenylosuccinate synthetase from rat skeletal muscle. J. Biochem. 81:859-869; 1977.

104. Paul, H.S.; Adibi, S.A. Assessment of effect of starvation, glucose, fatty acids and hormones on alpha-decarboxylation of leucine in skeletal muscle of rat. J. Nutr. 106:1079-1088; 1976.

105. Paxton, R.; Harris, R.A. Regulation of branched-chain alpha-ketoacid dehydrogenase kinase. Arch. Biochem. Biophys. 231:48-57; 1984.

106. Plante, R.I.; Houston, M.E. Exercise and protein catabolism in women. Ann. Nutr. Metab. 28:123-129; 1984.

107. Poortmans, J.R. Protein turnover and amino acid oxidation during and after exercise. Med. Sports Sci. 17:130-147; 1984.

108. Raggi, A.; Bergamini, C.; Ronca, G. Isozymes of AMP deaminase in red and white skeletal muscle. FEBS Lett. 58:19-23; 1975.

109. Raggi, A.; Ranieri-Raggi, M. Regulatory properties of AMP deaminase isoenzymes from rabbit red muscle. Biochem. J. 242:875-879; 1987.

110. Rahim, Z.H.A.; Perrett, D.; Lutaya, G.; Griffiths, J.R. Metabolic adaptation in phosphorylase kinase deficiency. Changes in metabolite concentrations during tetanic stimulation of mouse leg muscles. Biochem. J. 186:331-341; 1980.

111. Rennie, M.J.; Edwards, R.H.T.; Davies, C.T.M.; Krywawych, S.; Halliday, D.; Waterlow, J.C.; Millward, D.J. Protein and amino acid turnover during and after exercise. Biochem. Soc. Trans. 8:499-501; 1980.

112. Rennie, M.J.; Edwards, R.H.T.; Krywawych, S.; Davies, C.T.M.; Halliday, D.; Waterlow, J.C.; Millward, D.J. Effect of exercise on protein turnover in man. Clin. Sci. 61:627-639; 1981.

113. Rotto, D.M.; Kaufman, M.P. Effect of metabolic products of muscular contraction on discharge of group III and IV afferents. J. Appl. Physiol. 64:2306-2313; 1988.

114. Rundell, K.W.; Tullson, P.C.; Terjung, R.L. AMP deaminase binding in contracting rat skeletal muscle. Am. J. Physiol. 263:C287-C293; 1992.

115. Rundell, K.W.; Tullson, P.C.; Terjung, R.L. Altered kinetics of AMP deaminase by myosin binding. Am. J. Physiol. 263:C294-C299; 1992.

116. Sabina, R.L.; Swain, J.L.; Patten, B.M.; Ashizawa, T.; O'Brien, W.E.; Holmes, E.W. Disruption of the purine nucleotide cycle. A potential explanation for muscle dysfunction in myoadenylate deaminase deficiency. J. Clin. Invest. 66:1419-1423; 1980.

117. Sabina, R.L.; Swain, J.L.; Olanow, C.W. Myoadenylate deaminase deficiency. Functional and metabolic abnormalities associated with disruption of the purine nucleotide cycle. J. Clin. Invest. 73:720-730; 1984.

118. Sahlin, K.; Broberg, S.; Ren, J.M. Formation of inosine monophosphate (IMP) in human skeletal muscle during incremental dynamic exercise. Acta Physiol. Scand. 136:193-198; 1989.

119. Sahlin, K.; Katz, A.; Broberg, S. Tricarboxylic acid cycle intermediates in human muscle during prolonged exercise. Am. J. Physiol. 259:C834-C841; 1990.

120. Sans, R.M.; Jolly, W.W.; Harris, R.A. Studies on the regulation of leucine catabolism. Arch. Biochem. Biophys. 200:336-345; 1980.

121. Schwenk, W.F.; Haymond, M.W. Effects of leucine, isoleucine, or threonine infusion on leucine metabolism in humans. Am. J. Physiol. 253:E428-E434; 1987.

122. Sherwin, R.S.; Hendler, R.G.; Felig, P. Effect of ketone infusions on amino acid and nitrogen metabolism in man. J. Clin. Invest. 55:1382-1390; 1975.

123. Shiraki, H.; Ogawa, H.; Matsuda, Y.; Nakagawa, H. Interaction of rat muscle AMP deaminase with myosin: II. Modification of the kinetic and regulatory properties of rat muscle AMP deaminase by myosin. Biochim. Biophys. Acta 566:345-352; 1979.

124. Sinkeler, S.P.T.; Joosten, E.M.G.; Wevers, R.A.; Binkhors, R.A.; Oerleman, F.T.; Vanbenne, C.A.; Coerwink, M.M.; Oei, T.L. Ischaemic exercise test in myoadenylate deaminase deficiency and McArdle's disease: measurement of plasma adenosine, inosine, and hypoxanthine. Clin. Sci. 70:399-401; 1986.

125. Smith, K.; Rennie, M.J. Protein turnover and amino acid metabolism in human skeletal muscle. Clin. Endocrin. Metab. 4:461-498; 1990.

126. Snow, R.J.; McKenna, M.J.; Carey, M.F.; Hargreaves, M. Sprint training attenuates plasma ammonia accumulation following maximal exercise. Acta Physiol. Scand. 144:395-396; 1992.

127. Spriet, L.L.; MacLean, D.A.; Dyck, D.J.; Hultman, E.; Cederblad, G.; Graham, T.E. Caffeine ingestion and muscle metabolism during prolonged exercise in humans. Am. J. Physiol. 262:E891-E898; 1992.

128. Stayton, M.M.; Rudolph, F.B.; Fromm, H.J. Regulation, genetics, and properties of adenylosuccinate synthetase: a review. Curr. Top. Cell. Reg. 22:103-141; 1983.

129. Tawa, N.E., Jr.; Goldberg, A.L. Suppression of muscle protein turnover and amino acid degradation by dietary protein deficiency. Am. J. Physiol. 263:E317-E325; 1992.

130. Tessari, P.; Nissen, S.L.; Miles, J.M.; Haymond, M.W. Inverse relationship of leucine flux and oxidation to free fatty acid availability *in vivo*. J. Clin. Invest. 77:575-581; 1986.

131. Tullson, P.C.; Whitlock, D.A.; Terjung, R.L. Adenine nucleotide degradation in slow-twitch red muscle. Am. J. Physiol. 258:C258-C265; 1990.

132. Tullson, P.C.; Terjung, R.L. Adenine nucleotide metabolism in contracting skeletal muscle. Ex. Sports Sci. Rev. 19:507-537; 1991.

133. Wagenmakers, A.J.M.; Schepens, J.T.G.; Veldhuizen, J.A.M.; Veerkamp, J.G. The activity state of the branched-chain 2-oxo acid dehydrogenase complex in rat tissue. Biochem. J. 220:273-281; 1984.

134. Wagenmakers, A.J.M.; Brookes, J.H.; Coakley, J.H.; Reilly, T.; Edwards, R.H.T. Exercise-induced activation of the branched-chain 2-oxo acid dehydrogenase in human muscle. Eur. J. Appl. Physiol. 59:159-167; 1989.

135. Wagenmakers, A.J.M.; Coakley, J.H.; Edwards, R.H.T. Metabolism of branched-chain amino acids and ammonia during exercise. Clues from McArdle's disease. Int. J. Sports Med. 11:S101-S113; 1990.

136. Wagenmakers, A.J.M.; Beckers, E.J.; Brouns, F.; Kuipers, H.; Soeters, P.B.; van der Vusse, G.J.; Saris, W.H.M. Carbohydrate supplementation, glycogen depletion, and amino acid metabolism during exercise. Am. J. Physiol. 260:E883-E890; 1991.

137. Wahren, J.; Felig, P.; Hagenfeldt, L. Effect of protein ingestion on splanchnic and leg metabolism in normal man and in patients with diabetes mellitus. J. Clin. Invest. 57:987-999; 1976.

138. Watt, P.E.; Corbett, M.E.; Rennie, M.J. Stimulation of protein synthesis in pig skeletal muscle by infusion of amino acids during constant insulin availability. Am. J. Physiol. 263:E453-460; 1992.

139. Wheeler, T.J.; Lowenstein, J.M. Adenylate deaminase from muscle. Regulation by purine nucleotides and orthophosphate in the presence of 150 mM KCl. J. Biol. Chem. 254:8894-8899; 1979.

140. Whitlock, D.; Terjung, R.L. ATP depletion in slow-twitch red muscle of rat. Am. J. Physiol. 253:C426-C432; 1987.

141. Wibom, R.; Hultman, E. ATP production rate in mitochondria isolated from microsamples of human muscle. Am. J. Physiol. 259:E204-E209; 1990.

142. Wibom, R.; Hultman, E.; Johansson, M.; Matherei, K.; Constantin-Teodosiu, D.; Schantz, P.G. Adaptation of mitochondrial ATP production in human skeletal muscle to endurance training and detraining. J. Appl. Physiol. 73:2004-2010; 1992.

143. Wichser, J.; Kazemi, H. Ammonia and ventilation: site and mechanism of action. Resp. Physiol. 20:393-406; 1974.

144. Willhoft, N.M.; Pogson, C.I.; Rennie, M.J. Control of the size of the glutamine pool in rat skeletal muscle. FASEB J. 7:A396; 1993.

145. Winder, W.W.; Terjung, R.L.; Baldwin, K.M.; Holloszy, J.O. Effect of exercise on AMP deaminase and adenylosuccinase in rat skeletal muscle. Am. J. Physiol. 227:1411-1414; 1974.

146. Wolfe, R.R.; Goodenough, R.D.; Wolfe, M.H.; Royle, G.T.; Nadel, E.R. Isotopic analysis of leucine and urea metabolism in exercising humans. J. Appl. Physiol. 52:458-466; 1982.

147. Yeaman, S.J. The 2-oxo acid dehydrogenase complexes: recent advances. Biochem. J. 257:625-632; 1989.

Chapter 6

Metabolic Adaptations to Endurance Training: Substrate Metabolism During Exercise

ANDREW R. COGGAN AND BRADLEY D. WILLIAMS

Regularly performed endurance exercise (i.e., endurance training) induces profound adaptations in many physiological systems (e.g., cardiovascular, muscular, endocrine). One important effect of these adaptations is to modify the rates at which various fuels are used during exercise. Specifically, when compared with untrained subjects, endurance-trained individuals oxidize less carbohydrate and more fat during exercise performed at the same absolute intensity (i.e., at the same absolute power output or rate of oxygen uptake [$\dot{V}O_2$]) (12, 17, 18, 20, 45, 59, 74, 90, 94, 110, 129) and possibly even during exercise performed at the same relative intensity (i.e., at the same percentage of maximal oxygen uptake [$\dot{V}O_2$ max]) (21, 38, 60, 73, 81, 98, 121). Because depletion of the body's carbohydrate reserves is an important factor in the development of fatigue, this training-induced shift in substrate source undoubtedly plays a major role in the enhanced capacity for prolonged exercise that results from endurance training.

The metabolic adaptations to endurance training have been studied for many years, initially using indirect calorimetry (12) and subsequently using a wide variety of invasive and noninvasive techniques, including arteriovenous (a-v) balance measurements (59, 73, 110, 121), muscle biopsy sampling (20, 38, 45, 47, 48, 59, 60, 69, 73, 74), isotopic tracer infusion (10, 17, 18, 21, 22, 32, 58, 78, 82, 90, 94), and magnetic resonance spectroscopy (16, 93). Despite this scrutiny, a number of important questions remain. For example, although it is clear that trained individuals oxidize more fat during prolonged exercise, the specific tissue source (i.e., adipose vs. muscle) of these additional fatty acids remains uncertain. Similarly, although an increase in muscle mitochondrial respiratory capacity with training clearly plays a major part in this substrate shift, the biochemical mechanisms responsible have only been partially elucidated. The purpose of this chapter is, therefore, to review the metabolic adaptations to endurance training, with particular emphasis on recent literature in this area. Because conclusions drawn regarding the effects of training may depend in part on the experimental conditions employed, we begin by briefly examining the various models used to study the metabolic adaptations to endurance training.

Experimental Models

Over the years, a number of experimental approaches have been utilized to examine the effects of endurance training on substrate metabolism during exercise.

Animals vs. Humans

There are advantages to using animal models when studying the metabolic effects of frequent exercise. Perhaps the most obvious advantage is that researchers can perform invasive procedures (e.g., liver sampling) in animals that may not be feasible in humans. It may also be easier for researchers to demonstrate certain training adaptations using an animal model, because researchers can force cage-confined (i.e., deconditioned) laboratory animals to train strenuously by using noxious stimuli such as air jets or electrical shock. In addition, intersubject variability should be lower in studies of inbred animals than in studies of humans, although this particular advantage is negated when the same individual is examined both before and after training (see next section).

Caution must be used, however, when attempting to extrapolate from the results of animal studies to humans. As previously emphasized (19, 23), the metabolic responses to acute exercise may differ considerably between species. Consequently, the metabolic adaptations to exercise training may also differ. For example, endurance training markedly reduces plasma glucose clearance (18, 21, 73, 78, 94) and gluconeogenesis (22) during exercise in humans, but it does not affect glucose clearance (10, 32b) and actually enhances gluconeogenesis (32b, 116) in rats. This chapter, therefore, focuses on the adaptations of humans to endurance training and makes limited reference to studies of animals.

Cross-Sectional vs. Longitudinal Studies

The comparison of highly trained endurance athletes with untrained individuals provides a relatively time- and cost-efficient way of examining the physiological effects of training. Elite athletes also presumably represent the optimum of human adaptability for endurance exercise, and as such may be worth studying in their own right. A major disadvantage to such cross-sectional studies, however, is that it is impossible to be certain that any differences observed are due to endurance training per se and are not due to other factors, such as differences in genetic inheritance, body composition, habitual diet, etc.

By studying the same individual before and after completion of an endurance training program, it is possible to eliminate these potentially confounding influences. The resulting adaptations can therefore be more confidently ascribed to the exercise program itself. Furthermore, variability is reduced by having each subject serve as his or her own control, which increases statistical power. On the other hand, the training programs used in longitudinal studies are often limited in intensity and duration in comparison with training programs undertaken by elite athletes. Hence, longitudinal studies may still fail to reveal adaptations that might be elicited only by many years of extreme endurance training.

Information about the metabolic effects of endurance training can also be gained by following the regression of such adaptations when individuals cease exercising or "detrain" (25, 80, 89, 98). This approach also helps control for intersubject differences, but it enables larger and more rapid changes in activity level than can be achieved in a longitudinal training study. It must be assumed, however, that the physiological adaptations to training are lost at the same rate and to the same extent with detraining, which may or may not be a valid assumption.

Same Relative vs. Same Absolute Exercise Intensity

Most cross-sectional studies have compared untrained and trained subjects during exercise performed at the same percentage of $\dot{V}O_2$ max (8, 21, 29, 38, 54, 55, 60, 73, 98, 121). This approach arose from the classical idea that the metabolic responses to exercise were determined primarily by the ability to deliver O_2 to the exercising musculature (71). Because $\dot{V}O_2$ max was viewed as the major variable determining the physiological response to exercise, it was logical to control for the relative exercise intensity when examining the effects of training. It is now evident, however, that the hormonal and metabolic responses to exercise often differ between fit and unfit subjects even when exercise is performed at the same percentage of $\dot{V}O_2$ max (8, 21, 38, 54, 55, 60, 73, 81, 98, 121). This is probably because the factors that determine $\dot{V}O_2$ max are, in part, different from those that determine the physiological responses to exercise requiring less than 100% $\dot{V}O_2$ max. That is, while $\dot{V}O_2$ max appears to be limited primarily by the central circulation (cf. 108), substrate metabolism during submaximal exercise appears to be determined primarily by peripheral factors, especially the respiratory capacity of the exercising musculature (cf. 64). Hence, the rationale for comparing untrained and trained subjects during exercise at the same percentage of $\dot{V}O_2$ max has greatly diminished. This is particularly true because the resulting large difference in absolute energy expenditure makes interpretation of metabolic responses problematic at best.

In contrast, most (17, 18, 20-22, 45-49, 59, 69, 90, 94, 110, 131, 132), but not all (81, 98), longitudinal investigations have had subjects exercise at the same absolute intensity before and after training. In this way, the absolute demand for energy remains constant, making it is possible to directly compare absolute rates of substrate utilization. Such studies are clearly not intended to describe "real-life" patterns of substrate metabolism in trained and untrained individuals, because people are obviously capable of exercising at higher absolute and probably even higher relative intensities after training. Rather, the purpose of such a study design is to elucidate the mechanisms by which training improves exercise performance. For example, it is largely because training reduces the rate of carbohydrate utilization during exercise at any given absolute power output or $\dot{V}O_2$ that an individual is able to exercise more intensely in the trained state—if not, the greater metabolic demand would result in more rapid depletion of body carbohydrate stores and premature fatigue.

It has been suggested that training may increase the maximal capacity of some metabolic systems (e.g., gluconeogenesis; 32b, 116) and that such adaptations may not be evident during exercise performed at the same absolute submaximal intensity in the trained and untrained states. Although the former may be true, establishing the absolute maximum (i.e., a plateau) of an *in vivo* metabolic response is extremely difficult, especially during exercise. Furthermore, attempting to do so often results in differences in absolute exercise intensity and/or duration between trained and untrained subjects (77, 78, 91), making it difficult to determine mechanisms (i.e., what is cause and what is effect). This is not to say that such studies are not of value, but simply to emphasize that considerable caution must be used in designing and interpreting experiments intended to address such questions.

Effect of Training on Substrate Metabolism During Exercise

This section outlines the effect of training on various aspects of substrate metabolism during exercise.

Respiratory Exchange Ratio and Respiratory Quotient

Christensen and Hansen (12) appear to have been the first to demonstrate that training reduces the respiratory exchange ratio (RER; i.e., the ratio of $\dot{V}CO_2$ [CO_2 release] to $\dot{V}O_2$) during exercise, a finding that has been reproduced in numerous subsequent studies (17, 18, 20, 21, 38, 45, 46, 69, 73, 74, 90, 94, 119, 132). A similar effect of training is observed when the respiratory quotient (RQ) is measured directly across the exercising limbs (59, 73). This decrease in whole-body RER or local RQ with training has usually been interpreted to indicate a shift from carbohydrate toward fat as a source of energy during exercise. As will be discussed, this interpretation is supported by studies that have used other methods to examine substrate metabolism during exercise. However, because current concepts of the metabolic effects of training are still based, in part, on these changes in RER and/or RQ, it is important to consider possible limitations in the use of indirect calorimetry during exercise. This is especially true since it has been argued (45, 46, 119) that the decrease in $\dot{V}CO_2$ with training may be due to factors other than, or in addition to, a change in the mixture of substrates oxidized.

Quantification of substrate oxidation by indirect calorimetry relies on the assumption that $\dot{V}O_2$ and $\dot{V}CO_2$, as measured at the lungs or across a tissue bed, accurately reflect rates of O_2 consumption and CO_2 production by the mitochondria. This is almost certainly true for $\dot{V}O_2$, irrespective of the exercise intensity, because the O_2 stores of the body are quite small. During exercise above the lactate and/or ventilatory threshold, however, $\dot{V}CO_2$ may overestimate the actual rate of CO_2 production, due to release of CO_2 from bicarbonate stores (127). Conversely, during low- or moderate-intensity exercise (i.e., below the lactate or ventilatory threshold), $\dot{V}CO_2$ may significantly underestimate CO_2 production, due to retention of CO_2 in the bicarbonate pools (7, 113). The lower $\dot{V}CO_2$ during exercise after training, therefore, could simply be the result of reduced lactate accumulation and/or lower ventilation during exercise, rather than the result of alterations in substrate oxidation.

To address this issue, tracer-dilution methodology was used to determine the whole-body rate of appearance (R_a) of CO_2 in men performing cycle ergometer exercise at the same absolute power output before and after endurance training (17). Because R_aCO_2 measures CO_2 production, not CO_2 release, this method is not affected by changes in bicarbonate storage that could influence $\dot{V}CO_2$. R_aCO_2 also has the advantage of accounting for the small fraction of CO_2 production that is eliminated through nonrespiratory pathways (e.g., as urea), which cannot be detected by simply measuring $\dot{V}CO_2$. Although R_aCO_2 tends to overestimate net CO_2 production at rest (7, 35, 61), in part due to pyruvate carboxylation and subsequent isotopic exchange in the Kreb's cycle (35, 75), this problem is minimal during exercise, when the rate of CO_2 production is greatly increased and recovery of the tracer in expired breath approaches 100% (17, 50).

Using this technique, $\dot{V}CO_2$ during exercise was found to be highly correlated with R_aCO_2, both before (r = 0.98; P<0.001) and after (r = 0.99;

P<0.001) training (17). This was true even though for each subject the exercise intensity was above the lactate and/or ventilatory threshold before training, but not after training. Moreover, for each individual the training-induced reduction in $\dot{V}CO_2$ during exercise closely paralleled the training-induced reduction in R_aCO_2 (Figure 6.1). Hence, these data do not support the hypothesis that the decrease in $\dot{V}CO_2$, and therefore in RER or RQ, with training is simply the result of less lactate accumulation and/or lower ventilation during exercise (45, 46, 119). Instead, these data provide strong support for the long-held concept that training decreases the actual rate of mitochondrial CO_2 production during exercise. This decrease in CO_2 production is the result of a decrease in carbohydrate oxidation and an increase in fat oxidation, as discussed in detail in the next section.

Utilization of Muscle Glycogen and Plasma Glucose

The work of Christensen and Hansen (12) provided some of the first evidence that training reduces reliance on carbohydrate as a fuel during

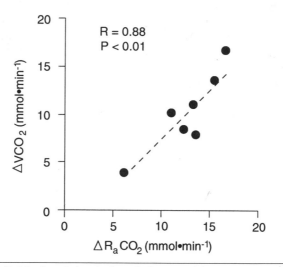

Figure 6.1   Individual training-induced changes (Δ) in the average rate of CO_2 appearance (i.e., R_aCO_2; determined using a primed, continuous infusion of $NaH^{13}CO_3$) and the average rate of CO_2 release (i.e., $\dot{V}CO_2$; determined using standard open circuit spirometry) during 120 min of cycle ergometer exercise at ~60% of pretraining $\dot{V}O_2$ max. ΔR_aCO_2 and $\Delta\dot{V}CO_2$ were closely correlated, supporting the concept that the lower $\dot{V}CO_2$ after training is the result of a slower rate of mitochondrial CO_2 production and is not simply the result of reduced ventilation and/or less metabolic acidosis during exercise. This training-induced reduction in CO_2 production can be due only to decreased reliance on carbohydrate and increased reliance on fat as an energy source during exercise (see text). Data are from Coggan et al. (17).

prolonged exercise. More direct support for this idea, however, awaited the re-introduction of the muscle biopsy procedure in the 1960s. Specifically, using this technique, Hermansen et al. (60) found that the rate of muscle glycogen utilization was similar in trained and untrained subjects exercising at the same relative intensity (i.e., at 75-80% of $\dot{V}O_2$ max). Because the absolute rate of energy expenditure was ~20% higher in the trained men, these data suggested a marked muscle glycogen-sparing effect of endurance training. This was soon confirmed in subsequent longitudinal studies of humans (74) and rats (4) performing exercise at the same absolute intensity before and after endurance training. Notably, when men trained only one leg and then were tested during two-legged exercise, glycogenolysis was slowest in the trained leg (59, 110), providing evidence that adaptations specific to the trained musculature were largely, if not entirely, responsible for this effect. In particular, the slower rate of glycogen utilization during exercise after training appears to be primarily the result of the training-induced increase in muscle mitochondrial content (see Muscle Respiratory Capacity, page 192). This is not to say, however, that this is the only mechanism by which training affects utilization of muscle glycogen or other substrates during exercise. Early on, for example, Baldwin et al. (4) noted that the training-induced reduction in glycogen utilization in the white vastus lateralis muscle of rats seemed out of proportion to the accompanying increase in mitochondrial content and suggested that this may have been due to reduced recruitment of this muscle following training. Support for this hypothesis came from the observation that citrate synthase activity in the white vastus rose by 50% in the first 2 weeks of training, but then subsequently fell as the more oxidative muscles (i.e., red vastus and soleus) progressively adapted to training (3). More recently, reduced recruitment of type II muscle fibers has been postulated to contribute to the glycogen-sparing effect of training in humans (121). The mechanisms by which training affects substrate utilization during exercise are considered in greater detail later in this chapter.

That endurance training reduces the rate of muscle glycogenolysis during exercise is widely recognized. It is less widely recognized that, at least in rats, training also slows the rate of liver glycogenolysis during exercise (4, 40). Indeed, although liver and muscle glycogen contribute roughly equally to the overall carbohydrate requirements of exercise in untrained rats, the slowing of liver glycogen utilization accounts for roughly two-thirds of the total training-induced reduction in carbohydrate utilization (4, 40). The reduced reliance on liver glycogen following training is due, at least in part, to a slower rate of glucose oxidation during both moderate-intensity and high-intensity exercise (10).

In contrast to the aforementioned studies of rats, early longitudinal studies of humans using the a-v balance technique failed to demonstrate any effect of training on leg glucose uptake during exercise (59, 110). As previously discussed (15, 18), however, this may have been due to an inadequate training stimulus and/or the difficulty in detecting a small absolute decrease in the already small a-v glucose difference. In support of the former possibility, Jansson and Kaijser (73) found that leg glucose uptake was substantially lower in highly trained cyclists than in untrained men during 1 hr of moderate-intensity (65-70% $\dot{V}O_2$ max) exercise. Kjær et al. (78), on the other hand, found no difference between trained athletes and untrained men in the tracer-determined rate of disappearance (R_d) of plasma glucose during a brief (12 min), high-intensity (up to 110% $\dot{V}O_2$ max) incremental exercise test. The latter results, however, may simply reflect the difficulty in accurately quantifying glucose R_d under such extreme non-steady state conditions (133).

Because of these uncertainties, a primed, continuous infusion of [U-^{13}C]glucose was used to determine the effects of endurance training on plasma glucose kinetics during 2 hr of exercise at 60% of pretraining $\dot{V}O_2$ max (18). As shown in Table 6.1, training markedly reduced steady state glucose R_a and R_d during the final 30 min of exercise. Glucose clearance (i.e., R_d/plasma glucose concentration) was also reduced, providing evidence that the lower R_d was due to diminished tissue (presumably muscle) glucose demand and was not due simply to decreased glucose availability resulting from the lower R_a. Essentially all the glucose taken up during exercise was eventually oxidized, both before and after training, as ~90% of the infused [U-^{13}C]glucose was recovered as breath $^{13}CO_2$. The estimated rate of oxidation (R_{ox}) of plasma-derived glucose therefore fell in parallel with the decrease in glucose R_d. Indeed, although R_{ox} represented only about one-third of total carbohydrate oxidation during exercise before training, the reduction in R_{ox} due to training accounted for just over one-half of the training-induced reduction in total carbohydrate oxidation.

The results of this study clearly demonstrated that endurance training in humans reduces the production, uptake, and oxidation of plasma glucose

Table 6.1   Effect of 12 weeks of Endurance Training on Plasma Glucose Kinetics During Prolonged Exercise at ~60% of Pretraining $\dot{V}O_2$ max

	Before training	After training
Plasma [glucose] (μmol/mL)	4.69 ± 0.13	4.93 ± 0.14
Glucose R_a and R_d (μmol·min^{-1}·kg^{-1})	44.6 ± 3.5	31.5 ± 4.3*
Glucose clearance (mL·min^{-1}·kg^{-1})	8.13 ± 0.53	5.54 ± 0.64*
% of R_d oxidized	92.2 ± 2.6	85.4 ± 4.5
Glucose R_{ox} (μmol·min^{-1}·kg^{-1})	41.1 ± 3.4	27.7 ± 4.8*

Values are $\bar{x}$ ± S.E. for 7 men. Glucose R_a, R_d, and R_{ox} were determined during the 90-120 min period of exercise using a primed, continuous infusion of [U–^{13}C]glucose. *P<0.001 vs. before training. Data from Coggan et al. (18).

during the later stages of prolonged exercise. Although analysis of the data using non-steady state equations suggested that this was also true early in exercise, this could not be determined with certainty, because the [U-^{13}C]glucose infusion was initiated with the onset of exercise. (This approach was chosen to avoid "pre-labeling" of body substrate stores, e.g., muscle glycogen, with ^{13}C, which can result in the overestimation of R_{ox} during exercise; 21.) The aforementioned study therefore was recently repeated using [6,6-^{2}H]glucose as the tracer (94). This allowed tracer to be infused before as well as during exercise, thereby enabling more accurate determination of the effects of endurance training on glucose R_a and R_d early in exercise, as well as at rest.

Endurance training did not affect glucose kinetics in the basal state. As in the initial study (18), however, training again markedly reduced glucose R_a and R_d during exercise (Figure 6.2). These differences were significant after only 15 min of exercise, and grew progressively larger as exercise continued. The overall rate of carbohydrate oxidation, as determined by indirect calorimetry, was also lower throughout exercise after training. Quantitatively, this decrease was greater than the accompanying reduction in glucose R_d, indicating that muscle glycogen utilization must also have been lower after training (Figure 6.2). In fact, during the first 30 min of exercise most (65-80%) of the carbohydrate-sparing effect of training appeared to have been due to a slowing of muscle glycogen utilization. After this time, however, differences in glucose utilization due to training again apparently accounted for slightly more than one-half of the overall training-induced reduction in carbohydrate oxidation.

The results of these two longitudinal investigations (18, 94) are consistent with recent cross-sectional studies (21, 73, 121) that have also quantified glucose uptake and total carbohydrate oxidation during exercise in untrained and trained subjects. Together, these data indicate that although sparing of muscle glycogen accounts for most of the overall training-induced reduction in carbohydrate utilization during the first ~30 min of moderate-intensity exercise, after this time reduced glucose turnover is quantitatively just as important. Recent data (22) demonstrate that although training significantly reduces the rate of gluconeogenesis, the lower glucose R_a during exercise is mostly due to a slower rate of hepatic glycogenolysis. Reductions in muscle glycogen utilization and liver glycogen utilization therefore contribute roughly equally to the overall carbohydrate-sparing effect of endurance training, at least during moderate-intensity exercise. This is so even though muscle glycogen is the major source of carbohydrate energy, both before and after training (18, 21, 73, 94, 121; Figure 6.2). Thus, in humans as in rats, endurance training results in a preferential sparing of liver glycogen during exercise. As a consequence, trained individuals are better able to maintain plasma glucose concentration during prolonged exercise (18, 21, 73, 94).

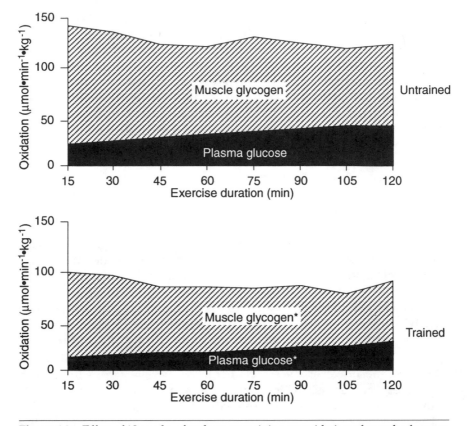

Figure 6.2 Effect of 12 weeks of endurance training on oxidation of muscle glycogen and plasma glucose during 120 min of cycle ergometer exericse at ~60% of pretraining $\dot{V}O_2$ max. Oxidation of plasma glucose was estimated from glucose R_d (determined using [6,6-^{2}H]glucose). Oxidation of muscle glycogen was estimated from the difference between glucose oxidation and total carbohydrate oxidation (determined using indirect calorimetry). During the first 30 min of exercise, the reduction in total carbohydrate oxidation appeared to be mostly (65-80%) due to reduced oxidation of muscle glycogen. After this time, however, the training-induced reduction in glucose oxidation accounted for slightly more than one-half of the overall carbohydrate-sparing effect of endurance training. Data are from Mendenhall et al. (94). Area under curve significantly lower than before training:*P<0.001.

It is now well established that training reduces utilization of both muscle glycogen and plasma glucose during exercise performed at the same absolute intensity before and after training. However, it is somewhat less clear whether this is also true when exercise is performed at the same relative intensity (i.e., at the same percentage of $\dot{V}O_2$ max). As indicated previously, Hermansen et al. (60) found no difference between untrained and trained subjects in the rate of muscle glycogen utilization during exercise at 75-80% $\dot{V}O_2$ max. Likewise, Kjær et al. (78) observed no difference between untrained and trained men in glucose R_d during high-intensity (up to 110% $\dot{V}O_2$ max) exercise. To our knowledge, however, no study of humans has ever found muscle glycogen or plasma glucose utilization to be *greater* in trained subjects than in untrained subjects during exercise at the same percentage of $\dot{V}O_2$ max. This is notable, because under such conditions the absolute demand for energy is significantly higher in trained subjects. Furthermore, other studies have demonstrated that trained individuals exhibit lower RER (73, 81, 98) or RQ (73) values and use less muscle glycogen (73, 121) and plasma glucose (21, 73, 121), even when the exercise is performed at the same relative intensity. In part, this may be due to the somewhat lower relative exercise intensities (i.e., 50-70% $\dot{V}O_2$ max) used in the latter studies. This would result in less stimulation of carbohydrate flux in both trained and untrained subjects, possibly making it easier to detect an effect of training. We have recently found, however, that RER and glucose R_d are lower in trained subjects than in untrained subjects, even during exercise at 80-85% $\dot{V}O_2$ max (19a). Thus, whether or not training reduces the rate of carbohydrate utilization during exercise at a given percentage of $\dot{V}O_2$ max more likely depends on the comparative extent of the cardiovascular and metabolic adaptations to training. That is, if training is accompanied by a large increase in $\dot{V}O_2$ max, then carbohydrate sparing may not be evident during exercise at the same relative exercise intensity, due to the resulting large increase in absolute substrate demand at any given percentage of $\dot{V}O_2$ max. With more intense or more prolonged training, however, the metabolic adaptations to training are apparently sufficient to reduce carbohydrate utilization even when exercise is performed at the same relative (and therefore a higher absolute) intensity (19a, 21, 73, 81, 98, 121).

Lactate Metabolism

The slowing of muscle glycogen and plasma glucose utilization with training is accompanied by a reduced accumulation of lactate in the exercising musculature (45, 47, 59, 73, 74, 110) and, consequently, a slower rate of lactate release into the circulation (59, 73, 110). Historically, such data have been interpreted as indicating that training reduces the actual rate of lactate production during exercise. Strong support for this hypothesis has come from studies demonstrating that training reduces the production of lactate by muscle during *in situ* electrical stimulation (24, 38a).

In contrast to this interpretation, Donovan and Brooks (32) have argued that training does not alter the rate of lactate production during exercise, but instead that the lower blood and muscle lactate concentration after training is the result of enhanced lactate clearance. This hypothesis is based primarily on isotopic tracer studies of lactate kinetics during exercise (32, 87a). Interpretation of these data is difficult, however, because labeled lactate equilibrates rapidly (but not instantaneously) with pyruvate (134), and therefore largely reflects pyruvate metabolism. The precise relationship between lactate and pyruvate kinetics is uncertain, though, because the extent of this equilibration probably depends in part on the circulation time between the site of tracer infusion and the site of sampling (133). Furthermore, even if this equilibration were complete, accurate determination of whole-body pyruvate/lactate R_a would require sampling from the compartment in which lactate/pyruvate production occurs (i.e., muscle) (133), which to date has not been done. Thus, the conclusion that training does not reduce lactate production during exercise (32) is probably incorrect.

It remains possible, however, that an enhanced rate of lactate clearance contributes to the lower blood and/or muscle lactate concentrations during exercise after training. Indeed, resting, trained rats demonstrated markedly lower blood and tissue lactate levels when infused with unlabeled lactate at high rates (32a, 32b). However, this training-induced enhancement of lactate clearance appears to be due, in part, to greater Cori cycle activity (32a-c), whereas, as previously mentioned, the rate of gluconeogenesis is lower in trained humans during exercise (22). Hence, whether training affects lactate clearance in exercising humans remains uncertain.

Utilization of Plasma Free Fatty Acids and Intramuscular Triglycerides

The training-induced reduction in carbohydrate oxidation during exercise is compensated for by an increase in fat oxidation. However, the source of the additional fatty acids is still uncertain.

Tracer infusion studies conducted in the 1960s and early 1970s using ^{14}C-labeled palmitate or oleate emphasized the importance of plasma free fatty acids (FFA) as an energy source during low- to moderate-intensity exercise (56, 57, 70, 71). These observations, in conjunction with the known training-induced increase in whole-body fat oxidation, led to the assumption that endurance training enhances reliance on plasma-borne FFA during exercise (62, 120). This notion was apparently reinforced by the observation that athletes (wrestlers) exercising on a treadmill at a $\dot{V}O_2$ of ~1.4 L/min (56) had higher R_a and R_d of plasma FFA than did nonathletes exercising on a cycle ergometer at a $\dot{V}O_2$ of ~1 L/min (57). Likewise, mongrel dogs classified as "trained," based on their blood lactate response to exercise, were observed to have a higher rate of plasma FFA turnover during exercise than did "untrained" dogs (71).

More controlled studies, however, have generally failed to support the notion that training increases the rate of plasma FFA utilization during exercise. For example, using a one-legged training model, Henriksson (59) observed no significant difference in net FFA uptake between the trained and untrained legs during 50 min of moderate-intensity, two-legged cycle ergometry. Similarly, Jansson and Kaijser (73) found no effect of training on leg extraction of plasma FFA (either gross or net) during 1 hr of cycling at 65% $\dot{V}O_2$ max. The plasma concentration and whole-body R_a, R_d, and clearance of FFA also did not differ between the trained and untrained subjects of this study. In addition, Martin et al. (90) recently demonstrated that training does not affect whole-body clearance of plasma FFA during prolonged (90-120 min) cycling at 60-65% of pretraining $\dot{V}O_2$ max. In this longitudinal investigation, the concentration, R_a, R_d, and R_{ox} of FFA were ~30% *lower* during exercise after training.

In contrast to the previously mentioned studies, Turcotte et al. (121) recently reported that thigh uptake of plasma FFA was significantly higher in trained men than in untrained men during the 3rd hr of single-leg knee-extension exercise. Whereas plasma FFA uptake rose linearly with increasing FFA concentration in the trained men, FFA uptake leveled off in the untrained men above a plasma concentration of ~700-800 µM. Turcotte et al. (121) interpreted these data as suggesting that FFA uptake by muscle is a carrier-mediated, saturable process and that training increases the maximal capacity for FFA transport into skeletal muscle, possibly by increasing the concentration of fatty acid binding proteins.

The results of Turcotte et al. (121) are not necessarily in conflict with the studies discussed earlier, but may simply be due to differences in exercise mode. In particular, muscle blood flow is much higher during knee-extension exercise than during cycle ergometry (1), and the corresponding increase in FFA delivery may have made it easier to demonstrate a plateau in FFA extraction by untrained subjects late in exercise. Furthermore, plasma FFA concentrations were similar in the untrained and trained men during knee-extension exercise, probably because lipolytic hormone concentrations were also similar. During exercise with a large muscle mass, however, the hormonal response to exercise is attenuated by training (see Hormonal Adaptations to Training, page 197), resulting in a lower R_a of FFA (90) and therefore lower plasma FFA concentrations (18, 20, 81, 90, 132). Because training does not affect FFA clearance (59, 73, 90), at least under these conditions, the rate of plasma FFA utilization is consequently also lower in trained subjects compared with untrained subjects during whole-body exercise performed at the same absolute intensity (90). Even when trained and untrained subjects exercise at the same percentage of $\dot{V}O_2$ max, plasma FFA use does not appear to be higher in the trained state (73), even though total energy expenditure and total fat oxidation are substantially greater.

The additional fat oxidized during whole-body exercise in trained subjects therefore appears to be derived primarily from some source other than adipose tissue triglycerides, possibly from intramuscular triglycerides. The triglyceride content of human muscle is much greater than that of some other species, such as the rat, and can serve as a significant source of energy during exercise (11, 13, 37, 41, 69). Hence, it seems possible that enhanced intramuscular lipolysis may account for the greater rate of fat oxidation after training. In keeping with this hypothesis, Hurley et al. (69) found that endurance training resulted in a much greater utilization of intramuscular triglycerides during prolonged exercise (Figure 6.3). This increase in intramuscular lipolysis could have supplied all the additional fatty acids oxidized during exercise after training, provided that the equivalent of ~8 kg of muscle was recruited during the exercise.

Endurance training has also been reported to increase the rate of hydrolysis of triglycerides circulating in very low-density lipoproteins (VLDL) (76). This effect appears to be mediated by an increase in muscle lipoprotein lipase activity accompanying the greater capillary endothelial surface area after training (2, 9, 76). Nevertheless, VLDL-triglycerides remain a relatively minor source of energy during exercise even after training, accounting for <10% of total energy expenditure (76). The increase in VLDL-triglyceride degradation with training is therefore probably more important for its potential long-term influence on blood lipid profiles (76) than in accounting for the higher rate of fatty acid oxidation during exercise after training.

Thus, the available evidence suggests that additional fatty acids oxidized during exercise in the trained state are derived primarily from the intramuscular triglyceride stores and not from adipose tissue triglycerides

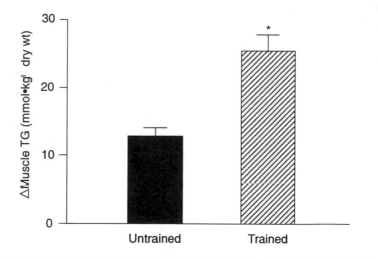

Figure 6.3   Effect of 12 weeks of endurance training on muscle triglyceride utilization (Δ muscle TG) during 120 min of cycle ergometer exericse at ~60% of pretraining $\dot{V}O_2$ max. The decrease in muscle triglyceride concentration during exercise was greater after training, suggesting that the additional fatty acids oxidized in the trained state are supplied by way of intramuscular lipolysis. Data are from Hurley et al. (69). Significantly higher than before training: *$P<0.001$.

(by way of plasma FFA) or from circulating triglycerides. Only one study, however, has directly tested this hypothesis, and it would be desirable for these results to be confirmed. Furthermore, almost all the aforementioned studies employed moderate-intensity, moderate-duration cycle ergometer exercise, and it is at least theoretically possible that the relative importance of adipose tissue and intramuscular triglycerides may differ between untrained and trained subjects, depending on the mode, intensity, or duration of exercise. This is especially true because the rate of utilization of plasma FFA is, in part, passively determined by plasma FFA concentration.

Utilization of Amino Acids

To date, no study of humans has directly examined the effects of endurance training on amino acid metabolism during exercise (although some studies have examined the effects of training on amino acid metabolism at rest [e.g., 82]). In rats, however, Henderson et al. (58) observed that training increased whole-body leucine turnover and oxidation during exercise at a given $\dot{V}O_2$. This could be due to a training-induced increase in muscle branched-chain ketoacid dehydrogenase activity (BCKADH, the rate-limiting enzyme for branched-chain amino acid catabolism) (31, 66). Hood and Terjung (66), however, found that training reduced the relative contribution of leucine oxidation to $\dot{V}O_2$ in electrically stimulated, perfused rat hindquarters, and they speculated that BCKADH may be activated less in trained muscle during exercise due to a smaller increase in free ADP concentration (see Muscle Respiratory Capacity, page 192). Hood and Terjung (66) therefore suggested that the training-induced increase in whole-body leucine oxidation observed previously (58) must have occurred in nonmuscle tissue (e.g., liver). This interpretation is consistent with the fact that, in rats, BCKADH activity is much greater in liver than in muscle (122).

It is difficult to extrapolate from these limited data to predict the effect of training on amino acid metabolism during exercise in humans. The possibility of species differences has been previously emphasized. This is particularly true for leucine metabolism, because the relative distribution of BCKADH activity in humans is exactly the opposite of that in rats (53). Furthermore, the metabolism of a single amino acid, such as leucine, is not representative of all amino acids, but is unique for that particular amino acid (135). Hence, considerable additional research will be required before this question can be adequately addressed.

Mechanisms by Which Training Affects Exercise Metabolism

Although the effects of endurance training on substrate metabolism have been well described, the underlying mechanisms responsible for these adaptations have been only partially identified. Most attention has focused on the training-induced increase in muscle respiratory capacity and hormonal adaptations to training.

Muscle Respiratory Capacity

For many years, the metabolic adaptations to endurance training were believed to be due simply to improvements in central cardiac function and, therefore, in muscle O_2 delivery and/or uptake (e.g. 71). However, in a landmark study published in 1967, Holloszy (63) reported that a strenuous program of endurance running doubled the capacity of the mitochondrial fraction of rat gastrocnemius muscle to oxidize pyruvate. Mitochondria from trained muscle were well coupled, indicating that this twofold increase in respiratory capacity was associated with a twofold increase in the capacity to generate ATP. Similar increases were observed in the cytochrome c content and succinate dehydrogenase, NADH dehydrogenase, cytochrome c reductase, cytochrome oxidase, and succinate oxidase activities of whole-muscle homogenates, demonstrating that the training-induced increase in pyruvate oxidation was not due simply to a more efficient isolation of mitochondria from trained muscle. Accompanying the increase in muscle respiratory capacity was a more than sixfold increase in exercise endurance.

These initial findings of a training-induced increase in muscle respiratory capacity were quickly confirmed in additional studies of rats (44) and other species (6), including humans (43, 99). Subsequent investigations demonstrated that training also increases the capacity of skeletal muscle to oxidize long-chain fatty acids (97) and ketone bodies (130), in addition to pyruvate (63). These adaptations are primarily the result of increases in the size and number of mitochondria (44, 67, 99). However, training-induced alterations in mitochondrial composition may also play a role. Citrate synthase activity, for example, increases by up to 100% with training when expressed per gram of muscle (5, 65), even though mitochondrial protein content increases by only ~60% (26, 63). Conversely, the activities of the mitochondrial isoforms of adenylate kinase, creatine kinase, and α-glycerophosphate dehydrogenase do not change with training when expressed relative to muscle wet weight, and therefore are reduced when expressed relative to total mitochondrial protein (100).

It is now widely recognized that the increase in muscle respiratory capacity is one of the primary mechanisms by which endurance training affects substrate utilization during exercise. However, because a greater muscle mitochondrial content should enhance the ability to oxidize acetyl CoA irrespective of the source (i.e., glycolysis versus β-oxidation), the question arises why this should result in the preferential utilization of lipid during exercise. Despite recent reports (126), it seems unlikely that this is due to a selective increase in the capacity of skeletal muscle mitochondria for fatty acid oxidation (26, 63, 97). Instead, the alterations in substrate utilization with training appear to be due largely to a lesser disturbance to energetic homeostasis during exercise. This theory has been eloquently developed elsewhere (63, 64), and this discussion will not be repeated in detail here. Briefly, however, with a greater mitochondrial volume after training, smaller decreases in ATP and phosphocreatine (PCr) and smaller increases in ADP and inorganic phosphate (P_i) are required during exercise to balance the rate of ATP synthesis with the rate of ATP hydrolysis (24, 33). The smaller increase in ADP, in turn, results in less of an increase in AMP formation by adenylate kinase and, therefore, also less of an increase in IMP and NH_4^+ formation by AMP deaminase (24, 33). These metabolic alterations, especially the smaller increases in P_i (106) and AMP (105), almost undoubtedly play a major role in accounting for the slower rate of glycogenolysis in muscle that has adapted to an endurance training program.

The slower rate of plasma glucose utilization during exercise after training also appears to be a function of the increase in muscle respiratory capacity (21). As previously discussed (15, 18, 21, 121), however, the precise mechanisms accounting for this effect are much less clear. Because training increases muscle hexokinase activity (20, 99) and attenuates the rise in muscle glucose-6-phosphate (G-6-P) concentration during exercise, it seems probable that the decrease in glucose use is the result of a reduction in glucose transport, not in glucose phosphorylation. However, exactly how an increase in muscle mitochondrial content with training might lead to less activation of the glucose transport process during exercise is not known.

Accompanying the decrease in muscle glycogen and plasma glucose utilization with training is, of course, an increased reliance on lipid as an energy source. Indeed, one long-standing hypothesis (62, 64) is that the greater utilization of fat during exercise after training helps to inhibit carbohydrate utilization through operation of the glucose-fatty acid cycle (i.e., through citrate-mediated inhibition of phosphofructokinase—PFK) (103, 104). Despite its long-standing nature, however, only a few attempts have been made to directly test this hypothesis (20, 24, 73). In support of this possibility, Jansson and Kaijser (73) observed that during moderate-intensity exercise, fat oxidation and muscle citrate concentration were higher and glycogen utilization and glucose uptake by muscle were lower in trained cyclists compared with untrained men. In contrast, Constable et al. (24) found that although training markedly attenuated the rate of glycogenolysis during brief (8-10 min), intense electrical stimulation of perfused rat hindlimbs, this did not appear to be due to inhibition of PFK, because G-6-P concentrations were actually lower, not higher, in the muscles of the trained rats. As previously discussed (20), however, these studies may not have been optimally designed to test the aforementioned hypothesis. For example, the higher muscle citrate concentration in the trained cyclists studied by Jansson and Kaijser (73) may have been due simply to their greater percentage of type I muscle fibers, and not to their higher rate of β-oxidation. Likewise, in the study of Constable et al. (24), substrate utilization was dominated by a large initial burst of glycogenolysis, which may have obscured any effect of training on *in vivo* PFK activity.

To avoid these interpretive difficulties, muscle citrate and G-6-P concentrations were measured in the same men performing prolonged submaximal exercise before and after endurance training (20). In support of the aforementioned hypothesis, muscle citrate concentration tended to be higher after training, both at rest and especially during exercise (Figure 6.4, *top*). This difference, however, only approached statistical significance ($P = 0.16$), even though the muscle biopsy samples were obtained at the end of a 2-hr exercise bout, which should have maximized muscle citrate concentration (73, 109). Furthermore, muscle G-6-P concentration was significantly *lower* during exercise after training (Figure 6.4, *middle*), and this training-induced reduction in G-6-P concentration closely paralleled the decrease in muscle glycogen degradation (Figure 6.4, *bottom*). These results provide evidence that during prolonged, moderate-intensity exercise, as during brief, *in situ* electrical stimulation (24), the training-induced reduction in carbohydrate utilization is due to a decrease in the rate of G-6-P production via glycogenolysis and/or glucose transport and phosphorylation, and is not due to inhibition of PFK by citrate or other metabolites (e.g., ATP). Therefore, operation of the classical glucose-fatty acid cycle does not appear to contribute to the training-induced inhibition of carbohydrate utilization during exercise. These data do not, however, rule out the possibility that the increase in β-oxidation with training reduces carbohydrate utilization during exercise through some mechanism other than inhibition of PFK. For example, both *in vitro* (51) and *in vivo* (52) experiments suggest that fatty acids may inhibit glucose transport in skeletal muscle. It is not clear, though, whether this is due to an enhanced rate of β-oxidation or represents a direct effect on the sarcolemma. Only the former would be relevant to the effects of training, because, as indicated previously, plasma FFA levels are usually lower during exercise in the trained state.

A possible alternative is that the increase in fatty acid oxidation with training is the result, not the cause, of the decrease in carbohydrate oxidation. That is, the increase in fat oxidation may be the result of less competition between acetyl CoA derived from carbohydrate and acetyl CoA derived from fat for entry into the tricarboxylic acid cycle. Of considerable interest in this context are recent studies suggesting that malonyl CoA, the first intermediate in fatty acid synthesis and a potent inhibitor of carnitine acyltransferase I (CAT I), may play an important role in regulating fatty acid oxidation in skeletal muscle during exercise (34, 128, 129). Muscle malonyl CoA concentrations decrease during prolonged exercise,

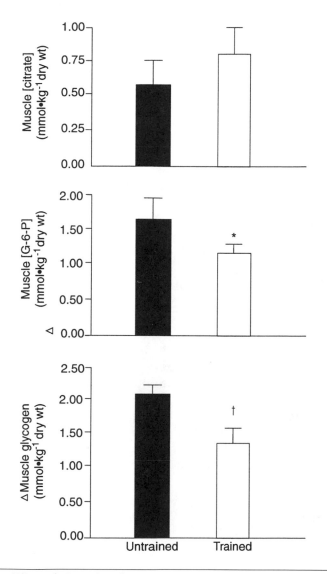

Figure 6.4   Effect of 12 weeks of endurance training on muscle citrate (*top panel*) and glucose-6-phosphate (G-6-P; *middle panel*) concentrations at the end of 120 min of cycle ergometer exericse at ~60% pretraining $\dot{V}O_2$ max. Also shown is net muscle glycogen utilization during the exercise bout (Δ muscle glycogen; *bottom panel*). Muscle citrate concentration during exericse was slightly, but not significantly (P=0.16), higher after training. Muscle G-6-P concentration, however, was lower in the trained state, and this training-induced reduction in G-6-P closely paralleled the reduction in muscle glycogen utilization. These data suggest that the slowing of carbohydrate utilization by training is not due to operation of the classical glucose-fatty acid cycle (i.e., citrate-mediated inhibition of phosphofructokinase and consequent accumulation of G-6-P), but must occur further up the glycolytic/glycogenolytic pathway. Data are from Coggan et al. (20). Significantly lower than before training: *P<0.05, †P<0.001.

generally paralleling carbohydrate availability, or, more specifically, the rate of carbohydrate flux (34, 129). It has been postulated that this decrease in malonyl CoA during exercise may be important in allowing entry of more long-chain fatty acids into the mitochondria for β-oxidation. It is therefore tempting to speculate that the slower rate of carbohydrate utilization after training may result in a greater fall in muscle malonyl CoA concentration during exercise, thereby relieving inhibition of CAT I and enhancing reliance on fatty acids as an energy source. Additional experiments will obviously be required to test this intriguing hypothesis. Regardless of the specific mechanism, however, additional attention should be directed toward the possibility that the increased utilization of fatty acids after training is causally related to the decrease in carbohydrate utilization.

The precise biochemical mechanisms by which training affects substrate metabolism during exercise have been only partially elucidated. Nevertheless, highly significant correlations have been demonstrated between muscle respiratory capacity and various indices of substrate use during exercise (e.g., RER) (98), blood lactate accumulation (72), muscle and liver glycogen depletion (40), P_i/PCr levels (16), and glucose R_d and R_{ox} (21) (Figure 6.5). Furthermore, the time course of training-induced alterations in substrate utilization during exercise (94) closely parallels the time course of the increase in mitochondrial enzyme levels (3; R.J. Spina and J.O. Holloszy, unpublished observations). A similar relationship is observed in the "off-response" (i.e., with detraining) (25). Therefore, it is clear that the increase in muscle respiratory capacity, with its concomitant influence on cellular energetics, is one of the most important means by which training alters substrate metabolism during exercise. Green et al., however, have been unable to detect a significant increase in muscle mitochondrial marker enzyme activities after either 5-7 days (47) or 10-12 days (45) of training, even though muscle glycogen utilization and (after 10-12 days of training) RER during exercise were reduced. Therefore, Green et al. (45, 47, 48) have suggested that, at least with short-term training, other mechanisms must be responsible for training-induced changes in substrate metabolism during exercise. However, after 10-12 days of training, succinate dehydrogenase activity had increased by 14% (P = 0.096), whereas citrate synthase activity had increased 23% (P = 0.111) (45). Although no such trend in maximal *in vitro* mitochondrial enzyme activities was evident after just 5-7 days of training (47), this shorter training program did diminish the rise in intramuscular free ADP concentration during exercise, providing evidence of a functional training-induced increase in *in vivo* mitochondrial respiratory capacity (33). Therefore, it seems likely that, as with long-term training, the metabolic effects of short-term training are due largely to an increase in muscle mitochondrial respiratory capacity.

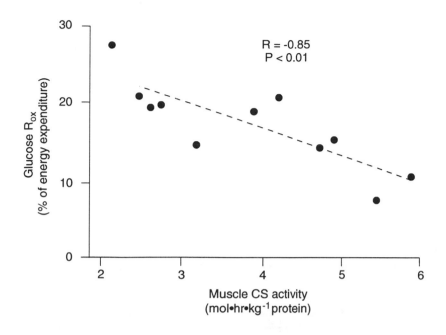

Figure 6.5   Relationship between citrate synthase (CS) activity in the vastus later-alis muscle and the rate of glucose oxidation (glucose R_{ox}; expressed as a percentage of total energy expenditure) during 90 min of exercise at 55% $\dot{V}O_2$ max. Glucose R_{ox} was highly and inversely correlated with muscle CS activity, supporting the hypothesis that muscle respiratory capacity plays an important role in determining the metabolic response to submaximal exercise. Adapted with permission from Coggan et al. (1992).

Hormonal Adaptations to Training

Although important, the augmentation of muscle respiratory capacity is not the only mechanism by which training affects substrate metabolism during exercise. Neuroendocrine responses play a major role in regulating substrate mobilization and utilization during exercise, and these responses are modified by endurance training. For example, plasma norepinephrine and epinephrine concentrations increase less during exercise performed at the same absolute intensity in the trained state, compared with the untrained state (8, 46, 48, 54, 55, 81, 94, 131, 132). Glucagon (8, 18, 49, 81, 94, 132), growth hormone (8, 54, 81), cortisol (87), and adrenocorticotropic hormone (87) levels also increase less during exercise in trained subjects. Conversely, insulin concentration, although lower at rest, decreases less during exercise and therefore tends to be higher in trained individuals (8, 18, 49, 54, 55, 94, 132).

The magnitude of the neuroendocrine response to dynamic exercise is usually viewed as being a function of the percentage of $\dot{V}O_2$ max elicited

(29, 87). Accordingly, it might be expected that training would attenuate changes in norepinephrine, etc., when exercise is performed at the same absolute $\dot{V}O_2$ before and after training. However, both cross-sectional (8) and longitudinal studies (49, 54, 55, 81, 131, 132) have demonstrated that training often minimizes hormonal responses even when exercise is performed at the same relative intensity in the untrained and trained states. Furthermore, the effects of training are evident only when the mode of exercise is the same as that used in training (92, 102), even though $\dot{V}O_2$ max may be identical under different conditions (92). Hence, these adaptations clearly represent a unique response to training and are not simply a function of the accompanying increase in $\dot{V}O_2$ max.

That training alters the plasma concentration of many hormones during exercise is well established. For the most part, however, the *quantitative* importance of these adaptations remains to be determined. Of necessity, the discussion that follows centers on the putative role played by alterations in four major hormones (i.e., norepinephrine, epinephrine, insulin, and glucagon).

Norepinephrine and Epinephrine. As mentioned, training significantly attenuates the sympathoadrenal response to acute exercise (8, 46, 48, 54, 55, 81, 94, 131, 132). This adaptation occurs very rapidly, with lower catecholamine levels evident after as little as 3 days of training (48). Indeed, essentially all the training-induced reductions in norepinephrine and epinephrine appear to occur in the first few weeks of training (94, 131, 132). In highly trained athletes, however, plasma norepinephrine and epinephrine concentrations during submaximal exercise were not altered by 3 weeks of detraining, although $\dot{V}O_2$ max fell significantly (25). These observations further emphasize the independence of training-induced changes in the hormonal response to exercise from changes in $\dot{V}O_2$ max and suggest that, at least for the catecholamines, the hormonal adaptations to training and detraining do not follow the same time course.

The metabolic significance of this reduced catecholamine response has not been clearly established. During intense exercise, however, circulating epinephrine concentrations often exceed levels that have been shown to affect carbohydrate and lipid metabolism in *resting* subjects (14, 42). Therefore, reduced epinephrine levels after training may contribute to many of the previously described alterations in substrate metabolism during exercise. For example, the slower rate of muscle glycogenolysis during exercise after training may be due, in part, to lower epinephrine concentrations. Similarly, lower epinephrine levels, in conjunction with less of a decline in insulin secretion, seem likely to contribute to the reduced rates of hepatic glucose production (18, 20, 22, 94) and adipose tissue lipolysis (90) during exercise after training. On the other hand, there is evidence that training may increase catecholamine action in a number of different tissues (84, 89, 114, 118). This makes it more difficult to predict the metabolic importance of lower epinephrine concentrations during exercise after training. For example, increased sensitivity and/or responsiveness of skeletal muscle to epinephrine could *theoretically* explain why intramuscular lipolysis during exercise (which appears to be due, at least in part, to β_2-receptor stimulation; 13) is greater in the trained state, even though epinephrine levels are markedly reduced. Unlike in rats (39, 127), however, endurance training in humans does not increase skeletal muscle β-adrenergic receptor density (88). Although the latter findings do not preclude changes in β-receptor distribution (i.e., externalization), agonist affinity, etc., due to training, the fact that muscle glycogenolysis (which is also activated by β_2-receptor stimulation) is lower during exercise in the trained state would also argue against a generalized training-induced increase in muscle epinephrine action.

Unlike epinephrine, which is derived almost exclusively from the adrenal medulla, almost all of the norepinephrine entering the circulation is due to "spillover" from sympathetic nerves (36, 111). Because release and uptake of norepinephrine occur simultaneously but at different rates in various tissues, and because activation of the various limbs of the sympathetic nervous system may occur independently of one another, assessment of overall sympathetic "tone" is quite difficult (36). Plasma norepinephrine concentrations, however, correlate reasonably well with more direct measures of sympathetic nervous system activity (123). The lower plasma norepinephrine levels during exercise after training have therefore been taken to reflect a generalized reduction in sympathetic nervous system outflow. This could not directly account for alterations in muscle glycogen or muscle triglyceride metabolism with training, because the adrenergic receptors of human muscle are exclusively of the β_2-subtype (86), which have little affinity for norepinephrine. However, reduced local norepinephrine release could contribute to the slower rates of FFA and glucose mobilization from adipose and liver tissue, respectively. Furthermore, a reduction in sympathetic outflow with training may also affect substrate metabolism indirectly, by altering the concentrations of other hormones (e.g., epinephrine and insulin). Direct measurements of norepinephrine spillover from various tissue beds during exercise before and after training will be required to confirm these hypotheses.

In contrast to the idea that activation of the sympathetic nervous system during exercise is attenuated by training, Kjær et al. (77, 78, 80) have reported that plasma epinephrine levels are higher in highly trained endurance athletes than in untrained men during intense (78) or prolonged (77) exercise. Increased epinephrine secretion was also observed in response to a number of non-exercise stimuli, such as insulin-induced hypoglycemia, glucagon infusion, or hypercapnia (79). Furthermore, plasma epinephrine levels during daily life (including training sessions) were found to be, on average, approximately twice as high in athletes than in non-athletes (27). It has therefore been proposed that prolonged, intense training leads to adrenal medullary hypertrophy, which results in increased epinephrine secretion in response to stress.

The hypothesis that training increases the secretion of epinephrine or other hormones is intriguing. Other studies, however, have not found epinephrine levels to be higher in trained subjects than in untrained subjects during maximal or near-maximal exercise (8, 19a, 29, 85). Furthermore, in well-trained athletes the epinephrine response to insulin-induced hypoglycemia was unaffected by 5 weeks of detraining, and therefore remained higher than that of untrained subjects (80). It is possible that 5 weeks was simply insufficient to reverse the effects of many years of training, because the sympathoadrenal adaptations to training appear to be lost at a slower rate with detraining. Alternatively, however, these cross-sectional observations (77-79) may simply reflect a selection phenomenon, in that individuals who show greater adrenal medullary responsiveness may be more likely to succeed, and therefore to continue to participate, in sports. This interpretation is consistent with studies of physiological "toughness," which suggest that humans or animals that display greater sympathoadrenal reactivity to an acute stress (such as cold exposure) are better able to cope with that stress (cf. 30). Longitudinal data are therefore required to determine whether endurance training of humans does in fact increase epinephrine secretory capacity, and if so, whether this is manifest during exercise. Unfortunately, such data are not yet available. It is interesting, however, that in rats, swim training increases the mass of the adrenal medulla but actually *reduces* the epinephrine response to insulin-induced hypoglycemia (115).

Insulin and Glucagon.   Although basal insulin concentrations are often lower in trained subjects, insulin levels typically decrease less during exercise in the trained state (8, 18, 49, 54, 55, 94, 132). As a result, circulating insulin concentrations tend to be higher during exercise in trained individuals, especially during the later stages of exercise. This appears to be due to less suppression of insulin secretion by the sympathetic nervous system, because C-peptide levels also decrease less during exercise after training (94).

As with the catecholamines, the quantitative significance of this training-induced difference in insulin concentration during exercise has yet to be firmly established. Insulin, though, is a potent inhibitor of both hepatic glucose production and adipose tissue lipolysis. Thus, relatively higher insulin levels after training seem likely to contribute to the slower rates of glucose and FFA release during exercise. However, significant differences in insulin (and C-peptide) concentration are usually evident only during later stages of exercise, whereas the R_a of glucose (94) and FFA (90) are lower throughout exercise. Furthermore, glucose production during exercise was lower after 12 weeks of training than after 10 days of training (94), even though insulin concentrations were similar. Thus, greater suppression of glucose production (95, 107) and lipolysis (83, 117) by insulin (i.e., enhanced insulin action) and/or differences in the concentrations of other hormones (e.g., epinephrine) probably also contribute to the training-induced alterations in glucose and FFA release during exercise.

Training also increases muscle insulin action (28, 95, 96), which, when coupled with a somewhat smaller decrease in insulin secretion during exercise, might be expected to result in a greater rate of insulin-stimulated glucose transport into muscle during exercise. Therefore, it is somewhat paradoxical that training reduces uptake of plasma glucose during exercise. Insulin concentrations are quite low during exercise, however, even after training, and are thus unlikely to play a significant role in directly stimulating glucose uptake. Indeed, it has been estimated (124) that in humans ~85% of the increase in glucose utilization during exercise is due to non-insulin-mediated mechanisms. Thus, the relatively higher insulin concentration during exercise after training is probably more important for its inhibitory effects on glucose production and adipose tissue lipolysis than for its potential influence on glucose utilization.

Endurance training also modifies (reduces) secretion of glucagon during exercise (8, 18, 49, 81, 94, 132). As with insulin, however, this effect is often evident only during the later stages of prolonged exercise and, therefore, appears to play only a secondary role in the training-induced reduction in glucose output during exercise.

Summary

Considerable progress has been made in describing the effects of training on substrate metabolism during exercise and in determining the mechanisms by which these effects are mediated. It is now quite clear that endurance-trained humans rely less on muscle glycogen and plasma glucose and more on fatty acids for energy during exercise at any given absolute intensity, and that this carbohydrate-sparing effect of training plays a major role in the training-induced improvement in exercise performance. However, the specific tissue source of the additional fatty acids remains uncertain, and the effects of endurance training on amino acid metabolism during exercise are unknown. Likewise, although it is evident that the metabolic adaptations to training are largely mediated by an increase in muscle respiratory capacity, the specific biochemical mechanisms involved have been only partially elucidated. The importance of changes in hormone concentrations and/or action during exercise and of other training-induced adaptations in muscle (e.g., increased glucose transporter number; 68, 101) also remain to be determined. Finally, the possibility that training increases the maximal amplitude of various physiological responses during prolonged or intense exercise requires further evaluation. Thus, although much is known, much also remains to be learned about the effects of endurance training on substrate metabolism during exercise.

References

1. Andersen, P.; Saltin, B. Maximal perfusion of skeletal muscle in man. J. Physiol. 366:233-249; 1985.

2. Bagby, G.J.; Johnson, J.L.; Bennett, B.W.; Shepherd, R.E. Muscle lipoprotein lipase activity in voluntarily exercising rats. J. Appl. Physiol. 60:1623-1627; 1986.

3. Baldwin, K.M.; Cooke, D.A.; Cheadle, W.G. Time course adaptations in cardiac and skeletal muscle to different training programs. J. Appl. Physiol. 42:267-272; 1977.

4. Baldwin, K.M.; Fitts, R.H.; Booth, F.W.; Winder, W.W.; Holloszy, J.O. Depletion of muscle and liver glycogen during exercise. Protective effect of training. Pflügers Arch. 354:203-212; 1975.

5. Baldwin, K.M.; Klinkerfuss, G.H.; Terjung, R.L.; Molé, P.A.; Holloszy, J.O. Respiratory capacity of white, red and intermediate muscle: adaptive response to exercise. Am. J. Physiol. 222:373-378; 1972.

6. Barnard, R.J.; Edgerton, V.R.; Peter, J.B. Effect of exercise on skeletal muscle. I. Biochemical and histochemical properties. J. Appl. Physiol. 28:762-766; 1970.

7. Barstow, T.J.; Cooper, D.M.; Sobel, E.M.; Landaw, E.M.; Epstein, S. Influence of increased metabolic rate on [^{13}C]bicarbonate washout kinetics. Am. J. Physiol. 259 (Regulatory Integrative Comp. Physiol. 28):R163-R171; 1990.

8. Bloom, S.R.; Johnson, R.H.; Park, D.M.; Rennie, M.J.; Sulaiman, W.R. Differences in the metabolic and hormonal responses to exercise between racing cyclists and untrained individuals. J. Physiol. 258:1-18; 1976.

9. Borensztajn, J.; Rone, M.S.; Babirak, S.P.; McGarr, J.A.; Oscai, L.B. Effect of exercise on lipoprotein lipase activity in rat heart and skeletal muscle. Am. J. Physiol. 229:394-397; 1975.

10. Brooks, G.A.; Donovan, C.M. Effect of endurance training on glucose kinetics during exercise. Am. J. Physiol. 244 (Endocrinol. Metab. 7):E505-E512; 1983.

11. Carlson, L.A.; Ekclund, L.G.; Fröberg, S.O. Concentration of triglycerides, phospholipids and glycogen in skeletal muscle and of free fatty acids and β-hydroxybutyric acid in blood in man in response to exercise. Eur. J. Clin. Invest. 1:248-254; 1971.

12. Christensen, E.H.; Hansen, O. Respiratorscher Quotient und O_2-Aufnahme. Skand. Arch Physiol. 81:180-189; 1939.

13. Cleroux, J.; Van Nguyen, P.; Taylor, A.W.; Leenen, F.H.H. Effects of β_1- vs. $\beta_1+\beta_2$- blockade on exercise endurance and muscle metabolism in humans. J. Appl. Physiol. 66:548-554; 1989.

14. Clutter, W.E.; Bier, D.M.; Shah, S.D.; Cryer, P.E. Epinephrine plasma metabolic clearance rates and physiologic thresholds for metabolic and hemodynamic actions in man. J. Clin. Invest. 66:94-101; 1980.

15. Coggan, A.R. Plasma glucose metabolism during exercise in humans. Sports Med. 11:102-124; 1991.

16. Coggan, A.R.; Abduljalil, A.M.; Swanson, S.C.; Earle, M.S.; Farris, J.W.; Mendenhall, L.A.; Robitaille, P.-M. Muscle metabolism during exercise in young and older untrained and endurance-trained men. J. Appl. Physiol. 75:2125-2133; 1993.

17. Coggan, A.R.; Habash, D.L.; Mendenhall, L.A.; Swanson, S.C.; Kien, C.L. Isotopic estimation of CO_2 production during exercise before and after endurance training. J. Appl. Physiol. 75:70-75; 1993.

18. Coggan, A.R.; Kohrt, W.M.; Spina, R.J.; Bier, D.M.; Holloszy, J.O. Endurance training decreases plasma glucose turnover and oxidation during moderate intensity exercise in men. J. Appl. Physiol. 68:990-996; 1990.

19. Coggan, A.R.; Mendenhall, L.A. Effect of diet on substrate metabolism during exercise. In: Lamb, D.R.; Gisolfi, C.V., eds. Perspectives in exercise science and sports medicine, vol. 5: energy metabolism in exercise and sport. Dubuque, IA: Brown and Benchmark; 1992: 435-464.

19a. Coggan, A.R.; Raguso, C.A.; Williams, B.D.; Sidossis, L.S.; Gastaldelli, A. Glucose kinetics during high-intensity exercise in endurance-trained and untrained humans. J. Appl. Physiol. In press.

20. Coggan, A.R.; Spina, R.J.; Kohrt, W.M.; Holloszy, J.O. Effect of prolonged exercise on muscle citrate concentration before and after endurance training in men. Am. J. Physiol. 264 (Endocrinol. Metab. 27):E215-E220; 1993.

21. Coggan, A.R.; Spina, R.J.; Kohrt, W.M.; Kirwan, J.P.; Bier, D.M.; Holloszy, J.O. Plasma glucose kinetics during exercise in subjects with high and low lactate thresholds. J. Appl. Physiol. 73:1873-1880; 1992.

22. Coggan, A.R.; Swanson, S.C.; Mendenhall, L.A.; Habash, D.L.; Kien, C.L. Effect of endurance training on hepatic glycogenolysis and gluconeogenesis during prolonged exercise in men. Am. J. Physiol. (Endocrinol. Metab.) In press.

23. Conlee, R.K. Muscle glycogen and endurance: a twenty-year perspective. In: Pandolf, K.P., ed., Exercise and sport sciences reviews, vol. 15. New York: Macmillan; 1987: 1-28.

24. Constable, S.H.; Favier, R.J.; McLane, J.A.; Fell, R.D.; Chen, M.; Holloszy, J.O. Energy metabolism in contracting rat skeletal muscle: adaptation to exercise training. Am. J. Physiol. 253 (Cell Physiol. 22):C316-C322; 1987.

25. Coyle, E.F.; Martin, W.H.; Bloomfield, S.A.; Lowry, O.H.; Holloszy, J.O. Effects of detraining on responses to submaximal exercise. J. Appl. Physiol. 59:853-859; 1985.

26. Davies, K.J.A.; Packer, L.; Brooks, G.A. Biochemical adaptation of mitochondria, muscle, and whole-animal respiration to endurance training. Arch. Biochem. Biophys. 209:539-554; 1981.

27. Dela, F.; Mikines, K.J.; Von Linstow, M.; Galbo, H. Heart rate and plasma catecholamines during 24 h of everyday life in trained and untrained men. J. Appl. Physiol. 73:2389-2395; 1992.

28. Dela, F.; Mikines, K.J.; Von Linstow, M.; Secher, N.H.; Galbo, H. Effect of training on insulin-mediated glucose uptake in human muscle. Am. J. Physiol. 264 (Endocrinol. Metab. 26):E1134-E1143; 1992.

29. Deuster, P.A.; Chrousos, G.P.; Luger, A.; Bernier, L.L.; Trostmann, U.H.; Kyle, S.B.; Montgomery, L.C.; Loriaux, D.L. Hormonal and metabolic responses of

untrained, moderately trained, and highly trained men to three exercise intensities. Metabolism 38:141-148; 1989.

30. Dienstbier, R.A. Behavioral correlates of sympathoadrenal reactivity: the toughness model. Med. Sci. Sports Exerc. 23: 846-852; 1991.

31. Dohm, G.L.; Hecker, A.L.; Brown, W.E.; Klain, G.J.; Puente, F.R.; Askew, E.W.; Beecher, G.R. Adaptation of protein metabolism to endurance training. Increased amino acid oxidation in response to training. Biochem. J. 164:705-708; 1977.

32. Donovan, C.M.; Brooks, G.A. Endurance training affects lactate clearance, not lactate production. Am. J. Physiol. 244 (Endocrinol. Metab. 7): E83-E92; 1983.

32a. Donovan, C.M.; Pagliasotti, M.J. Enhanced efficiency of lactate removal after endurance training. J. Appl. Physiol. 68:1053-1058; 1990.

32b. Donovan, C.M.; Pagliasotti, M.J. Endurance training enhances lactate clearance during hyperlactatemia. Am. J. Physiol. 257 (Endocrinol. Metab. 20):E782-E789; 1989.

32c. Donovan, C.M.; Sumida, K.D. Training improves glucose homeostasis in rats during exercise via glucose production. Am. J. Physiol. 258 (Regulatory Integrative Comp. Physiol. 27):R770-R776; 1990.

33. Dudley, G.A.; Tullson, P.C.; Terjung, R.L. Influence of mitochondrial content on the sensitivity of respiratory control. J. Biol. Chem. 262:9109-9114; 1987.

34. Elayan, I.M.; Winder, W.W. Effect of glucose infusion on muscle malonyl-CoA during exercise. J. Appl. Physiol. 70:1495-1499; 1991.

35. Elia, M. Estimation of short-term energy expenditure by the labeled bicarbonate method. In: Whitehead, R.G.; Prentice, A., eds. New techniques in nutritional research. New York: Academic; 1991: 207-227.

36. Esler, M.; Jennings, G.; Korner, P.; Blombery, P.; Sacharias, N.; Leonard, P. Measurement of total and organ-specific norepinephrine kinetics in humans. Am. J. Physiol. 247 (Endocrinol. Metab. 10):E21-E28; 1984.

37. Essén, B.; Hagenfeldt, L.; Kaijser, L. Utilization of blood-borne and intramuscular substrates during continuous and intermittent exercise in man. J. Physiol. 265:489-506; 1977.

38. Evans, W.J.; Bennett, A.S.; Costill, D.L.; Fink, W.J. Leg muscle metabolism in trained and untrained men. Res. Q. 50:350-359; 1979.

38a. Favier, R.J.; Constable, S.H.; Chen, M.; Holloszy, J.O. Endurance training reduces lactate production. J. Appl. Physiol. 61:885-889; 1986.

39. Fell, R.D.; Lizzo, F.H.; Cervani, P.; Crandall, D.I.. Effects of contractile activity on rat skeletal muscle β-adrenoceptor properties. Proc. Soc. Exp. Biol. Med. 180:527-532; 1985.

40. Fitts, R.H.; Booth, F.W.; Winder, W.W.; Holloszy, J.O. Skeletal muscle respiratory capacity, endurance, and glycogen utilization. Am. J. Physiol. 228:1029-1033; 1975.

41. Fröberg, S.O.; Mossfeldt, F. Effect of prolonged strenuous exercise on the concentration of triglycerides, phospholipids and glycogen in muscle of man. Acta Physiol. Scand. 82:167-171; 1971.

42. Galster, A.D.; Clutter, W.E.; Cryer, P.E.; Collings, J.A.; Bier, D.M. Epinephrine plasma thresholds for lipolytic effects in man. J. Clin. Invest. 67:1729-1738; 1981.

43. Gollnick, P.D.; Armstrong, R.B.; Saubert, C.W.; Piehl, K.; Saltin, B. Enzyme activity and fiber composition in skeletal muscle of untrained and trained men. J. Appl. Physiol. 33:312-319; 1972.

44. Gollnick, P.D.; King, D.W. Effect of exercise and training on mitochondria of rat skeletal muscle. Am. J. Physiol. 216:1502-1509; 1969.

45. Green, H.J.; Ball-Burnett, M.E.; Smith, D.; Livesey, J.; Farrance, B.W. Early muscular and metabolic adaptations to prolonged exercise training in humans. J. Appl. Physiol. 70:2032-2038; 1991.

46. Green, H.J.; Coates, G.; Sutton, J.R.; Jones, S. Early adaptations in gas exchange, cardiac function, and haematology to prolonged exercise training in man. Eur. J. Appl. Physiol. 63:17-23; 1991.

47. Green, H.J.; Helyar, R.; Ball-Burnett, M.; Kowalchuk, N.; Symon, S.; Farrance, B. Metabolic adaptations to training precede changes in muscle respiratory capacity. J. Appl. Physiol. 72:484-491; 1992.

48. Green, H.J.; Jones, L.L.; Houston, M.E.; Ball-Burnett, M.E.; Farrance, B.W. Muscle energetics during prolonged cycling after exercise hypervolemia. J. Appl. Physiol. 66:622-631; 1989.

49. Gyntelberg, F.; Rennie, M.J.; Hickson, R.C.; Holloszy, J.O. Effect of training on the response of plasma glucagon to exercise. J. Appl. Physiol. 43:302-305; 1977.

50. Habash, D.L.; Kien, C.L.; Horswill, C.A.; Lamb, D.R. Isotopic dilution of CO_2: index of CO_2 production (VCO_2) during brief periods of physical activity. FASEB J. 4:A654; 1990.

51. Hardy, R.W.; Ladenson, J.H.; Henriksen, E.J.; Holloszy, J.O.; McDonald, J.M. Palmitate stimulates glucose transport in rat adipocytes by a mechanism involving translocation of the insulin sensitive glucose transporter (GLUT4). Biochem. Biophys. Res. Comm. 177:343-349; 1991.

52. Hargreaves, M.; Kiens, B.; Richter, E.A. Effect of increased plasma free fatty acid concentrations on muscle metabolism in exercising men. J. Appl. Physiol. 70:194-201; 1991.

53. Harper, A.E.; Miller, R.H.; Block, K.P. Branched-chain amino acid metabolism. Ann. Rev. Nutr. 4:409-454; 1984.

54. Hartley, L.H.; Mason, J.W.; Hogan, R.P.; Jones, L.G.; Kotchen, T.A.; Mougey, E.H.; Wherry, F.E.; Pennington, L.L.; Ricketts, P.T. Multiple hormonal responses to graded exercise in relation to physical training. J. Appl. Physiol. 33:602-606; 1972.

55. Hartley, L.H.; Mason, J.W.; Hogan, R.P.; Jones, L.G.; Kotchen, T.A.; Mougey, E.H.; Wherry, F.E.; Pennington, L.L.; Ricketts, P.T. Multiple hormonal responses to prolonged exercise in relation to physical training. J. Appl. Physiol. 33:607-610; 1972.

56. Havel, R.J.; Naimark, A.; Borchgrevink, C.F. Turnover rate and oxidation of free fatty acids of blood plasma in man during exercise: studies during continuous infusion of palmitate-1-C^{14}. J. Clin. Invest. 42:1054-1063; 1963.

57. Havel, R.J.; Carlson, L.A.; Ekelund, L.-G.; Holmgren, A. Turnover rate and oxidation of different free fatty acids in man during exercise. J. Appl. Physiol. 19:613-618; 1964.

58. Henderson, S.C.; Black, A.L.; Brooks, G.A. Leucine turnover and oxidation in trained rats during exercise. Am. J. Physiol. 249 (Endocrinol. Metab. 12): E137-E144; 1985.

59. Henriksson, J. Training induced adaptation of skeletal muscle and metabolism during submaximal exercise. J. Physiol. 270:661-667; 1977.

60. Hermansen, L.; Hultman, E.; Saltin, B. Muscle glycogen during prolonged severe exercise. Acta Physiol. Scand. 71:129-139; 1967.

61. Hoerr, R.A.; Yu, Y.-M.; Wagner, D.A.; Burke, J.F.; Young, V.R. Recovery of ^{13}C in breath from $NaH^{13}CO_3$ infused by gut and vein: effect of feeding. Am. J. Physiol. 257 (Endocrinol. Metab. 20): E426-E438; 1989.

62. Holloszy, J.O. Biochemical adaptations to exercise: aerobic metabolism. Exerc. Sports Sci. Rev. 1:45-71; 1973.

63. Holloszy, J.O. Biochemical adaptations in muscle. Effects of exercise on mitochondrial oxygen uptake and respiratory enzyme activity in skeletal muscle. J. Biol. Chem. 242:2278-2282; 1967.

64. Holloszy, J.O.; Coyle, E.F. Adaptations of skeletal muscle to endurance exercise and their metabolic consequences. J. Appl. Physiol. 56:831-838; 1984.

65. Holloszy, J.O.; Oscai, L.B.; Don, I.J.; Molé, P.A. Mitochondrial citric acid cycle and related enzymes: adaptive response to exercise. Biochem. Biophys. Res. Commun. 40:1368-1373; 1970.

66. Hood, D.A.; Terjung, R.L. Effect of endurance training on leucine metabolism in perfused rat skeletal muscle. Am. J. Physiol. 253 (Endocrinol. Metab. 16): E648-E656; 1987.

67. Hoppler, H.; Lüthi, P.; Claassen, H.; Weibel, E.R.; Howald, H. The ultrastructure of normal human skeletal muscle. A morphometric analysis of untrained men, women, and well-trained orienteers. Pflügers Arch. 344:217-232; 1973.

68. Houmard, J.A.; Egan, P.C.; Neufer, P.D.; Friedman, J.E.; Wheeler, W.S.; Israel, R.G.; Dohm, G.L. Elevated skeletal muscle glucose transporter levels in exercise-trained middle-aged men. Am. J. Physiol. 261 (Endocrinol. Metab. 24): E437-E443; 1991.

69. Hurley, B.F.; Nemeth, P.M.; Martin, W.H.; Hagberg, J.M.; Dalsky, G.P.; Holloszy, J.O. Muscle triglyceride utilization during exercise: effect of training. J. Appl. Physiol. 60:562-567; 1986.

70. Issekutz, B.; Miller, H.I.; Rodahl, K. Lipid and carbohydrate metabolism during exercise. Fed. Proc. 25:1415-1420; 1966.

71. Issekutz, B.; Miller, H.I.; Paul, P.; Rohahl, K. Aerobic work capacity and plasma FFA turnover. J. Appl. Physiol. 20:293-296; 1965.

72. Ivy, J.L.; Withers, R.T.; Van Handel, P.J.; Elger, D.H.; Costill, D.L. Muscle respiratory capacity and fiber type as determinants of the lactate threshold. J. Appl. Physiol. 48:523-527; 1980.

73. Jansson, E.; Kaijser, L. Substrate utilization and enzymes in skeletal muscle of extremely endurance-trained men. J. Appl. Physiol. 662:999-1005; 1987.

74. Karlsson, J.; Nordesjö, L.-O.; Saltin, B. Muscle glycogen utilization during exercise after physical training. Acta Physiol. Scand. 90:210-217; 1974.

75. Kien, C.L. Isotopic dilution of CO_2 as an estimate of CO_2 production during substrate oxidation studies. Am. J. Physiol. 257 (Endocrinol. Metab. 20): E296-E298; 1989.

76. Kiens, B.; Lithell, H. Lipoprotein metabolism influenced by training-induced changes in human skeletal muscle. J. Clin. Invest. 83:558-564; 1989.

77. Kjær, M.; Christensen, N.J.; Sonne, B.; Richter, E.A.; Galbo, H. Effect of exercise on epinephrine turnover in trained and untrained male subjects. J. Appl. Physiol. 59:1061-1067; 1985.

78. Kjær, M.; Farrell, P.A.; Christensen, N.J.; Galbo, H. Increased epinephrine response and inaccurate glucoregulation in exercising athletes. J. Appl. Physiol. 61:1693-1700; 1986.

79. Kjær, M.; Galbo, H. Effect of physical training on the capacity to secrete epinephrine. J. Appl. Physiol. 64:11-16; 1988.

80. Kjær, M.; Mikines, K.J.; Linstow, M.V.; Nicolaisen, T.; Galbo, H. Effect of 5 wk of detraining on epinephrine response to insulin-induced hypoglycemia in athletes. J. Appl. Physiol. 72:1201-1204; 1992.

81. Koivisto, V.; Hendler, R.; Nadel, E.; Felig, P. Influence of physical training on the fuel-hormone response to prolonged low intensity exercise. Metabolism 31:192-197; 1982.

82. Lamont, L.S.; Patel, D.G.; Kalhan, S.C. Leucine kinetics in endurance trained humans. J. Appl. Physiol. 69:1-6; 1990.

83. Lavoie, J.-M.; Bongbélé, J.; Cardin, S.; Bélisle, M.; Terrettaz, J.; Van De Werve, G. Increased insulin suppression of plasma free fatty acid concentration in exercise-trained rats. J. Appl. Physiol. 74:293-296; 1993.

84. LeBlanc, J.; Boulay, M.; Dulac, S.; Jobin, M.; Labrie, A.; Rousseau-Migneron, S. Metabolic and cardiovascular responses to norepinephrine in trained and nontrained human subjects. J. Appl. Physiol. 42:166-173; 1977.

85. Lehmann, M.; Keul, J.; Huber, G.; Da Prada, M. Plasma catecholamines in trained and untrained volunteers during graduated exercise. Int. J. Sports Med. 2:143-147; 1981.

86. Liggett, S.B.; Shah, S.D.; Cryer, P.E. Characterization of β-adrenergic receptors of human skeletal muscle obtained by needle biopsy. Am. J. Physiol. (Endocrinol. Metab. 17): E795-E798; 1988.

87. Luger, A.; Deuster, P.A.; Kyle, S.B.; Gallucci, W.T.; Montgomery, L.C.; Gold, P.W.; Loriaux, D.L.; Chrousos, G.P. Acute hypothalamic-pituitary-adrenal responses to the stress of treadmill exercise. Physiologic adaptations to physical training. New Eng. J. Med. 616:1309-1315; 1987.

87a. MacRae, H.S.-H.; Dennis, S.C.; Bosch, A.N.; Noakes, T.D. Effects of training on lactate production and removal during progressive exercise in humans. J. Appl. Physiol. 72:1649-1656; 1992.

88. Martin, W.H.; Coggan, A.R.; Spina, R.J.; Saffitz, J.E. Effects of fiber type and training on β-adrenoceptor density in human skeletal muscle. Am. J. Physiol. 257 (Endocrinol. Metab. 20): E736-E742; 1989.

89. Martin, W.H.; Coyle, E.F.; Joyner, M.; Santeusanio, D.; Ehsnai, A.A.; Holloszy, J.O. Effects of stopping exercise training on epinephrine-stimulated lipolysis in humans. J. Appl. Physiol. 56:845-848; 1984.

90. Martin, W.H.; Dalsky, G.P.; Hurley, B.F.; Matthews, D.E.; Bier, D.M.; Hagberg, J.M.; Rogers, M.A.; King, D.S.; Holloszy, J.O. Effect of endurance training on plasma free fatty acid turnover and oxidation during exercise. Am. J. Physiol. 265 (Endocrinol. Metab. 28): E708-E714; 1993.

91. Mazzeo, R.S.; Grantham, P. Norepinephrine turnover in various tissues at rest and during exercise: evidence for a training effect. Metabolism 38:479-483; 1989.

92. Mazzeo, R.S.; Marshall, P. Influence of plasma catecholamines on the lactate threshold during graded exercise. J. Appl. Physiol. 67:1319-1322; 1989.

93. McCully, K.K.; Boden, B.P.; Tuchler, M.; Fountain, M.R.; Chance, B. Wrist flexor muscles of elite rowers measured with magnetic resonance spectroscopy. J. Appl. Physiol. 67:926-932; 1989.

94. Mendenhall, L.A.; Swanson, S.C.; Habash, D.L.; Coggan, A.R. Ten days of exercise training reduces glucose production and utilization during moderate-intensity exercise. Amer. J. Physiol. 266 (Endocrinol. Metab. 29):E136-E143; 1994.

95. Mikines, K.J.; Sonne, B.; Farrell, P.A.; Tronier, B.; Galbo, H. Effect of training on the dose-response relationship for insulin action in men. J. Appl. Physiol. 66:695-703; 1989.

96. Mikines, K.J.; Sonne, B.; Farrell, P.A.; Tronier, B.; Galbo, H. Effect of acute exercise and detraining on insulin action in trained men. J. Appl. Physiol. 66:704-711; 1989.

97. Molé, P.A.; Oscai, L.B.; Holloszy, J.O. Adaptation of muscle to exercise. Increase in levels of palmityl CoA synthetase, carnitine palmityltransferase, and palmityl CoA dehydrogenase, and the capacity to oxidize fatty acids. J. Clin. Invest. 50:2323-2330; 1971.

98. Moore, R.L.; Thacker, E.M.; Kelley, G.A.; Musch, T.I.; Sinoway, L.I.; Foster, F.L.; Dickinson, A.L. Effect of training/detraining on submaximal exercise responses in humans. J. Appl. Physiol. 63:1719-1724; 1987.

99. Morgan, T.E.; Short, F.A.; Cobb, L.A. Effect of long-term exercise on human muscle mitochondria. In: Pernow, B.; Saltin, B., eds. Muscle metabolism during exercise. New York: Plenum; 1971: 87-95.

100. Oscai, L.B.; Holloszy, J.O. Biochemical adaptations in muscle. II. Response of mitochondrial adenosine triphosphatase, creatine phosphokinase, and adenylate kinase activities in skeletal muscle to exercise. J. Biol. Chem. 246:6968-6972; 1971.

101. Ploug, T.; Stallknecht, B.M.; Pedersen, O.; Kahn, B.B.; Ohkuwa, T.; Vinten, J.; Galbo, H. Effect of endurance training on glucose transport capacity and glucose transporter expression in rat skeletal muscle. Am. J. Physiol. 259 (Endocrinol. Metab. 22):E778-E786; 1990.

102. Powers, S.K.; Howley, E.T. Exercise physiology. Theory and application to fitness and performance. Dubuque, IA: Wm. C. Brown; 1990: 281-283.

103. Randle, P.J.; Garland, R.B.; Hales, C.N.; Newsholme, E.A. The glucose-fatty acid cycle: its role in insulin sensitivity and the metabolic disturbances of diabetes mellitus. Lancet 1:785-789; 1963.

104. Randle, P.J.; Newsholme, E.A.; Garland, P.B. Regulation of glucose uptake by muscle. 8. Effect of fatty acids, ketone bodies and pyruvate, and of alloxan diabetes and starvation, on the uptake and metabolic fate of glucose in rat heart and diaphragm muscles. Biochem. J. 93:652-665; 1964.

105. Ren, J.M.; Hultman, E. Regulation of phosphorylase a activity in human skeletal muscle. J. Appl. Physiol. 69:919-923; 1990.

106. Ren, J.M.; Gulve, E.A.; Cartee, G.D.; Holloszy, J.O. Hypoxia causes glycogenolysis without an increase in % phosphorylase a in rat skeletal muscle. Am. J. Physiol. 263 (Endocrinol. Metab. 26):E1086-E1091; 1992.

107. Rodnick, K.J.; Haskell, W.L.; Swislocki, A.L.M.; Foley, J.E.; Reaven, G.M. Improved insulin action in muscle, liver, and adipose tissue in physically trained human subjects. Am. J. Physiol. 253 (Endocrinol. Metab. 16):E489-E495; 1987.

108. Rowell, L.B. Human cardiovascular adjustments to exercise and thermal stress. Physiol. Rev. 54:75-159; 1974.

109. Sahlin, K.; Katz, A.; Broberg, S. Tricarboxylic acid cycle intermediates in human muscle during prolonged exercise. Am. J. Physiol. 259 (Cell Physiol. 28):C834-C841; 1990.

110. Saltin, B.; Nazar, K.; Costill, D.L.; Stein, E.; Jansson, E.; Essén, B.; Gollnick, P.D. The nature of the training response: peripheral and central adaptation to one-legged exercise. Acta Physiol. Scand. 96:289-305; 1976.

111. Savard, G.; Strange, S.; Kiens, B.; Richter, E.A.; Christensen, N.J.; Saltin, B. Noradrenaline spillover during exercise in active versus resting skeletal muscle in man. Acta Physiol. Scand. 131:507-515; 1987.

112. Silverberg, A.B.; Shah, S.D.; Haymond, M.W.; Cryer, P.E. Norepinephrine: hormone and neurotransmitter in man. Am. J. Physiol. 234 (Endocrinol. Metab. Gastrointest. Physiol. 3): E252-E256; 1978.

113. Slanger, B.H.; Kusubov, N.; Winchell, H.S. Effect of exercise on human CO_2-HCO_3^- kinetics. J. Nucl. Med. 11:716-718; 1970.

114. Spina, R.J.; Ogawa, T.; Coggan, A.R.; Holloszy, J.O.; Ehsani, A.A. Exercise training improves left ventricular contractile response to β-adrenergic agonist. J. Appl. Physiol. 72:307-311; 1992.

115. Stallknecht, B.; Kjær, M.; Mikines, K.J.; Maroun, L.; Ploug, T.; Ohkuwa, T.; Vinten, J.; Galbo, H. Diminished epinephrine response to hypoglycemia despite enlarged adrenal medulla in trained rats. Am. J. Physiol. (Regulatory Integrative Comp. Physiol. 28):R998-R1003; 1990.

116. Sumida, K.D.; Urdiales, J.H.; Donovan, C.M. Enhanced gluconeogenesis from lactate in perfused livers after endurance training. J. Appl. Physiol. 74:782-787; 1993.

117. Suda, K.; Izawa, T.; Komabayashi, T.; Tsuboi, M.; Era, S. Effect of insulin on adipocyte lipolysis in exercise-trained rats. J. Appl. Physiol. 74:2935-2939; 1993.

118. Svendenhag, J.; Martinsson, A.; Ekblom, B.; Hjemdahl, P. Altered cardiovascular responsiveness to adrenaline in endurance-trained subjects. Acta Physiol. Scand. 126:539-550; 1986.

119. Taylor, R.; Jones, N.L. The reduction by training CO_2 output during exercise. Eur. J. Cardiol. 9:53-62; 1979.

120. Terjung, R.L.; Kaciuba-Uscilko, H. Lipid metabolism during exercise: influence of training. Diabetes/Metabolism Rev. 2:35-51; 1986.

121. Turcotte, L.P.; Richter, E.A.; Kiens, B. Increased plasma FFA uptake and oxidation during prolonged exercise in trained vs. untrained humans. Am. J. Physiol. 262 (Endocrinol. Metab. 25):E791-E799; 1992.

122. Wagenmakers, A.J.M.; Schepens, J.T.G.; Veerkamp, J.H. Effect of starvation and exercise on total activity of the branched-chain 2-oxo acid dehydrogenase complex in rats. Biochem. J. 223:815-821; 1984.

123. Wallin, B.G.; Sundlöf, G.; Eriksson, B.-M.; Dominiak, P.; Grobecker, H.; Linblad, L.E. Plasma noradrenaline correlates to sympathetic muscle nerve activity in normotensive man. Acta Physiol. Scand. 111:69-73; 1981.

124. Wasserman, D.H.; Geer, R.J.; Rice, D.E.; Bracy, D.; Flakoll, P.J.; Brown, L.L.; Hill, J.O.; Abumrad, N.N. Interaction of exercise and insulin action in humans. Am. J. Physiol. 260 (Endocrinol. Metab. 23):E37-E45; 1991.

125. Wasserman, K. The anaerobic threshold: definition, physiological significance, and identification. Adv. Cardiol. 35:1-23; 1986.

126. Wibom, R.; Hultman, E.; Johansson, M.; Matherei, K.; Constantin-Teodosiu, D.; Schantz, P.G. Adaptation of mitochondrial ATP production in human skeletal muscle to endurance training and detraining. J. Appl. Physiol. 73:2004-2010; 1992.

127. Williams, R.S.; Bishop, T. Skeletal muscle β-adrenergic receptors: variations due to fiber type and training. Am. J. Physiol. 246 (Endocrinol. Metab. 9): E160-E167; 1984.

128. Winder, W.W.; Arogyasami, J.; Barton, R.J.; Elayan, I.M.; Vehrs, P.R. Muscle malonyl-CoA decreases during exercise. J. Appl. Physiol. 67:2230-2233; 1989.

129. Winder, W.W.; Arogyasami, J.; Elayan, I.M.; Cartmill, D. Time course of exercise-induced decline in malonyl-CoA in different muscle types. Am. J. Physiol. 259 (Endocrinol. Metab. 22):E266-E271; 1990.

130. Winder, W.W.; Baldwin, K.M.; Holloszy, J.O. Exercise-induced increase in the capacity of rat skeletal muscle to oxidize ketones. Can. J. Physiol. Pharmacol. 53:86-91; 1975.

131. Winder, W.W.; Hagberg, J.M.; Hickson, R.C.; Ehsani, A.A.; Holloszy, J.O. Time course of sympathoadrenal adaptation to endurance training in man. J. Appl. Physiol. 45:370-374; 1978.

132. Winder, W.W.; Hickson, R.C.; Hagberg, J.M.; Ehsani, A.A.; McLane, J.A. Training-induced changes in the hormonal and metabolic response to submaximal exercise. J. Appl. Physiol. 46:766-771; 1979.

133. Wolfe, R.R. Radioactive and stable isotope tracers in biomedicine. New York: Wiley-Liss; 1992: 133-142.

134. Wolfe, R.R.; Jahoor, F.; Miyoshi, H. Evaluation of the isotopic equilibration between lactate and pyruvate. Am. J. Physiol. 254 (Endocrinol. Metab. 17): E532-E535; 1988.

135. Wolfe, R.R.; Wolfe, M.H.; Nadel, E.R.; Shaw, J.H.F. Isotopic determination of amino acid-urea interactions in exercise in humans. J. Appl. Physiol. 56:221-229; 1984.

Chapter 7

Metabolic Determinants of Activity Induced Muscular Fatigue

HOWARD J. GREEN

Mammalian skeletal muscles are capable of generating enormous forces and power outputs when appropriately activated (6). However, repeated attempts to reproduce equivalent mechanical expressions are invariably met with failure, as characterized by an early and progressive deterioration in performance. In its simplest form, this deterioration is what we have come to recognize as fatigue, or more precisely in the case of the voluntary exercising mammal, neuromuscular fatigue. Although the occurrence of varying degrees of neuromuscular fatigue is an unavoidable reality experienced by most of us during the course of our daily activities, surprisingly little is known about the specific mechanisms involved. Until relatively recently, most experimental investigations have been focused on describing the manifestations of fatigue and the factors modifying its onset and progression. For example, we now know the relative importance of different variables constituting the task itself, such as the muscle mass involved, the intensity of the contraction, the velocity of movement, the range of muscle lengths at which the task is performed, and the temporal characteristics of the contraction and relaxation schedule. There also appear to be large differences between individuals in the vulnerability to fatigue. Sex, age, health status, body composition, and genetic endowment in terms of the structure, organization, and composition of the neural and muscular systems all represent significant variables. Endurance and fatigability are also critically dependent on the physical and chemical composition of the environment in which the task is performed. Few would dispute the premature exhaustion that results from exercising in the heat and humidity or at altitude, particularly in the unacclimatized state.

But what is the underlying basis for the failure of the neuromuscular system to allow performance to be maintained at a desired level? The collective impression that generally persists and is frequently invoked to explain fatigue is based on the energy state of the muscle. Muscles that are fatigued, it is reasoned, are low in ATP. This position is not without credibility. Contracting muscles greatly accelerate the utilization of ATP, and because ATP concentration in muscle is very low (estimated at 5 mM · kg^{-1} wet wt, enough for only a few seconds), a slight imbalance in ATP regenerating mechanisms could result in an energy crisis. However, at least in the voluntary exercising human, low ATP levels do not appear to be the cause of fatigue (53, 55). Although it is generally accepted that in many types of fatigue, energy state is probably implicated, the mechanistic basis is far more complicated and elusive than previously realized. In spite of many obstacles, progress is being made. Modern researchers, armed with an impressive array of analytical tools, are now capable of probing defective processes at a number of levels of organization ranging from the muscle itself to the cell and to the molecular structure of the diverse range of proteins constituting the organelles involved in excitation and contraction. For these tools to be applied successfully, however, a clear understanding of the mechanical basis of fatigue is a prerequisite. How the alterations in specific mechanical properties are coupled with the metabolic state of the muscle then becomes researchable.

How Might Metabolism Induce Fatigue?

Because it is generally agreed that it is impossible to deplete ATP stores more than 20 to 25% in voluntary exercise, regardless of the characteristics of the task, and because the affinity of the ATPase for ATP is so high, depletions of this order do not affect the saturation of the enzyme with ATP (60). Consequently, it is generally agreed that ATP is not the direct cause of what is being commonly referred to as metabolic fatigue. Instead, investigations are being increasingly focused on the metabolic by-products (30, 90) and, in particular, the phosphate energy system (28). Increases in contractile activity result in the recruitment of the ATPase enzyme systems in the muscle and in the rate of ATP hydrolysis. Attempts to satisfy cellular ATP requirements result from mobilization of ATP regenerating metabolic pathways such as oxidative phosphorylation, glycolysis, and high-energy phosphagen transfer. The increased flux results in an increase in the concentration of metabolic by-products. The high-energy phosphagen subsystem, which includes the reactions catalyzed by creatine phosphokinase (CPK) and adenylate kinase (AK), given its equilibrium nature, is capable of rapid and responsive changes to protect ATP levels, particularly at the initiation of activity (47). Creatine phosphate (PCr), as an example, exists in concentrations approximately threefold higher than

ATP and can serve as an effective, albeit brief, buffer for ATP when ATP utilization is abruptly increased. These high-energy phosphagen transfer reactions generate by-products. Near stoichiometric increases in creatine (Cr) and phosphate (P_i) occur with decreases in PCr (28). Closely related to the high-energy phosphagen system is the purine nucleotide cycle. One arm of this cycle, which involves the AMP deaminase reaction, uses AMP for the production of inosine monophosphate (IMP) and ammonia (NH_3). Collectively, these metabolites are increasingly being recognized as causal agents in fatigue, as they interact with one or more processes involved in excitation and contraction of the muscle (48). Increases in mitochondrial respiration and glycolysis also generate intermediates, and it is conceivable that increases in those metabolites could also be implicated at some level. For example, elevations in hydrogen ion concentration, generated in part from glycolysis, appear to have a significant role in fatigue (97).

Interestingly, most, if not all, of the metabolites increase with the ATP requirements of the task. Modern attempts to explain metabolic control stress the integrated nature of the metabolic systems and the common signals directing their activation (28, 47). Metabolites generated from high-energy phosphagen reactions are viewed as critical in coordinating the activation of the oxidative and glycolytic systems (28, 64). The dilemma, however, is identifying which metabolites represent the key modulators and to what degree other factors may be involved (66).

A similar dilemma also exists with identifying specific metabolites involved in muscular fatigue. At moderate levels of exercise, where ATP synthetic rates are rigorously matched to ATP utilization rates and where pH changes minimally, the total pool of reactants involved in high-energy phosphagen metabolism remains constant. As a result, all of the individual metabolites are interrelated and consequently are functions of each other (27). Under such circumstances, isolation of a single reactant species as a mediator of fatigue is difficult, if not impossible. With more intense exercise, which results in metabolic acidosis and reductions in the high-energy phosphagen pool as a consequence of IMP accumulation, the ability to discriminate between different potential putative modulators involved in fatigue is improved, which is similar to what has been suggested in metabolic control models (26). However, as emphasized in the voluntary exercising human, the reductions in ATP and in the total phosphagen pool appear to be relatively modest. Without unphysiological interventions, attempts to target specific reactants or metabolites as primary candidates will continue to prove elusive.

Isolation of a specific metabolic species as the definitive cause of fatigue poses additional challenges. The intracellular environment can conventionally be viewed as a "soup" containing a number of cations, such as potassium (K^+), sodium (Na^+), magnesium (Mg^{2+}), calcium (Ca^{2+}), and hydrogen (H^+) ions, and anions such as bicarbonate (HCO_3^-), chloride (Cl^-), and lactate (La^-). These electrolytes have potentially important roles to play in fatigue for several reasons. First, some metabolic reactions are influenced by the concentrations of specific ions. Second, ions such as Ca^{2+} bind to specific proteins such as troponin C, one of the regulatory proteins of the myofibrillar apparatus. The binding of Ca^{2+} is an essential step in initiating the sequence of events that eventually culminates in actin and myosin moving to the strong binding, force generating state (97). Third, ion movement is critical to maintaining electrical neutrality and, consequently, functional integrity. The sarcolemma, T tubule, and sarcoplasmic reticulum (SR), as examples, have elaborated special channels to permit counter ion movements (113). Finally, ions can bind to high-energy phosphagens and in so doing become a more reactive substrate for ATPase reactions (113). ATP and ADP, as examples, bind both Mg^{2+} and H^+, the balance between the two determining the net negative charge on the substrate. Cations and anions also complex with each other. Hydrogen phosphate can exist in the monoprotonated (HPO_4^{2-}) or diprotonated form ($H_2PO_4^-$), the balance between the two forms being determined by the pH. The effect of phosphate on selected processes such as actomyosin cycling may depend on the form the phosphate exists in (30, 105). Finally, the intracellular ionic environment can alter the free energy realized from high-energy hydrolysis reactions (113). For example, increases in H^+ can depress the free energy of ATP hydrolysis, potentially threatening the energy dependent processes involved in excitation and contraction.

For increases in contractile activity to occur, the sarcolemma and the T tubules must be able to conduct a regenerative action potential, and the sarcoplasmic reticulum must be able to release and sequester Ca^{2+}. These excitation events in conjunction with the metabolic reactions, which occur to provide the needed energy, result in alterations in the intracellular ionic environment. The change in the intracellular environment occurs because of shifts in ionic species between different compartments, alterations in substrate concentrations, shifts in the free and bound forms, and the generation of specific ions by metabolic processes (113). One of the most conspicuous effects of an increase in contractile intensity is the generation of reducing equivalents, namely H^+ ions. During maximal exercise the pH in muscle can decline from a rest value of approximately 7.0 to values in the range of 6.3 to 6.5 (75). This large increase in H^+ accumulation can affect not only metabolism and metabolic reactions directly, but in addition it can greatly disturb the entire intracellular ionic milieu, resulting in different proportions of free and bound forms of certain ionic species such as Mg^{2+} (113). In addition, H^+ may compete directly with other cations such as Ca^{2+} for access to the Ca^{2+} binding sites on troponin C or disrupt counter ion movements at the level of specific organelles. When metabolic acidosis, which results from intense activity, also occurs in conjunction with large changes in metabolic products such as P_i, ADP, and AMP from high-energy phosphagen transfer reactions, a "soup" of a decidedly different flavor is produced.

What are the Mechanical Manifestations of Fatigue?

In its most conspicuous form, fatigue can be identified by a failure to maintain a desired level of performance or work. For example, if the activity involves cycling or running, the point at which the individual can no longer sustain the power output is defined as the threshold heralding the onset of fatigue. Identifying the underlying basis for the deterioration is not so simple. Basically, the ultimate goal is to specify what intracellular process in excitation and contraction represents the primary site of failure. To achieve this objective, a number of different levels of investigation is necessary. In the work modalities cited, the coordination of multiple muscles is needed to produce the activity. In cycling, some seven different muscles in each side of the lower body contribute to the production of power generated during the thrust phase (58). The first objective is to identify, if possible, the muscle that appears to be unable to sustain its contribution. Direct measurements of the absolute contribution of specific muscles are not possible. To perform these determinations, electromyography is employed, and measurements of the integrated activity (IEMG) are used to calculate power output. Even under the best of circumstances, identification of a primary failing muscle may not be possible, because the activated muscles are synergistic in nature, possessing to some degree the ability to readily compensate for each other (107). Moreover, the physical output of a given muscle represents the interaction of the mechanical output of each of the recruited motor units. Because the output of each motor unit would be expected to change in a time-dependent fashion, the composite output must be viewed as depending on the cumulative changes occurring in the entire motor neuron pool that is activated (107).

Most mechanical performances are complex entities composed of a number of fundamental attributes. A failure in one attribute may disrupt the mechanical output. Tasks range in complexity in terms of the number and the levels of interaction of the basic elements. Isometric activity, given the fact that the contraction is performed at constant muscle length and consequently occurs without any observable shortening or lengthening, is the easiest to model. If the contraction is relatively intense, a tetanus or a fused contraction is produced. In this situation, identifying the site of fatigue is relatively easy because only one mechanical parameter is involved. However, at lower intensities of muscle contraction, where force is oscillatory because of the non-fused contractions, additional factors are involved that might impair performance. Both the contraction time (CT) and relaxation time (RT) are important in the peak force attained. Decreases in CT and decreases in RT can be independent events controlled by different intracellular processes, but both are capable of reducing the peak force transient. On the other hand, prolongation of these properties with repeated activity might serve as an important tactic in maintaining force output (12, 123). Before changes in a specific intracellular process can be hypothesized as a contributor to fatigue, care must be exercised in defining the mechanical parameters of interest.

The contraction schedule must also be considered as an additional modifying variable. Contractions are frequently performed intermittently with different activation and relaxation periods. In such circumstances, particularly where forces must be generated instantaneously and repeatedly, even greater emphasis is placed on the kinetics of the processes involved in activation and relaxation and their ability to sustain a given force transient.

When it is recognized that tasks are commonly performed at different muscle lengths and defined by very precise activation and relaxation histories, it is easy to see how disturbances can develop at a number of levels. The possibility that a singular process can be identified as a primary cause of fatigue under such complex circumstances appears remote.

Voluntary activity also creates additional problems for the enterprising researcher preoccupied with fatigue mechanisms. Muscles are composed of motor units, and each motor unit is recruited in an apparently stereotyped and ordered fashion, depending on the requirements of the task (62). This recruitment property introduces the possibility that fatigue recorded at the whole muscle may be due to a subpopulation of the active motor units. Indeed, even if all of the motor units are recruited, as occurs in many types of tasks, large differences exist in the fatigability of the muscle fibers innervated by different motor axons (15). Because most muscles, particularly in the human, are composed of a mixture of different fiber types, fatigability may be more exaggerated in some motor units than in others. Differences in fatigability between motor units may also be exaggerated by the demands imposed by the task (14). The possibility exists that failure in specific fiber types and motor units has a different mechanistic basis and that the specific site of failure may be task dependent (41).

Most of the physical tasks that one performs routinely and repetitively on a daily basis are dynamic, involving shortening and lengthening of the muscle and producing work, both positive and negative. Fatigue mechanisms identified on the basis of isometric activity may have limited relevance to tasks where work is involved (121). In dynamic activity, force generation at variable velocities depends not only on the appropriate timing of activation of the muscle, but also on the behavior of the contractile elements. The actin-myosin must be able to quickly oscillate not only in and out of attached and detached states, but also in and out of strong and weak binding configurations while in the attached state (97). To sustain similar mechanical output with repeated contractions, the force histories at different muscle lengths must be accurately reproduced as well. It is possible that given the specific intracellular adjustments that must be made, failure may be due to an inappropriate response more at one length than another.

Collectively, these considerations emphasize the multiple mechanical expressions that may occur when the muscle contracts. To a large degree, these different parameters emphasize different intracellular processes for their expression. Fatigue may occur at different rates, depending on the mechanical complexity of the task performed. Isotonic activity, as an example, results in a more rapid fatigue than isometric activity (4, 115). The implications of identifying the fundamental processes responsible for fatigue in a dynamic activity such as cycling are enormous. Because the force and work transients developed during cycling depend on elements of both isometric and dynamic behavior occurring at different lengths and velocities, the combinations are almost limitless.

These considerations focus on the unreality of attempting to elucidate the primary causes of fatigue in complex tasks involving multiple muscle groups performed voluntarily. Advances in isolating specific intracellular processes under such circumstances depend on the knowledge generated by more fundamental preparations and designs. Ultimately, these findings can be used to construct models on which one can hypothesize as to the specific mechanisms of fatigue in complex tasks and then elaborate creative strategies to investigate these hypotheses experimentally.

Models Used to Examine Fatigue Mechanisms

A large collection of different approaches ranging from *in vitro* studies to *in vivo* studies at the whole animal level have been used to advance our understanding as to why the neuromuscular system cannot sustain a criterion level of task performance. Although many of these models are unphysiological, they are essential building blocks in our quest to relate intracellular organization and composition with function. The key is to make sure that the results from these experiments are appropriately interpreted and applied.

One level of study involves the use of *in vitro* models. In these investigations, an attempt is made to study function by simulating different intracellular environments in the test tube. Muscle tissue is fractionated, usually by differential centrifugation, to obtain a sample that is enriched in a specific organelle. In general, these preparations have been used to examine the function of specific organelles, such as the sarcolemma, the sarcoplasmic reticulum, or the myofibrillar apparatus. Researchers have used *in vitro* procedures extensively to study energy metabolic behavior in terms of pathway recruitment and control. Typically these studies attempt to manipulate one variable, such as ATP, ADP, P_i, pH, Ca^{2+}, etc., and to systematically examine the effect of the metabolite over a range of physiological concentrations characteristic of the working state (26, 47). These metabolites have also been used to investigate the metabolic basis of fatigue (106). Frequently, these studies will also incorporate a fatigued muscle with a fresh muscle in order to characterize potential differences between the two as a result of the exercise (10). These studies may address the function of a specific organelle directly (e.g., ionic exchange across the sarcolemma, 77; Ca^{2+} release by the sarcoplasmic reticulum, 93, 94) or examine the enzymatic activity of one of the ATPases that has a major responsibility for the functional status of the organelle (106). In this regard, three major ATPases in the muscle, the sarcolemma Na^+-K^+ ATPase, the sarcoplasmic reticulum Ca^{2+}-ATPase, and the actomyosin ATPase, have received much attention in fatigue studies performed *in vitro* (Figure 7.1). Theoretically, the alterations in function that are observed in a specific organelle should be accounted for, at least in part, by the activity of the ATPase.

Although *in vitro* studies are viewed as important building blocks, the interpretation and application of the results must be tempered with the realization that the organelle may be substantially disrupted by the preparation or only partially recovered. Furthermore, attempts to recreate what is undoubtedly a complex and dynamic intracellular environment may be simplistic.

At another level, the muscle tissue itself, without disruption, may be studied directly by *in vitro* techniques. With this approach, either the whole muscle, a bundle of muscles, or single fibers dissected from the muscle are placed in a physiological medium and connected to a force transducer. The tissue can be stimulated with different protocols and different mechanical parameters monitored over time. The single fiber technique has proved to be extremely popular, particularly with the advent of very sensitive transducers for accurate force measurements in very low ranges. Single fibers may be examined with their sarcolemma intact or with the sarcolemma removed. The "skinned fiber" technique provides the added advantage of allowing direct manipulation of the intracellular environment. These studies allow artificial control of free intracellular Ca^{2+} levels and permit the examination of mechanical behavior at different levels of activation and with selected changes in the intracellular environment (30). In studies using intact fibers or whole muscle preparations, manipulation of the intracellular environment must be, by and large, attempted by pharmacological agents (103). However, intact preparations have the advantage of allowing examination of the effect of changes in the extracellular environment on the progress and recovery from activity induced fatigue (86).

As with all *in vitro* studies, the physiological relevance remains an issue. Studies with intact tissue are a step closer to reality because the intracellular organization of the fiber is presumably not disturbed. With these preparations, the contractile patterns are induced or imposed. This

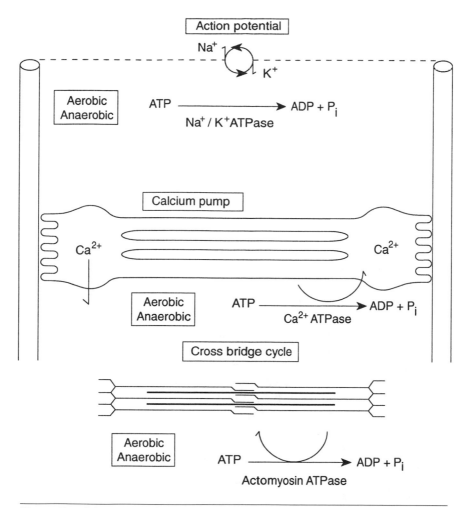

Figure 7.1   Major sites of ATP utilization used to sustain excitation and contraction in the muscle cell. Represented on the figure are the sarcolemma Na^+-K^+ ATPase, the sarcoplasmic reticulum Ca^{2+} ATPase, and the actomyosin ATPase.

stereotyped activation protocol denies an inherent flexibility that *in vivo* neuromuscular systems have when voluntarily activated, namely the ability for a flexible recruitment strategy to help defend against fatigue (11, 107). In general, induced activation results in an earlier and more pronounced fatigue than during voluntary activity at the same mechanical demands (74).

Studies performed *in vivo* using whole animal preparations have long represented the basic reference for the examination of fatigue. At one level, the experimental animal is anaesthetized, the limb of concern is stabilized, and the muscle is isolated and prepared for stimulation and mechanical measurements. As in other preparations, the muscle can be stimulated with different protocols, and the fatigue manifestations can be characterized. Furthermore, with *in vitro* techniques, the muscle can be rapidly sampled and examined for functional alterations in specific organelles (9, 16). Manipulation of the extracellular environment can be realized by changing the composition of the blood. A very popular preparation now used extensively, is to perfuse the hindlimb with an artificial blood containing ingredients of experimental interest (83). Fatigue studies have also been performed at the single motor unit level (15). To isolate single motor units, dorsal root dissection is performed in the anaesthetized animal until a single motor nerve is isolated. This nerve can then be stimulated, the muscle frozen, and the active fibers identified on the basis of histochemically determined glycogen depletion patterns. Because many analyses at both the organelle and metabolic levels can be performed on sections of single fibers, it is possible to relate specific alterations in motor unit function with changes at the level of the single fiber.

A primary concern with these *in situ* studies is the physiological viability of the preparations because experimental protocols typically take several hours. Fatigue patterns with *in situ* studies, as with the *in vitro* preparations, are created with induced contractile protocols, which allow precise control of the activity history, but do not allow any opportunity for fatigued fibers to be sporadically rested according to their fatigue state.

Understanding the mechanistic basis of fatigue in voluntary activity is usually the ultimate quest. In voluntary exercise experiments in both humans and other species, it is difficult to gain access to the tissue before the transient intracellular changes induced by the activity recover. It is also difficult to establish objective measurements of fatigue and to isolate the fatigue to specific muscles. One advantage of studying humans or other large species is that samples of tissue can be rapidly obtained with the needle biopsy technique (40). Recent advances in nuclear magnetic resonance procedures (^{31}P-NMR) now make it possible to study metabolism in exercising muscle noninvasively (90, 100). Voluntary exercise studies allow specific hypotheses to be tested based on models derived from the results of more controlled *in situ* and *in vitro* research. Such evidence will always be correlational, because extensive interactions between muscle fibers, motor units, and muscles are potentially possible at all levels of organization. Extreme caution must be exercised in extrapolating the results of such experiments to definitive fatigue mechanisms. When these studies are properly designed, however, they address reality in its uncontaminated form, and the results can increase the confidence that certain events in fatigue can be implicated. The predicative power of models generated to explain fatigue in voluntary exercise is dependent on an ongoing interaction between the knowledge generated from all experimental approaches.

The Identification of Specific Fatigue Sites

If there is a metabolic basis for fatigue, the metabolic effects must operate at one or more of the processes involved in force production. In voluntary activity, these processes can be outside the muscle or in the muscle. Processes outside the muscle, collectively referred to as central processes, include events leading to recruitment of the fibers (11, 40). Disturbances in higher motor centers or in reflex feedback from the muscle potentially can alter the excitability of the alpha motoneuron (11). In addition, the impulses generated in the motor nerve may be distorted because of branch point fatigue or inhibition at the level of the neuromuscular junction (11). As a consequence of central failure, the activation of the motor unit and muscle fiber is compromised, resulting in an altered and undesirable mechanical behavior that has been identified as fatigue. Central failure may also have a metabolic basis, either as a result of metabolic changes in the muscle altering reflex feedback or by direct effects of the by-products released from the muscle carried by the blood and acting at one or more central locations (54). Although experimental evidence linking metabolism to central fatigue remains tenuous, the existence of a central basis for fatigue in certain types of tasks and in certain types of muscles appears to be well established (54).

Peripheral sites classically identified as being potentially limiting where repetitive activity is involved have been categorized on the basis of function into excitation, excitation-contraction coupling, and contraction processes. Excitation sites include the sarcolemma and the T tubule system. Functionally, these organelles are specialized to conduct the electrical signals into the interior of the muscle fiber. When the excitation signal is conducted into the interior of the fiber, it must result, if contractions are to ensue, in the opening of the Ca^{2+} channels in the sarcoplasmic reticulum, which leads to a release of stored Ca^{2+} into the cytosol. To do this, the excitation signal in the T tubule membrane must be able to communicate with the Ca^{2+} channels in the terminal cisternae of the sarcoplasmic reticulum, which involves transversing a gap estimated at between 10 and 15 nm (125). This process is called excitation-contraction coupling. The manner in which the excitation signal is communicated across the gap, whether mechanical, chemical, or electrical remains uncertain (35). However, disruptions in excitation-contraction coupling, which are suspected in certain types of fatigue (36), would effectively alter the cytosolic Ca^{2+} transient. The final site involved in activation is the sarcoplasmic reticulum. The primary functions of the sarcoplasmic reticulum are to release Ca^{2+} into the cytosol and to sequester the Ca^{2+} back into the sarcoplasmic reticulum. With the opening of the Ca^{2+} release channel, Ca^{2+} rapidly floods into the cytosol, producing an elevation in the level of free Ca^{2+}. The level of free Ca^{2+} determines the degree of activation of the myofibrillar apparatus (97). When excitation is terminated, Ca^{2+} sequestration predominates, cytosolic

Ca^{2+} levels are lowered, and relaxation ensues. Alterations in either Ca^{2+} release or Ca^{2+} uptake may impact on mechanical behavior and may represent a cause of fatigue.

The myofibrillar complex, composed of the regulatory proteins troponin and tropomyosin and the contractile proteins actin and myosin, represents the contractile apparatus. Disturbances in the ability of the regulatory proteins to respond to the Ca^{2+}-activating signal or in the ability of the actin and myosin to move to different states—strong binding, weak binding, detached—might also be implicated in force impairment.

By and large, research strategies have attempted to identify the one or more sites that appear to be the locus of the problem in activity induced fatigue. Studies on the role of metabolism would be facilitated considerably if such sites could be unambiguously identified. Although some progress is being made, much uncertainty remains.

Differentiation between central and peripheral failure in the neuromuscular system has been accomplished with a number of techniques. In voluntary activity, one approach has been to compare the difference between the maximal voluntary force (MVC) that can be generated with the force that is artificially induced by electrical stimulation (12). Discrepancies between the two (e.g., where artificially induced force exceeds MVC) are recognized as having a component of central fatigue. The "interpolated twitch" is another application of this technique (129). In the interpolated twitch, an impulse is superimposed on an MVC. Increases in force are indicative of a central involvement in fatigue. Electromyographic measurements (EMG) also appear useful in differentiating between central and peripheral sites. Declines in the integrated EMG (IEMG) with force reductions suggest an attenuation in central drive. If the integrity of the neuromuscular junction and the sarcolemma can be established, as is frequently possible with the intervention of stimulation to the motor nerve of the muscle and the recording of a mass action potential (M-wave), then the diagnosis is more certain. In some preparations, particularly where *in vitro* or *in situ* techniques are used, force output from motor nerve stimulation is compared with stimulation through intracellular electrodes. Although this procedure does not include higher centers, it does enable examination of the role of the neuromuscular junction in the force decay that occurs with repeated nerve stimulation (12).

Examining the role of the sarcoplasmic reticulum (SR) and T tubule-sarcoplasmic reticulum coupling as potential fatigue sites is even more difficult. Recent advances in the use of fluorescent dyes such as Fura-2 and Indo-1 have permitted direct monitoring of cytosolic Ca^{2+} transients in single fiber preparations with different stimulation protocols (135). When these measurements are combined with force measurements, associations can be made between failure in the force generating capabilities and the reduction in the cytosolic Ca^{2+} concentration. Care must be taken, however, in the interpretation of results, because these experiments cannot provide information as to whether changes have also occurred in the Ca^{2+} sensitivity of the myofibrillar apparatus and the regulatory Ca^{2+} binding protein, troponin C, in particular.

Another approach that has been used in an attempt to isolate the role of the SR is the application of pharmacological agents such as the methylxanthines, which bind to the Ca^{2+} channel and stimulate the release of Ca^{2+} sequestered in the SR. The use of these agents, caffeine being one of the most popular, provides the opportunity to examine the role of the SR in the intact voluntary exercising mammal, such as the human, because caffeine can be administered orally or intravenously (40). However, the interpretation of the findings remains problematic. Restoration of force following activity and caffeine administration is strongly supportive of increased SR Ca^{2+} release. However, the mechanism underlying a fatigue-induced reduction in SR Ca^{2+}-release could conceivably be due to improper sarcolemma and T tubule signal conduction or a problem in coupling the excitation signal in the T tubule to the Ca^{2+}-release channel (36, 135).

Investigation of the role of the myofibrillar apparatus in fatigue has by and large been restricted to *in vitro* preparation of skinned fibers. Skinned fibers allow the systematic manipulation of Ca^{2+} levels and therefore the level of activation. Simulation of the chemical and physical environments typically found in the contracting muscle allows insight into the potential role of the myofibrillar apparatus (30). Techniques for the selective removal or modification of one or more of the regulatory proteins have also been developed, and these offer the opportunity to localize the failure to specific components of the myofibrillar complex (102).

One of the major problems in fatigue research is the general inability to ascribe undesirable alterations in specific types of mechanical output to one or more sites in excitation and contraction. Individual sites can be investigated; however, alterations in the integrity of the site, particularly when measured under *in vitro* conditions and in the absence of what has happened at other sites, do not necessarily indicate cause. A desirable goal in fatigue research is to indicate with reasonable confidence that given certain contractile demands, a predictable pattern of disturbance will occur in certain mechanical parameters and that this disturbance is site specific. In addition, the ultimate accomplishment would be to diagnose the mechanistic basis of a failing process and how the dysfunction is induced by the intracellular environment and, in particular, the metabolic changes that occur with repeated activity.

The Sarcoplasmic Reticulum and Fatigue

The sarcoplasmic reticulum, by virtue of its control over cytosolic free Ca^{2+} [$(Ca^{2+})_i$] levels, is an inviting candidate among the various organelles involved in excitation and contraction to be implicated in fatigue. In the absence of changes in the sensitivity of the myofibrillar apparatus to the Ca^{2+} signal, the activation level and, consequently, the mechanical response are intimately dependent on the Ca^{2+} transient. Changes in the $(Ca^{2+})_i$ transient can alter the mechanical response in a number of ways. At the simplest level, reductions in steady state Ca^{2+}, below a critical threshold, will result in a reduction in isometric tetanic force (97). Because most coordinated movement depends on force transients with varying rates of force development and decay, alterations in the time dependent character of $(Ca^{2+})_i$ concentration with excitation can have serious consequences. Muscle fiber and motor unit contributions to mechanical tasks frequently depend on submaximal or subtetanic contractions. In such cases, changes in the rate at which $(Ca^{2+})_i$ accumulates or the rate at which it decreases can result in serial alterations in the force profile, which may be beneficial or detrimental depending on the task requirements. For example, a reduction in the rate of decline in $(Ca^{2+})_i$ at low frequencies of stimulation can result in incomplete relaxation. Incomplete relaxation could enhance or help defend subsequent force levels in a manner independent of changes in the peak $(Ca^{2+})_i$ with repeated excitation (12).

Because much of human activity is dynamic, meaning that muscle fibers are required to shorten or lengthen for varying distances and at varying velocities and force outputs, highly sophisticated and precise control of $(Ca^{2+})_i$ levels is a requirement. For example, in movements of high velocity, the $(Ca^{2+})_i$ must not only be saturating for maximal actin-myosin cycling, but it must also be spatially distributed to all of the troponin C sites in the thin filaments in all of the sarcomeres. Because a typical muscle fiber contains many thousands of sarcomeres, the logistics associated not only with distribution of $(Ca^{2+})_i$, but also with the timing constraints that are imposed, are difficult to contemplate. High velocity movements also require instantaneous and precise control over concentrations of $(Ca^{2+})_i$, both during activation and following activation. A reduction in the rate of $(Ca^{2+})_i$ decline following activation could result in a counterforce when agonistic muscles are activated to return the muscle to the original position. Under such circumstances, incomplete relaxation could result not only in inefficiency, but also in some impairment to the task itself.

As is intuitively obvious, the best way to understand the role of changes in $(Ca^{2+})_i$ in fatigue is to measure the concentration directly in conjunction with the mechanical history. With the advent of dyes such as aequorin, Fura-2, and Indo-1, which fluoresce when combined with free Ca^{2+}, and the development of very sensitive transducers for measuring force levels in single fibers, these experiments are now possible (135). Indeed, a number of recent publications have examined the role of $(Ca^{2+})_i$ in fatigue in both *Xenopus* fibers and mouse fibers (2, 131, 134). In these experiments, the single fiber is isolated, dissected from the animal, placed in a physiological solution, and connected to a transducer. The fiber is injected with one of the fluorescent dyes and then subjected to a specific stimulation protocol.

Results published to date, which have been obtained from repetitive stimulation and isometric force measurements, have consistently implicated low $(Ca^{2+})_i$ as part of the fatigue that is observed (131). To date, these data represent the most compelling evidence that the sarcoplasmic reticulum might be implicated in the failure to maintain force with repeated activation. As the authors emphasize, however, the apparent inability of the SR to maintain a desired $(Ca^{2+})_i$ level has been observed only after the first 10 to 20 tetanic contractions and with a very specific stimulation protocol (135). It remains to be determined how vulnerable the SR is to different activation protocols that require more complex and diverse mechanical behavior. Indeed, as previously emphasized, the observation that force failure may be explained at the level of SR with artificially contrived *in vitro* protocols does not necessarily mean that the SR is a failure site in voluntary movement, given the apparent flexibility in the neural recruitment strategies that are possible (12, 41).

A reduction in $(Ca^{2+})_i$ concentration with sustained activation would, in all probability, be a direct result of altered Ca^{2+} cycling at the level of the SR. A failure of the SR to maintain $(Ca^{2+})_i$ homeostasis could arise directly from an impairment to the SR itself or as a consequence of a disturbance in external control of this organelle by the excitatory stimulus. To appreciate either possibility and the potential role of metabolism, some characterization of the structure, organization, and function of the SR is necessary.

The SR is an extremely elaborate membranous network that envelops each myofibril in a muscle fiber. Structurally, the SR has been divided into regions. These regions consist of the longitudinal tubules (LT), which run parallel to the myofibrils, and the terminal cisternae (TC), which are continuous with the LT but oriented at right angles. In the mammalian sarcomere, two TCs exist in opposition to each other but are separated by a transverse tubular system (T tubules). These structures, referred to as a triad because they contain one T tubule and two TCs, represent the site of excitation-contraction coupling (110). For the SR to become activated, the inward spread of the action potential, which is conducted by the T tubules, must be communicated to the SR across a gap that separates these two structures and is estimated to be some 10 to 15 nm in width (125).

Control of cytoplasmic levels by the SR depends on three separate properties or functions. First of all the SR must have a storage capability for Ca^{2+}, which remains sequestered during the period when the muscle is quiescent. Although there still remains some uncertainty, the general consensus is that proteins, such as calmodulin, exist in the lumen of the SR, and these proteins have a high binding affinity for Ca^{2+}. These proteins are believed to maintain the Ca^{2+} in storage, pending excitation of the cell (110). Second, upon excitation, the stored Ca^{2+} must be released into the cytoplasm from the lumen of the SR. This function occurs primarily at the terminal cisternae, the Ca^{2+} storage site, where a large concentration of proteins exist that are specialized for Ca^{2+} channel function. These proteins are called Ca^{2+} channel proteins or ryanodine receptors because they have been found to bind the plant alkaloid, ryanodine (85, 110).

The third property of the SR, namely Ca^{2+} sequestration function, occurs primarily in the longitudinal tubules, where rich concentrations of the Ca^{2+}-ATPase exist. The Ca^{2+}-ATPase is a Ca^{2+}-transporting enzyme that binds with free Ca^{2+} in the cytosol and is capable of transporting the Ca^{2+} into the lumen of the SR against an electrochemical gradient. Unlike the Ca^{2+} release property of the SR, Ca^{2+} uptake requires energy. In a normal functioning Ca^{2+}-ATPase, two Ca^{2+} ions are transported into the SR per ATP molecule (110). Sequestration of the released $(Ca^{2+})_i$ is obligatory for relaxation of the fiber following excitation.

In simplest terms, the SR may be viewed as a specialized structure that enhances the speed with which a fiber may respond to different excitation patterns. By having the activator Ca^{2+} stored within the cell in the immediate vicinity of the contractile proteins and by communicating with the SR electrically, a much faster mechanical response can be elicited than by depending on the extracellular entry and diffusion of Ca^{2+}. Skeletal muscle cells display wide extremes in mechanical function. For example, fast-twitch fibers contract and relax much more rapidly than slow-twitch fibers. These differences between the two fiber types are dependent, in part, on the composition of the SR. The SR in fast fibers is much more extensive, containing a higher density of both Ca^{2+} channels and Ca^{2+}-ATPase enzymes (109). Although there are differences in isoforms of these proteins between the different fiber types, the density of the protein is probably the primary factor underlying functional differences (59, 109).

Reductions in $(Ca^{2+})_i$, as have been found in single fiber preparations subjected to repeated stimulation (2, 131, 132, 134), could be due to direct disturbances in either the Ca^{2+}-releasing function or the Ca^{2+}-sequestering function of the SR. Reductions in Ca^{2+} release through the Ca^{2+} channels, in the absence of compensatory adjustments in Ca^{2+} uptake by the SR, will result in a depressed $(Ca^{2+})_i$. Although this is suspected (135), direct measurements of amount of Ca^{2+} released with activation have been difficult to accomplish analytically, even in the single fiber preparation. However, given that the Ca^{2+}-uptake function may occur independently of Ca^{2+} release, impairment in Ca^{2+} release would appear to be the primary mechanism underlying depressed $(Ca^{2+})_i$ levels (135). More recent work with single fibers of mouse skeletal muscle supports this hypothesis (44, 132).

Hypotheses directed at explaining the mechanistic basis of a depressed SR Ca^{2+}-release function have been formulated primarily on the basis of experiments performed *in vitro* with Ca^{2+} channels synthetically inserted into the phospholipid bilayers (94). The results of these studies suggest a metabolic basis for the progressive failure of the SR to release adequate

Ca^{2+}. The Ca^{2+}-release channel has been purified and biochemically characterized (118). It is believed to be inserted into the membrane of the terminal cisternae and to exist primarily as a large foot protein extending into the triadic gap. The foot protein not only contains vestibules, central and radial channels ostensibly for Ca^{2+} storage and transport, but also contains cytoplasmic orientated receptor regions for binding specific ligands and modulating the channel state (110). Caffeine, as an example, is a widely known and used compound, capable of holding the channel in an open state and eliciting large releases of Ca^{2+} into the cytoplasm (95).

Calcium release in synthetic preparations appears to be regulated, at least in part, by different species of the adenine nucleotides. High ATP levels and micromolar increases in free ADP [$(ADP)_f$] and free AMP [$(AMP)_f$], operating in conjunction with low Mg^{2+} and using Ca^{2+} to initiate release, all appear to stimulate increased release (93-95). These modulators have important implications for SR Ca^{2+}-release function during contractile activity and fatigue. In general, nonfatiguing activity would stimulate Ca^{2+} release. With increases in the intensity of contraction and increases in ATP turnover, decreases in ATP and increases in $(AMP)_f$ and $(ADP)_f$ occur. Given the fact that the reduction in ATP is, at best, modest with voluntary activity, the effect on Ca^{2+} release should be minimal (94). Increases in the adenine nucleotides, however, should facilitate high release rates. With more intense activity, however, other changes occur that could have deleterious effects on Ca^{2+} release. The metabolic acidosis that accompanies intense activity would appear to have an inhibitory effect (95). Decreases in pH levels also increase the concentration of free Mg^{2+}, and because increases in Mg^{2+} have also been shown to be inhibitory, the collective impact could be a reduction in Ca^{2+} release (95).

A missing and important component in modeling SR Ca^{2+}-release function during fatigue is the uncertainty regarding the primary initiating stimulus in Ca^{2+} release. Although the Ca^{2+}-induced Ca^{2+} release hypothesis has received much credibility as the triggering mechanism, other mechanisms have also been proposed (35, 110). In this context, because the adenine nucleotides are believed to have modulating functions, the most significant event could be what is happening to the triggering mechanism in fatigue induced by repetitive activity.

Changes in Ca^{2+} sequestration by the SR could also play a crucial role in altering mechanical behavior. Time-dependent increases in the rate of Ca^{2+} uptake with activity, although generally acknowledged not to occur, could effectively lower $(Ca^{2+})_i$ levels and consequently force generation. Conversely, and more likely, decreases in the rate of Ca^{2+} uptake could have detrimental or facilitatory consequences, depending on the nature of the task. It has also been suggested that reductions in Ca^{2+} uptake during repeated stimulation also impair Ca^{2+} release because of decreases in intraluminal Ca^{2+} content (135). However, it is difficult to envisage how this would occur, because $(Ca^{2+})_i$ would build up in the cytosol, and providing the high values did not reduce release, no impairment should result. However, if Ca^{2+} buffering were increased by cytosolic binding proteins such as parvalbumin, or if some of the Ca^{2+} is sequestered to sites other than the SR, such as the T tubules, Ca^{2+} loading could potentially be a limiting factor in Ca^{2+} release. What is not known is how much reserve is available and how much Ca^{2+} could reasonably be diverted to other locations without impairing the Ca^{2+}-release function by the SR.

Although at present still controversial, evidence from *in vitro* experiments suggests that Ca^{2+} uptake in both homogenate and SR fractions is substantially depressed after both prolonged (17) and intense (18, 50) activity. Although some element of uncertainty exists with regard to changes in Ca^{2+} uptake properties by the SR with acute exercise, chronic stimulation of skeletal muscle for more sustained periods has been repeatedly documented to impair Ca^{2+} uptake (38, 82, 87). There is also evidence, obtained from both short-term (18) and long-term periods of activity (82), that the total Ca^{2+} sequestered by the SR may be seriously impaired. Reductions in Ca^{2+} storage resulting from impairment in total Ca^{2+} uptake could potentially compromise the amount of Ca^{2+} released with activation.

The reductions in Ca^{2+} sequestration properties by the SR appear to result from alterations in the Ca^{2+}-ATPase enzyme, at least where extended periods of contractile activity occur (82). The Ca^{2+}-ATPase enzyme, primarily localized in the longitudinal tubules of the SR, is believed to consist of at least three specialized regions: a head and a stalk, which are located in the cytosol, and a base piece region, which is embedded in the phospholipid membrane of the SR (72). The head is believed to contain three globular subunits, each specialized for a specific function. One subunit has a nucleotide binding site for ATP, a second subunit is involved in phosphorylation, and the third appears to be involved in energy transduction (72). Calcium binding is believed to occur within the transmembrane domain (22). The steps involved in Ca^{2+} transport have been extensively studied and appear to involve the binding of ATP, complexed with Mg^{2+} and two Ca^{2+} ions. A phosphoenzyme intermediate is formed ($E-P_1$), which on release of energy undergoes a conformational change to a lower energy state ($E-P_2$), and in the process, Ca^{2+} is translocated into the lumen and released (110). Upon release of Ca^{2+}, the original conformational $E-P_1$ state is reestablished, and in the process, P_i and Mg AMP are released into the cytosol (110).

Impairment in Ca^{2+} uptake by the SR appears to result in modifications of the activity of the ATPase enzyme (82). Because Ca^{2+} ATPase transport is an energy dependent process, changes in the by-products of ATP hydrolysis, such as ADP and P_i, appear to impair Ca^{2+} ATPase activity and Ca^{2+} uptake properties. This may occur as a direct result of increasing ADP and P_i concentrations and impairing return to the $E-P_1$ state (33) or as a result of accumulation of metabolic by-products effecting reductions in the amount of free energy released on hydrolysis of ATP (31, 33). Reductions in pH also appear to have a potent effect on Ca^{2+} accumulation by the SR (81). Because increases in the products of ATP hydrolysis, such as ADP and P_i, are most often accompanied by increases in H^+ ionic concentration with intense exercise, an accumulative effect of these metabolites collectively contributing to a profound depression of SR Ca^{2+} sequestering properties would be expected. Such appears to be the case (18). However, prolonged exercise, which results in only modest alterations in the adenine nucleotides and P_i and minimal change in pH, also appears to depress Ca^{2+} uptake function (17). Changes in SR function under these circumstances would not appear to have a metabolic basis.

Changes in maximal Ca^{2+}-ATPase activity have, with some exceptions, corroborated the changes in Ca^{2+}-sequestering properties of the SR (17, 82). Using the chronic stimulation model in rabbit fast-twitch muscles, researchers have established that the alteration in Ca^{2+}-ATPase activity results from an impairment in the nucleotide binding site on the enzyme, rendering it inactive (38, 82, 88). The inactivation appears to affect only a subpopulation of the ATPase enzymes that are confined to a specific region of the SR vesicles (87). Why only specific regions appear to be susceptible and what underlying mechanisms are responsible for alterations in the nucleotide binding site are uncertain.

Changes in Ca^{2+} uptake and Ca^{2+}-ATPase activity by the SR following contractile activity have been assessed under *in vitro* conditions, with the reaction conditions optimized to maximize the response. Under such conditions, changes strongly suggest disturbances *in vivo*. However, the absence of changes measured *in vitro* does not imply that changes have not occurred *in vivo*. Transient changes in SR function no doubt occur in response to changes in the intracellular environment, for example, during metabolic by-product accumulation (31). Changes measured in SR function *in vitro* must be construed as a more persistent effect induced, for example, by changes in the adenine nucleotide binding site on the enzyme (38).

A fundamental issue yet to be elucidated experimentally relates to the physiological significance of depression in Ca^{2+} uptake by the SR with repetitive activity. Relaxation would appear to be the fundamental property affected; however, care must be exercised in assigning all phases of relaxation to alterations in Ca^{2+} uptake. Recent work has suggested that other processes, such as altered crossbridge kinetics, may be implicated as well (19, 133). In some tasks, a slowing of Ca^{2+} sequestration may be desirable, helping to minimize force loss by slowing relaxation and allowing subsequent activations to be superimposed on a residual level of force (123). Such a compensation may also permit firing frequency to be reduced without loss of force, potentially minimizing the chance for failure to occur at the sarcolemma (12). However, the implication of these findings across a wider spectrum of mechanical tasks must be viewed skeptically. The results of these studies have been obtained with relatively short and intense activation periods where large depressions in pH would be expected, where large depressions in force exist, and where isometric force is the only mechanical property of interest. More diverse tasks where dynamic behavior is involved at different forces and velocities would not be expected to benefit from prolongations in relaxation time. The possibility that Ca^{2+}-cycling rates may be slowed with potentially minimal impact in certain types of mechanical behavior, however, is exciting from the standpoint of efficiency. Because Ca^{2+} uptake by the SR is energetically costly, representing some 30-50% of ATP utilization in certain situations (31), reducing the Ca^{2+} cycling rate would be expected to reduce ATP hydrolysis rates and help stabilize ATP concentration. The implications of alterations in Ca^{2+}-sequestration or Ca^{2+}-release function, however, remain to be examined.

A direct metabolic effect on SR function (Ca^{2+} release and Ca^{2+} uptake), at least with a specific type of sustained contractile activity, seems extremely likely. The difficulty, however, in accepting a specific role is the general lack of experimental evidence. Indeed, a number of mechanisms have also been hypothesized as underlying SR functional alterations, with metabolic factors assuming an indirect or secondary role. These mechanisms have ranged from alterations in the physical environment, such as temperature (71), to ionic changes (1, 81, 92, 114), damage induced by free radicals (16, 80, 112), and proteolytic digestion (16, 96). Studies aimed at identifying mechanisms must concentrate not only on the ATPase pump protein itself, but also on the phospholipid environment in which the protein is embedded. For example, increased activity levels result in changes in the intracellular ionic composition. Substantial amounts of potassium (K^+) can be lost from the cell (117). At least in isolated SR fractions, K^+ has been shown to stimulate both Ca^{2+} transport and ATP hydrolysis (114). The stimulatory effect of K^+ could occur in two ways. Potassium could directly affect the activity of the enzyme itself by accelerating the decomposition of the phosphate intermediate in the reaction cycle of the ATPase, an event that may result from reductions in fluidity of the phospholipid membrane. Secondly, the longitudinal tubules, which contain the major portion of the ATPase enzymes, contain channels for monovalent cations, and this allows for counter ion exchange during net Ca^{2+} uptake. Given that exercise alters not only K^+, but also a range of other cations, including Na^+, H^+, and Mg^{2+}, and that changes are interdependent (83), it is possible that the effects of alterations in the ionic environment may be more profound than previously acknowledged.

The Sarcolemma-T Tubule System and Fatigue

For muscle contraction to occur, the neural signal must be transmitted to the interior of the fiber to open the Ca^{2+} release channels of the sarcoplasmic reticulum (SR) and induce an increase in free $[Ca^{2+}]_i$. The structures involved in conducting the impulse to the interior of the fiber are the sarcolemma and the T tubules. The sarcolemma membrane is composed of a phospholipid bilayer embedded with several different types of proteins that envelop the fiber. The T tubule system is, in effect, an extension of the sarcolemma that exists as invaginations at regular intervals along the sarcolemma (two per sarcomere) and extends inwardly and becomes flanked by the terminal cisternae of the sarcoplasmic reticulum (SR). Both the sarcolemma and the T tubules possess the property of excitability in that they contain a resting membrane potential and are capable of becoming depolarized and of conducting an action potential. In simplest terms, the sarcolemma and T tubules represent an electrical pathway whereby the excitation received from the motor nerve, via the neuromuscular junction and the motor end plate, can be transported to specific intracellular sites. The force developed by a muscle fiber is closely dependent on the frequency of the impulses conducted in the nerve and consequently the frequency with which action potentials can be regenerated in the sarcolemma and T tubules. With increasing frequency of stimulation, force increases proportionately up to approximately 100 impulses per second (100 Hz) where a saturation effect is observed. In the absence of any intracellular compensation within the fiber, an inability of the sarcolemma or T tubule system to transmit at an impulse frequency at which it is activated by the nerve can result in an impairment in force output, particularly at discharge frequencies below 100 Hz. A disturbance in the electrical properties of the fiber is particularly important in dynamic activities where neural impulse patterns must be precisely transmitted to the SR to ensure appropriate contraction and relaxation schedules necessary for coordinated movement. It is a common practice in fatigue studies to construct force-stimulus frequency curves in order to evaluate the frequency dependency of the force loss that occurs. Terms such as high-frequency fatigue and low-frequency fatigue are descriptive of the range of stimulus frequencies over which the force loss is conspicuous (40).

As with all potential peripheral fatigue studies, a major challenge is to identify definitively that the sites involved in fiber excitation represent failure points and, consequently, are the cause of an inability to generate a desired mechanical response. At least in the voluntary exercising human, much of the evidence linking the sarcolemma with fatigue is indirect and comes from electromyographic (EMG) recordings. For example, an inability of the sarcolemma to generate the number of action potentials directed by the nerve and neuromuscular junction would result in changes in selected properties of the EMG, such as the integrated EMG (12) and the power spectrum EMG (61). A reduction in the integrated EMG (IEMG) could indicate a reduction in the number of the motor unit action potentials (MUAP), whereas a shift in the power spectrum toward low frequency might indicate an inability to generate action potentials at a high rate. Changes in both the surface IEMG and the surface power spectrum

EMG have been frequently observed with fatiguing activity. The problem, however, has been in determining the relevance of these changes when explaining the force decrement that is observed and whether the sarcolemma is the primary site responsible for the EMG abnormalities.

Changes in the properties of the surface EMG could conceivably not result from a problem at the level of the sarcolemma, but from a problem in the neural command to the muscle or in the transmission of the neural signals across the neuromuscular junction (12). At present, at least in voluntary exercise, there is no effective way of isolating these sites. In some muscles, an M wave, defined as a muscle surface action potential, can be elicited by subjecting the motor nerve to a single supramaximal stimulus. A change in the amplitude or area of the M wave, although suggestive of a problem of the sarcolemma, could also be due to an impaired neuromuscular activation (12). If the M wave is not compromised, however, sites more peripheral to the sarcolemma would appear to underlie the loss of force. A similar conclusion also follows if the nerve or muscle is stimulated at different frequencies during the progression of fatigue induced by voluntary activity. This procedure can eliminate the role of the neuromuscular junction and the sarcolemma as sites of failure only if the EMG is normal.

Other problems also occur in the interpretation of the EMG changes that occur with exercise. The surface integrated EMG could be affected by changes in the muscle conduction velocity and/or by changes in both the population and synchronization of recruited motor units (12). Much of the same considerations apply to the power spectrum EMG (61).

The aforementioned considerations notwithstanding, a failure of the sarcolemma to sustain an excitation pattern is strongly suspected (74, 135), at least in some fatiguing tasks. The tasks most often implicated are those performed continuously at high intensity, where relatively high frequencies of stimulation are needed to elicit the force required for the task (74, 135). Under these conditions, reductions in the integrated EMG have been noted in conjunction with reductions in force output (11). However, it has also been noted that, in spite of the apparent reduction in neural drive (as evident in the IEMG), the excitation is sufficient to fully exploit the force residual remaining in the muscle (11). The reduction in neural drive is hypothesized as a compensatory strategy that occurs secondary to disturbances in excitation-contraction coupling in the muscle cell which, in fact, minimizes the chance of excitation failure at the level of the sarcolemma and T tubule systems (12). Although the concept of "muscle wisdom" is provocative, depending on reflex mechanisms and mediated by intracellular changes, much remains to be determined regarding task specificity, muscle selectivity, and motor unit type (41).

In tasks at submaximal force outputs performed for extended periods of time, the surface IEMG has been reported to increase (46, 61). This increase, interpreted as an exaggerated neural drive, has been proposed as a mechanism to defend against excitation-contraction failure in the muscle cell (46). Because the task is performed at submaximal force outputs, potential neural compensations include increasing the firing frequency to motor units already recruited or expanding the motor unit pool recruited. Surface IEMG measures are not capable of differentiating between these strategies and consequently are not capable of implicating the significance of excitation failure in the mechanical impairment that occurs. However, recent work has suggested that in prolonged submaximal voluntary contractions, increased motor unit recruitment, synchronization of motor unit activity, and lowering of motor unit firing frequencies occur (78). The reduction in firing frequency may be an example of muscle wisdom, which was previously alluded to.

The most compelling evidence linking fatigue with excitation failure comes from artificial patterns of stimulation induced to the nerve or muscle of *in vitro* or *in vivo* preparations. In these experiments, high-frequency stimulation has been shown to dramatically alter the IEMG and the properties of the action potential (74). Recovery from fatigue induced by high-frequency stimulation is rapid, supporting the suggestion that the neuromuscular junction or muscular structures involved in excitation are involved in recovery (74). The involvement of muscle excitation structures, the sarcolemma and T tubules, is being increasingly implicated in this type of failure based on electrophysiologic and ion exchange measures.

Changes in the excitation properties of the sarcolemma, although frequently documented in a variety of tasks but infrequently verified as the definitive site of force failure, appear to occur because of ionic imbalances between the intracellular and interstitial compartments. Like most excitable membranes, the sarcolemma has a transmembrane potential that is maintained by precise control over a number of monovalent ions. This control is provided by a variety of intrinsic proteins inserted into the lipid bilayer of the sarcolemma, which either form channels for the co-transport and exchange of selected ionic species or enable the active transport of specific ions. As examples, in the sarcolemma and, to some extent, in the T tubules, channels have been identified for K^+, Na^+, Cl^-, and Ca^{2+} transport and for Na^+/H^+, Na^+/Ca^{2+}, and Cl^-/HCO_3^- co-transport and exchange (113). Given the apparent role of K^+ in stabilizing resting membrane potential, it is not surprising that at least four channels (Inward Rectifier, Delayed Rectifier, ATP-dependent, Ca^{2+}-dependent) are involved in maintaining K^+ gradients (113).

The generation of an action potential depends on the opening of the Na^+ and K^+ channels with a consequent flow of Na^+ to the interior of the cell and K^+ to the interstitial space. An inability to quickly reestablish Na^+ and K^+ gradients across the membrane could alter the membrane potential and compromise the ability to generate a repetitive action potential with a normal configuration. The reduction in action potential frequency that results in the alteration in the size of the action potentials could impair the ability of the T tubule to effectively signal the sarcoplasmic reticulum, and in particular, the ability of the Ca^{2+}-channel to open and release sufficient quanta of Ca^{2+}. The reestablishment of ionic gradients for Na^+ and K^+ is controlled primarily by the ATPase pump (24). Activation of the Na^+-K^+ ATPase pump is triggered by the concentrations of K^+ and Na^+ on the exterior and interior of the cell, respectively, resulting in increased cycling. With each cycle, three Na^+ ions are transported out of the cell and two K^+ ions are transported into the cell, a process that is electrogenic and depends on the use of energy generated by the hydrolysis of ATP (24).

It has been repeatedly confirmed (83) in a variety of repetitive tasks, regardless of intensity, that K^+ is lost from the cell and Na^+ is increased in the cell. An inability of the Na^+-K^+ pump to cycle at a high enough rate has been repeatedly implicated as the fundamental problem (25, 117). Evidence in support of the suggestion that the activity of the Na^+-K^+ pump is limiting comes from *in vitro* stimulated muscle preparations in which Na^+-K^+ pump activity has been increased by the β_2-selective adrenoceptor agonist terbutaline. In these preparations K^+ and Na^+ imbalances are reduced and fatigue resistance is increased (76).

Assuming that the cycling rate of the Na^+-K^+ ATPase pump is limiting, a hypothesis with which there remains some disagreement (113), it is not entirely clear whether the problem resides with an insufficient Na^+-K^+ ATPase activity that is conspicuous at the outset of the task or whether a time dependent suppression in Na^+-K^+ ATPase activity occurs with repetition of the task. An insufficient Na^+-K^+ ATPase activity could occur because of an inadequate pump concentration or because of an inability to fully activate the enzyme. Clausen (25) has calculated that even at modest stimulation frequencies and full activation of the pump, the limitation appears to be in the concentration of the Na^+-K^+ ATPase enzyme. However, recent work (42) suggests that there are differences between fast muscles and slow muscles in their ability to activate the Na^+-K^+ pump during stimulation. Soleus muscles were found to be more sensitive to intracellular increases in Na^+ and consequently experienced minimal gain in Na^+ and loss of K^+ from the cell. In contrast, the EDL showed marked intracellular K^+ loss and Na^+ increases, which was consistent with the lower activation of Na^+-K^+ ATPase. The differences between muscle types could not be explained on the basis of differences in pump concentration or isoform type (42). It is possible that differences between the fast and slow muscles in the ability to activate the Na^+-K^+ ATPase may underlie, at least in part, the differences in fatigability that has been observed.

It is conceivable that repeated activity could also result in a suppression of Na^+-K^+ ATPase activity, as has been demonstrated for the Ca^{2+} ATPase of the sarcoplasmic reticulum (16). Reductions in Na^+-K^+ ATPase activity could have a metabolic basis, mediated either by reductions in ATP concentration or by an increase in the products of ATP hydrolysis. Reductions in ATP concentration do not appear as a probable cause, however, because in many types of activities ATP concentration is relatively well protected and because the Na^+-K^+ ATPase can operate very effectively at low concentrations of ATP (113). Some individuals would argue, however, and quite appropriately, that regional reductions in ATP could occur in the subsarcolemmal area and not be detected when global ATP measurements are made. The concept of compartmentalization and specialization of muscle metabolic pathways and substrates, particularly with regard to the needs of the sarcolemma, remains controversial.

A suppression in Na^+-K^+ ATPase activity could result from an increase in the by-products of ATP hydrolysis, such as phosphate (P_i) and hydrogen (H^+) ions. Both of these ions would be expected to alter the Na^+-K^+ ATPase activity once certain concentration levels are attained (34, 68). If the task requirements exceed a certain intensity, both of these metabolites would increase progressively over time. If such is the case, this could explain the impairment in neuromuscular propagation as evidenced by the decline in M wave amplitude that was recently observed (46) during tasks requiring submaximal force levels sustained to fatigue. Whether the neuromuscular failure is specific to fast-twitch fibers, as speculated by Everts and Clausen (42), remains to be determined.

In contrast to the SR Ca^{2+} ATPase enzyme, it has been very difficult to document acute reductions in Na^+-K^+ ATPase with activity because of analytical problems. In homogenate preparations, the specificity of the sarcolemma Na^+-K^+ ATPase reaction has not been well established. Preparations of sarcolemmal membrane demand substantial masses of tissue given the low sarcolemmal yield. Problems also exist with the purity of the preparations when sarcolemmal fractionation, which yields highly variable results, is attempted (24).

It should also be emphasized that the cycling rate of Na^+ and K^+ across the sarcolemma can also be modified by changes in the phospholipid moiety in the absence of changes in the Na^+-K^+ ATPase protein. In addition, the sarcolemma Na^+-K^+ ATPase, at least in the myocardium, has been shown to be highly susceptible to free radical induced lipid peroxidation, resulting in a depression in Na^+-K^+ ATPase activity (77). Prolonged activity could potentially result in sarcolemmal damage as a result of free radical formation (124).

Indirect evidence that the Na^+-K^+ ATPase may be limiting in protecting the integrity of sarcolemmal excitation processes comes from experiments when changes in Na^+-K^+ ATPase expression have been examined with chronic activity. In rabbit fast muscle, chronic stimulation at low frequency (10 Hz) results in an approximate twofold increase in Na^+-K^+ pump concentration within 4 days after the onset of stimulation (56). Increases in Na^+-K^+ pump concentration have also been documented in human skeletal muscle, with both sprint training (91) and prolonged cycle training (57). In both of the studies in humans, the increase in the Na^+-K^+ ATPase concentration has been linked to a reduction in K^+ released from the exercising muscle (57, 91).

In summary, changes in the muscle EMG have been repeatedly documented to occur in a wide variety of tasks, and these changes have been commonly linked to neuromuscular disturbances. Measurements employing electron probe technology, instrumental neutron activation analyses, and ionic selective electrodes have documented imbalances in intracellular Na^+ and K^+ homeostasis, suggesting alterations in sarcolemma membrane excitability. In high-frequency stimulation of the muscle, depressions in the excitability of the sarcolemma and/or T tubules appear to be a primary cause of force failure. In maximal voluntary contractions, however, such may not be the case because reductions in M wave amplitude appear to be accompanied by parallel reductions in the EMG (46). Indeed, the reductions in force with repetitive subtetanic stimulation, which have been attributed to excitation-contraction failure (135), may not apply to voluntary held submaximal contractions. In these tasks, neuromuscular mechanisms may dominate.

Myofibrillar Determinants of Fatigue

It has long been suspected that, at least with certain types of repetitive activity, fatigue results from an inability of the myofibrillar apparatus to translate the calcium signal into an expected force. A number of sites may be implicated in myofibrillar failure, beginning with alterations in the regulatory proteins, troponin and tropomyosin, and extending to disturbances in actin and myosin and crossbridge interaction.

In the intact muscle fiber, however, it has been literally impossible to isolate myofibrillar failure from failure in excitation or excitation-contraction coupling. This is because it is difficult to know what is happening to free cytosolic calcium concentration $(Ca^{2+})_i$, the signal involved in activating the myofibrillar apparatus, during contractile induced fatigue. Historically, studies examining myofibrillar function during fatigue have had to rely on skinned fiber preparations with manipulation of the $(Ca^{2+})_i$ signal. In these experiments, an intracellular environment, thought to be representative of fatigue, is mimicked, and mechanical performance is examined at different levels of $(Ca^{2+})_i$. It has also become possible with this approach to independently alter specific metabolites or metabolic end products and to study their impact either in isolation or in combination with other metabolites (30, 97). This approach has been complemented by *in vitro* experiments where the dependency of the myofibrillar ATPase activity to different concentrations of the metabolic by-products (75) or, indeed to exercise itself, is investigated (9). Reductions in myofibrillar

ATPase activity are assumed to result in perturbations, at least in some types of contractile performance.

More recently, the development of techniques using fluorescent dyes with a high affinity for Ca^{2+} has enabled $(Ca^{2+})_i$ levels to be measured in intact, contracting single fibers with membranes intact (135). Coincident measurement of force levels with intracellular $(Ca^{2+})_i$ measurements has allowed determination of the role of the myofibrillar apparatus. As with the other experimental procedures, these studies form the building blocks upon which to construct models and form hypotheses regarding the mechanisms of fatigue in physiological settings and particularly where voluntary tasks are of interest.

The best evidence for myofibrillar failure comes from experiments in stimulated frog (*Xenopus*) or mouse single fibers where reductions in force with repetitive stimulation have been observed in excess of what can be accounted for by reductions in intracellular $(Ca^{2+})_i$ concentration. These experiments have indicated that myofibrillar involvement in fatigue is largely dependent on the specifics of the stimulation protocol (135). As previously emphasized, consensus is gradually emerging that with high frequencies of stimulation, fatigue results from disturbances in excitation, mediated by a failure to reestablish ionic gradients across the sarcolemmal and/or T tubule membranes (135). At lower tetanic frequencies, myofibrillar failure can be observed and is characterized by a shift to the right in the force-$(Ca^{2+})_i$ relationship (97, 135). This means that at a given $(Ca^{2+})_i$, force is depressed. It should be noted that in these experiments reductions in $(Ca^{2+})_i$ are also observed, implying that disturbances in sarcoplasmic reticulum function occur in conjunction with alterations in the myofibrillar response to a given Ca^{2+} level (135). It has also been noted that where myofibrillar Ca^{2+} sensitivity is depressed, maximal Ca^{2+}-activated force is also depressed (135).

Recently, other investigators using a variety of creative techniques have implicated the myofibrils of intact fibers in fatigue without direct assessment of intracellular $(Ca^{2+})_i$. Edman and Lou (39), using different contractile schedules in single fibers of frog tibialis anterior muscle in conjunction with caffeine, a known stimulator of Ca^{2+}-release from the sarcoplasmic reticulum, have dissociated myofibrillar from non-myofibrillar fatigue. They found that by providing a sufficiently long interval between tetanic stimuli, fatigue could be induced that could not be overcome by caffeine. In contrast, when only short recovery intervals were provided, a procedure designed to maximize activation failure, caffeine could overcome the contractile induced fatigue. Yet another intriguing approach has been provided by Barclay et al. (8), who attempted to isolate myofibrillar from non-myofibrillar failure by measuring heat generated by ATP splitting associated with the crossbridges and Ca^{2+} turnover. They found that after the first few tetani, Ca^{2+} turnover heat remained relatively stable, whereas crossbridge heat and force declined progressively. These results were interpreted to mean that reductions in the Ca^{2+} sensitivity of the myofilaments had occurred, or that there was a reduction in the average force generated per crossbridge, or both.

Collectively, these studies support the general consensus that in certain types of fatigue, the myofibrils become incapacitated and are unable to translate a given Ca^{2+} signal into an expected mechanical response.

The results obtained from experiments on skinned single fibers are consistent with a role for the myofibrillar complex in the etiology of fatigue (30, 97). These experiments have also extended our understanding, not only with regard to the potential role of different metabolic by-products in crossbridge behaviour, but also to how specific metabolites selectively alter different mechanical parameters. Of the wide range of metabolic end-products examined, two have been shown to have the most profound affect on mechanical function, namely phosphate (P_i) and hydrogen (H^+) ions. During activity, P_i increases approximately stoichiometrically with the reduction in creatine phosphate (PCr). Given the relatively high concentration of PCr relative to ATP, a thirtyfold increase in P_i is not unrealistic (31). A number of investigators (21, 29, 48) have repeatedly demonstrated that increases in P_i result in a pronounced rightward shift in the isometric force-calcium concentration relationship, illustrating that at both submaximal and maximal activation levels, force is depressed. Increases in P_i in skinned fibers, however, do not affect the maximal velocity of shortening (V_{max}) (30). Although there is still uncertainty, the effect of increases in P_i are thought to occur directly at the level of the contractile proteins, actin and myosin.

Increases in P_i are believed to depress the rate at which P_i is released from the actomyosin $\cdot$ ADP $\cdot$ P_i complex, reducing the number of crossbridges moving from a weakly bound to a strongly bound force generating state (97). Because V_{max} is determined not by the number of strongly bound crossbridges but by the rate at which actomyosin can dissociate, an event which appears to be dependent on ADP release from the actomyosin ADP complex, V_{max} behaviour would not be expected to be altered substantially (30).

A controversial issue is whether it is the monoprotonated (HPO_4^-) or the diprotonated ($H_2PO_4^-$) form that affects crossbridge behaviour (105). At physiological pH, the P_i is relatively equally distributed between the monoprotonated and diprotonated forms (pK = 6.81). However, as pH is reduced, as it is with heavy exercise, the diprotonated form predominates. In skinned fibers, the depression in the calcium-activated force by P_i correlates closely with the concentration of the diprotonated species (105). This finding has been taken as evidence of the greater significance of the diprotonated form in depressing force. However, it has been pointed out (30) that these experiments have been unable to isolate the relative roles of the monoprotonated and diprotonated forms because P_i has the same relative effect at different levels of pH when different forms predominate.

The increases in the concentration of hydrogen ions (H^+) appear to be another potent modulator of myofibrillar behaviour (21, 29, 98). During heavy exercise, the H^+ ions generated from ATP hydrolysis and glycolysis can lower the pH from 7.0 to 6.2 (97). At low pH values, both the peak isometric force (P_o) and the maximal velocity of shortening (V_{max}) are substantially depressed (30). The mechanistic basis of the pH effect is unknown; however, both the regulatory and the contractile proteins are believed to be involved. For example, the rightward shift in the force-calcium concentration relationship, at low pH, could be due to a reduction in Ca^{2+}-binding to troponin C, because H^+ ions are known to compete for the Ca^{2+}-binding sites on this protein (43). Alternatively, H^+ ions could act directly at the level of actomyosin behaviour, effectively reducing the weak to strong binding complexes, reducing the force generated per crossbridge, or affecting dissociation of the actin and myosin (30, 98). The potential sites at which H^+ can regulate contractile behaviour at the myofibrillar level appear numerous and may, in addition, involve modification of the cooperative interactions between the different regulatory and contractile proteins (97). The refinement of different techniques for interchanging selected regulatory protein isoforms would appear to represent a major step in advancing our understanding in this area.

The roles of numerous other by-products have also been studied with the skinned fiber preparation. These include lactate, ADP, AMP, creatine, IMP, adenosine, and inosine (30). In general, all of these metabolites have been found to have little or no effect at concentrations thought to be physiologically relevant to heavy exercise (21, 48). Increases in ADP, as an example, appear to elicit a small decrease in V_{max} and a small increase in P_o. This paradoxical effect has been interpreted on the basis of the strongly bound force generating crossbridge state. With increased ADP, the rate of dissociation of the strongly bound state is slowed, thereby increasing P_o but reducing V_{max} (97).

Collectively, the experiments with skinned fibers suggest that at the myofibrillar level, the primary metabolic modulators of crossbridge behaviour are H^+ and P_i, with a secondary effect from ADP. Because both P_i and H^+ can increase coincidentally during heavy exercise, the combined effects would be to induce a profound depression in mechanical function. Interestingly, the impact of different metabolic end products, with the exception of H^+, appear to be specific in terms of the mechanical property affected.

Few individuals would dispute the substantive contribution that has resulted from the skinned fiber experiments to advancing our understanding of the potential role of the myofibrillar complex in fatigue and the mechanisms involved. However, care must be exercised in extrapolating the results of these experiments to physiological settings. For purposes of stability, skinned fiber experiments are conducted at very low temperatures with an artificial environment thought to reflect the live fiber. A great deal remains to be known about the contents of the cytosol *in vivo*, particularly in regard to the role of low molecular weight inorganic compounds and ionic strength (30, 135). Neither of these factors has been incorporated into the skinned fiber model.

A different but complementary approach to those previously described has been to examine the effects of metabolic end products on the myofibrillar ATPase activity measured *in vitro*. Reductions in the myofibrillar ATPase activity would be expected to affect one or more of the kinetic steps involved in weak to strong binding and consequently crossbridge behaviour. In a recent comprehensive study examining a range of metabolites in carp white muscle, Parkhouse (106) has found that myofibrillar ATPase activity was reduced by more than 50%, at relatively low levels of P_i, within a range that would be expected in activity of moderate intensity. Similarly, reductions in pH to levels that might be expected in heavy activity (pH 6.0) elicited a dramatic reduction in myofibrillar ATPase activity. This investigator also found that the combined effects of P_i and pH did not appear to be additive and that it was the monoprotonated form and not the diprotonated form of P_i that elicited the depression in myofibrillar ATPase activity. Surprisingly, reductions in ATP concentration also suppressed ATPase activity, a finding not supported by others (30), at least in the physiological range of concentrations. Although some discrepancies exist with regard to the *in vitro* findings of Parkhouse (106) and the findings from the skinned fiber preparation (30, 97), discrepancies that could conceivably be explained by the unique behaviour of carp muscle, two findings are consistent. The results of both the *in vitro* and skinned fiber studies support a major role for both P_i and H^+ in myofibrillar failure.

The *in vitro* determined myofibrillar ATPase activity has also been examined in homogenates prepared from exercised tissue. The rationale for these studies is that activity induced reductions in myofibrillar ATPase activity would suggest a potential site for impaired performance. However, both high-frequency stimulation of rat plantaris muscle (126, 127) and prolonged running (9, 45) have failed to elicit changes in myofibrillar ATPase activity in skeletal muscle of various fiber type composition. Although interesting, these findings do not establish a role for myofibrillar ATPase activity during the exercise because the measurements are made *in vitro* under supposedly optimal conditions. As previously noted, changes in myofibrillar ATPase activity would most likely occur *in vivo* in concert with changes in the intracellular metabolites and most notably P_i and H^+ (30, 97). When changes in myofibrillar ATPase occur when measured *in vitro* following exercise, an alteration in the structure of the enzyme is implied. In this regard, a pronounced shift to the right in the relationship between calcium and myofibrillar ATPase activity has been noted in heart muscle (9).

In summary, all the evidence obtained from intact single muscle fibers, skinned muscle fibers, and *in vitro* measurements of myofibrillar ATPase activity is consistent with a role of the myofilaments in the etiology of fatigue. Extrapolating these findings to voluntary tasks, however, is not without risk.

Energy Metabolism and Fatigue

It seems clear that metabolic end product accumulation, and not reductions in ATP concentration, represents a component of fatigue during repetitive activity. This conclusion has also been corroborated in physiological settings where simultaneous measurements of force and ^{31}P-nuclear magnetic spectroscopic (^{31}P-NMR) determinations of selected metabolic parameters (20, 101, 130) were made. Measurements of muscle metabolic behaviour taken with ^{31}P-NMR are particularly well suited for fatigue studies because spectra can be obtained for determinations of PCr, ATP, H^+, and P_i (including the proportion in the diprotonated form) (111). As such, this technique offers the opportunity for examining two of the prime metabolic by-products (P_i, H^+) that have been consistently implicated in force failure with the skinned fiber and *in vitro* procedures. Reductions in the time needed to resolve ^{31}P-NMR spectra have now made it possible to examine changes in selected metabolites and force decrements much more frequently and within a much shorter time frame (32).

Recent work with improved ^{31}P-NMR resolution techniques has established that force loss occurring in response to a sustained maximal voluntary contraction (MVC) is much more closely related to P_i and specifically $H_2PO_4^-$ than to H^+ accumulation (32). The recovery of force following activity was also much better correlated with P_i and $H_2PO_4^-$ than with H^+ alone. Although H^+ continues to be acknowledged as an important metabolite in fatigue, the conditions under which it alters mechanical performance and the H^+ concentration required to exert an effect at least *in vivo* are uncertain. One possibility is that the role of H^+ in fatigue may become more emphasized during longer periods of heavy activity, after P_i has peaked and progressive increases in H^+ occur (13, 101).

One of the major obstacles to investigating the independent role of H^+, and indeed any metabolite, in fatigue induced *in vivo* is the associated changes that occur in other metabolites. One experimental approach that has been employed to induce acidosis in muscle without changes in other metabolites is to increase the carbon dioxide (CO_2) concentration (86, 99). Meyer et al. (99) used such an approach in perfused cat muscles and reported that intracellular acidification as low as pH 6.5 had little effect on peak tetanic force development in muscles composed of a predominance of either fast- or slow-twitch fibers. Collectively, these results support a conclusion arrived at earlier by Mainwood and Renaud (86), that pH may not be the major factor in promoting disturbances in mechanical function. If such is the case, the conclusions obtained from skinned fiber preparations, at least with regard to pH and performance, may not apply *in vivo*. It should be noted, however, that many protocols examining pH disturbances have investigated only a very specific mechanical property, namely isometric or static force. It is possible that pH may exert its greatest influence in dynamic activity where kinetic behaviour is challenged. Indeed, there is impressive evidence to indicate that such is the case (120).

Although ^{31}P-NMR techniques offer the exciting opportunity to examine intracellular alterations in selected metabolites and fatigability in physiological settings, the procedure is not without limitations. These studies are essentially associative in nature and do not address causality. Another problem has to do with localization of the ^{31}P-NMR signal within the contracting muscle. It is possible that changes in specific metabolites could be localized or compartmentalized within the muscle cell, which are obscured using ^{31}P-NMR (32).

In spite of the impressive advances that have been made in recent years regarding metabolic fatigue and its causes, much remains to be done. Notwithstanding the potential problems associated with extrapolating the results obtained with skinned fiber experiments to *in vivo* settings, we continue to have only a rudimentary understanding of the effects of metabolic end product accumulation on excitation and excitation-contraction coupling. The skinned fiber preparation has permitted examination of metabolic changes at the level of myofibril function only. No such model exists for investigating the metabolic factors affecting sarcolemma Na^+-K^+ ATPase activity and sarcoplasmic reticulum Ca^{2+} uptake and release. It is possible that dependencies on specific metabolic by-products may be substantially different between the different ATPases located at different sites, resulting in much different functional alterations. Compartmentalization of ATP supply mechanisms may also occur regionally in association with the major ATPase enzymes of the fiber. At present, it is unclear to what extent metabolic ATP regenerative pathways differ between the different regions and whether or not differences exist in the accumulation of selected metabolites. Changes in the ionic balance within the fiber must also be considered, both in terms of the interdependency with metabolic changes and in terms of the role of ions in channel and enzyme function (113). As an example, the pronounced K^+ loss that occurs with activity could conceivably alter a wide range of processes within the muscle cell (84).

Fatigue and the Defense
of ATP Concentration: A Model

Given that ATP concentration appears to be highly protected in working muscle, at least during voluntary effort, an association with fatigue is suggested. Muscle ATP concentration represents a balance between ATP synthesis rates and ATP utilization rates (Figure 7.2). With increases in activity, ATP utilization rates, mediated by increases in the activity of the major ATPases in the muscle, increase dramatically. To prevent significant reductions in ATP concentration, ATP regenerative pathways must be sensitively poised to react to any perturbation in ATP. High energy phosphate transfer mechanisms, and in particular PCr hydrolysis, seem to be perfectly equipped as a first line of defense. Relative to ATP, PCr concentration is high, the activity of creatine phosphokinase (CPK) is high, and the equilibrium constant for ATP formation by CPK is large (63). Collectively, these properties enable PCr to be almost completely responsive to fluctuations in ATP concentration. Increases in glycolysis and oxidative phosphorylation are also rapidly activated to protect ATP levels. Current theory on metabolic control stresses a close interrelationship between the change in phosphorylation potential, mediated by changes in the by-products of high energy phosphate transfer and recruitment of both oxidative phosphorylation and glycolysis (28).

In the model presented, fatigue is construed as a protective strategy designed to protect ATP levels when ATP regenerative pathways are incapable of meeting demand. Reductions in ATPase activity reduce ATP utilization rates, and this prevents excessive reductions in ATP levels. Physiologically, the reduction in ATP utilization rates results in fatigue or an inability to generate a desired force. It is interesting, but not surprising, that metabolic by-product accumulation such as increases in P_i appear to couple the severity of the exercise and the metabolic demands that occur to fatigue (28, 32). At least with short-term activity, both the progress of and recovery from fatigue are closely associated with P_i and in particular $H_2PO_4^-$ concentration (32).

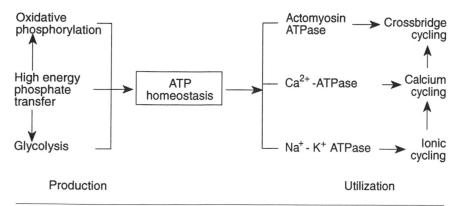

Figure 7.2 Mechanisms used to defend cellular ATP concentration during increased activity. Schema depicts metabolic pathways used to increase ATP production and major processes involved in ATP utilization. ATP homeostasis occurs when ATP synthetic rates balance ATP utilization rates.

The association between metabolic by-product accumulation (in particular, P_i increases) and fatigue onset and recovery may only apply to situations where the activity is relatively brief, lasting for 1 or 2 min. In such circumstances, rapid and full recovery of MVC has been noted, suggesting that the metabolic component is fully responsible for the impairment in performance (7). If the activity is sustained, however, a non-metabolic component also appears to exist, because metabolic recovery precedes force recovery. At present it is unknown what intracellular process is impaired, although excitation-contraction coupling is strongly suspected (7, 135). In this regard it is unclear whether the impairment occurs as a result of prolonged exposure to the accumulated metabolic by-products or whether it occurs independently and as a consequence of the repetitive activity per se. Mainwood and Renaud (86) have hypothesized that it is the incubation of the muscle cell in the environment containing accumulated metabolic by-products such as H^+ that induces the persistent weakness that follows more prolonged activity.

An intriguing issue is whether during the course of fatigue, intracellular changes might modify ATP regenerative mechanisms, thereby creating a greater strain on protective strategies designed to defend ATP balance. As an example, Gollnick et al. (49) have found that high-intensity intermittent running in horses induced significant impairment in skeletal muscle mitochondrial respiratory capacity when measured *in vitro*. This finding supports earlier work in which changes in mitochondrial ultrastructure were found after multiple bouts of exercise (104). Other studies using measures of maximal enzymatic activity have also found a down regulation of some of the mitochondrial enzymes following exercise (73). Alterations in glycolytic potential have also been examined following short-term intense activity. Interestingly, *in vitro* studies have demonstrated reductions in maximal phosphofructokinase (PFK) activity, a key regulator of glycolysis at pH ranges typical of heavy exercise, but a depression in glycolytic flux does not appear to result during *in situ* and *in vivo* conditions (119). However, a reduction in glycolytic flux rate can be demonstrated during intense, short-term activity with an occluded circulation which prevents lactate removal from the contracting muscle. The significance of these results on ATP regenerative mechanisms remains unknown. It has been estimated that flux potential via oxidative phosphorylation and glycolysis is far in excess of what can be recruited during maximal activity. If such is the case, the depression in flux potential that occurs in certain conditions may merely compromise the reserve. If the reduction in flux potential impinges on the flux rate needed to sustain ATP synthesis, ATP homeostasis could be seriously challenged unless a down regulation in ATP utilization rates occurs.

A down regulation in ATP utilization rates does appear to occur as evidenced by the reductions in ATPase activity and reductions in force

(30). However, other strategies may operate to downregulate ATP utilization rates while attempting to preserve muscular performance. Previous investigators have determined that in muscles composed of a high proportion of fast fibers ATP utilization rates during intense activity can be reduced with only minimal changes in the tension-time index (21). Such an increase in efficiency does not appear to extend to muscles of essentially slow-twitch composition.

A potential intracellular strategy to downregulate ATP costs may occur via myosin light chain phosphorylation, a phenomenon that is also restricted to fast-twitch fibers (122). It seems clear that myosin light chain phosphorylation results in a potentiation of twitch force and in force below approximately 50% of peak tetanic contraction (122). Under such conditions, myosin light chain phosphorylation, which would occur soon after the initiation of activity, could serve to defend force in the face of reductions in myofibrillar ATPase activity and ATP turnover (30).

Yet another strategy may be operative during voluntary activity. During intense short-term activity, the frequency of stimulation needed to fully activate the fatiguing muscle is reduced (12). The reduction in the stimulation frequency is perceived as being a compensatory adjustment designed to minimize excitation failure in the sarcolemma and T tubule system. According to this hypothesis, the prolongation in relaxation time that accompanies this form of exercise allows for a reduction in stimulation frequency, while still exploiting the residual force potential remaining in the muscle (12).

The reductions in calcium cycling by the sarcoplasmic reticulum may also contribute to the increased efficiency that has been observed in fatiguing muscle. Calcium uptake by the sarcoplasmic reticulum can represent an expensive component of the energy requirement of the contracting muscle, estimated at upwards of 30% in some types of activity (110). For example, in isometric activity force may be preserved by decreasing Ca^{2+} uptake and Ca^{2+} release while maintaining cytosolic Ca^{2+} levels. Consequently, a depression in SR ATPase activity could be construed as a beneficial accommodation design to protect the force remaining in the muscle at reduced Ca^{2+} cycling rates and reduced energy costs.

All of the potential strategies would appear to be most effective only in isometric type activity and only in fast fibers where both SR Ca^{2+} ATPase and myofibrillar ATPase activities are very high relative to slow-twitch fibers. However, these strategies would appear to negatively impact dynamic performance, where ATP hydrolysis rates are critical in supporting rapid cycling of crossbridges.

Training and Metabolic Fatigue

Regular exercise is known to result in profound increases in fatigue resistance. At least part of the increase in work capacity following training appears to be mediated by reducing the metabolic component of fatigue. With training, a tighter metabolic control results such that at a given submaximal work intensity, oxidative phosphorylation is preserved with lower concentrations of the metabolites, such as AMP, ADP, Cr, and P_i, which are involved in high energy phosphate transfer reactions (90). Muscle lactate concentration and consequently H^+ levels are also reduced (67, 90). The reductions in both P_i and H^+ would be expected to result in a greater fatigue resistance.

Another conspicuous adaptation resulting from training is a pronounced reduction in the rate at which glycogen is depleted from the muscle during prolonged exercise. Numerous previous studies (as reviewed by Green, 55) have established a dependency between the availability of muscle glycogen and the ability to perform prolonged exercise. Conceivably, the glycogen sparing effect of training would be expected to contribute to the enhancement of work performance.

Differences in the metabolic response to exercise may also underlie the differences that have been observed in fatigability between the different fiber types and subtypes (15). Fast fibers with low oxidative potential (FG) are rapidly fatigable and are characterized by large changes in metabolic end product accumulation (65). Both slow-twitch (SO) and fast-twitch-oxidative-glycolytic (FOG) fibers, on the other hand, are much less fatigable than FG fibers. Both of these fiber types also display a much tighter metabolic control, demonstrating substantially less change in phosphorylation potential at a given level of ATP turnover (37).

The common denominator differentiating loose versus tight metabolic control responses and fatigability appears to be the oxidative potential of the fiber (37, 51, 67). With a high mitochondrial potential, sensitivity is increased and a given level of respiration can be obtained with lower levels of the postulated effectors, such as P_i and ADP. The lower levels of these metabolic by-products also appear to impact on glycogenolysis and glycolysis, resulting in less lactic acid and a higher pH. The difference in metabolic response could be responsible for the increased fatigue resistance in fibers with high oxidative potential (79). It has also been hypothesized that increases in fatigue resistance consequent to training are closely associated with increases in mitochondrial potential (67, 90). However, this hypothesis does not appear to be totally valid from at least two perspectives.

Training can induce a tighter metabolic response without increases occurring in mitochondrial potential (52), and the tighter metabolic response appears to be accompanied by improved work tolerance (57). Furthermore, substantive increases in fatigue resistance can occur independently of increases in oxidative potential (3, 89, 116). These observations suggest that more than the oxidative potential might be involved in determining the fatigue resistant nature of the fiber. In this regard, regular activity can induce extensive adaptations at all levels of organization (108). These adaptations could serve to decrease the sensitivity of the excitation-concentration processes to given metabolic end product perturbations in the intracellular environment with repetitive activity. Alternatively, the changes in the content and composition of the organelle involved in translating the neural signal into force may be better able to withstand the challenges that occur with repetitive activation, independent of any metabolic consideration.

Summary

Identification of the mechanisms underlying neuromuscular fatigue during repetitive, voluntary activity remains the ultimate quest for investigators engaged in research in this area. Although impressive advances have been made and continue to be made, definitive conclusions will continue to prove elusive. There are many reasons for this. In the first case, tasks are generally very complex, containing varying proportions of a number of physical parameters, the importance of which may change during different phases of the task. Further tasks may vary in the intensity, the velocity, and the muscle length at which they are performed. Many tasks also involve recruitment of more than one muscle with highly individualized recruitment and decruitment profiles. The muscles involved in the task may be composed of different fiber types, with different synergistic muscles depending on one fiber type more than another. All of these considerations influence both the onset and the progress of fatigue.

Many sites also exist as potential failure points within the contracting muscle cell. Which site becomes limiting and under what conditions remain uncertain. Tasks differ in the challenge placed on the different excitation and contraction processes, and it is possible that this may be an important consideration in the loss of functional integrity experienced by a given process. However, it is not at all clear whether different sites have different tolerances to combat the repeated challenges induced by the task.

Impressive progress is being made in understanding activity induced disturbances in selected excitation-contraction processes. In general, the cause of such disturbances has been dichotomized into metabolic and nonmetabolic factors. Metabolic factors address the role of energy potential and the deleterious effects induced by alterations in energy state and by-product accumulation. Using a variety of techniques, investigators are gaining increasing evidence that changes in selected by-products can have a potent influence on a number of intracellular processes (69, 70, 128). At least with brief acute exercise, these metabolic by-products appear to underlie force failure, the specific mechanical effect depending to some degree on the metabolite species (30).

Nonmetabolic fatigue, or fatigue that occurs in the absence of a significant metabolic disturbance, is also well documented (5). This type of fatigue is most readily apparent after eccentric exercise where the energy demands are low but the force production is high (23). Although this type of exercise is accompanied by disruptions in the internal organization of the fiber, it is not clear whether force impairment is due to a specific site or involves a combination of several sites. Nonmetabolic fatigue can also be demonstrated in a variety of tasks and is characterized by a persistent weakness after metabolic recovery has occurred. An intriguing yet unproved hypothesis is that changes in the intracellular environment, mediated by metabolic factors, if allowed to persist for a critical period, induce structural or compositional changes in membranes and proteins at selected intracellular sites.

In the voluntary exercising human, identification of a failing site within the muscle may also be complicated by central considerations. It is generally recognized that some degree of neural compensation is possible to offset failure in the muscle cell. This compensation would appear to involve changing the activation pattern to specific motor units. The degree to which this is possible would depend on the characteristics of the activity. More intense activities reduce the possible strategies that can be invoked because firing frequency and motor unit recruitment are near maximal at the onset of the task. Indeed, with this degree of strain imposed on the excitation and contraction process, changes in the intracellular environment may only have to change minimally to effect deterioration in performance (69).

Acknowledgments

This work was supported by the Natural Sciences and Engineering Research Council (Canada) and Sport Canada.

References

1. Abramcheck, C.W.; Best, P.M. Physiological role and selectivity of the in situ potassium channel of the sarcoplasmic reticulum in skinned frog skeletal muscle fibers. J. Gen. Physiol. 93:1-22; 1989.

2. Allen, D.C.; Lee, J.A.; Westerblad, H. Intracellular calcium and tension during fatigue in isolated single muscle fibres from Xenopus Laevis. J. Physiol. 415:433-458; 1989.

3. Alway, S.E. Is fiber mitochondrial volume density a good indicator of muscle fatigability to isometric exercise? J. Appl. Physiol. 70:2111-2119; 1991.

4. Amerides, B.T.; Clanton, T.L. Increased fatigue of isovelocity vs. isometric contractions of canine diaphragm. J. Appl. Physiol. 69:740-746; 1990.

5. Armstrong, R.B.; Warren, G.L.; Warren, J.A. Mechanisms of exercise-induced muscle fibre injury. Sports Med. 12:184-207; 1991.

6. Astrand, P.O.; Rodahl, K. Textbook of work physiology. New York: McGraw-Hill; 1986: 523-576.

7. Baker, A.J.; Kostov, K.G.; Miller, R.G.; Weiner, M.W. Slow force recovery after long duration exercise: metabolic and activation factors in muscle fatigue. J. Appl. Physiol. 74:2294-2300; 1993.

8. Barclay, C.J.; Cureton, N.A.; Woledge, R.C. Changes in crossbridge and non-crossbridge energetics during moderate fatigue of frog muscle fibres. J. Physiol. 468:543-555; 1993.

9. Belcastro, A.; Parkhouse, W.; Dobson, G.; Gilchrist, J.S. Influence of exercise on cardiac and skeletal muscle myofibrillar proteins. Mol. Cell. Biochem. 83:27-36; 1988.

10. Belcastro, A.N.; MacLean, I.; Gilchrist, J. Biochemical basis of muscle fatigue associated with repetitious contractions of skeletal muscle. Int. J. Biochem. 17:447-453; 1985.

11. Bigland-Ritchie, B. Muscle fatigue and its influence on changing neural drive. Clin. Chest Med. 5:21-34; 1984.

12. Bigland-Ritchie, B.; Woods, J.J. Changes in muscle contractile properties and neural control during human muscle fatigue. Muscle & Nerve 7:691-699; 1984.

13. Boska, M.D.; Moussavi, R.S.; Carson, P.J.; Weiner, M.W.; Miller, R.G. The metabolic basis of recovery after fatiguing exercise in human muscle. Neurol. 40:240-244; 1990.

14. Brooks, S.V.; Faulkner, J.A. Forces and powers of slow and fast skeletal muscles in mice during repeated contractions. J. Physiol. 436:701-710; 1991.

15. Burke, R.E.; Levine, D.N.; Tsairis, P.; Zajac, F.E. Physiological types and histochemical profiles in motor units of the cat gastrocnemius. J. Physiol. (London) 234:723-748; 1973.

16. Byrd, S.K. Alterations in the sarcoplasmic reticulum: a possible link to exercise-induced muscle damage. Med. Sci. Sports Ex. 24:531-536; 1992.

17. Byrd, S.K.; Bode, A.K.; Klug, G.A. Effects of exercise of varying duration on sarcoplasmic reticulum function. J. Appl. Physiol. 66:1383-1388; 1989.

18. Byrd, S.K.; McCutcheon, L.J.; Hodgson, D.R.; Gollnick, P.D. Altered sarcoplasmic reticulum function after high intensity exercise. J. Appl. Physiol. 67:2072-2077; 1989.

19. Cady, E.B.; Elshoue, H.; Jones, D.A.; Moll, A. The metabolic causes of slow relaxation in fatigued human skeletal muscle. J. Physiol. 418:327-337; 1989.

20. Cady, E.B.; Jones, D.A.; Lynn, J.; Newham, D.J. Changes in force and intracellular metabolites during fatigue of human skeletal muscle. J. Physiol. (London) 418:311-325; 1989.

21. Chase, P.B.; Kushmerick, M.J. Effects of pH on contraction of rabbit fast and slow skeletal muscle fibers. Biophysical J. 53:935-946; 1988.

22. Clarke, D.M.; Loo, T.W.; MacLennan, D.H. Functional consequences of alterations of amino acids located in the nucleotide-binding domain of Ca^{2+}-ATPase of sarcoplasmic reticulum. J. Biol. Chem. 265:14088-14092; 1990.

23. Clarkson, P.M.; Nosaka, K.; Braun, B. Muscle function after exercise-induced muscle damage and rapid adaptation. Med. Sci. Sports Ex. 24:512-520; 1992.

24. Clausen, T. Regulation of active Na⁺-K⁺ transport in skeletal muscle. Physiol. Rev. 66(3):542-580; 1986.

25. Clausen, T. Significance of Na⁺-K⁺ pump regulation in skeletal muscle. News in Physiol. Sci. 5:148-151; 1990.

26. Connett, R.J. Analysis of metabolic control: new insights using a scaled creatine kinase model. Am. J. Physiol. 254:R949-R959; 1988.

27. Connett, R.J.; Honig, C.R. Reply: Letter to the editor. J. Appl. Physiol. R289-R290; 1990.

28. Connett, R.J.; Honig, C.R.; Gayeski, T.E.J.; Brooks, G.A. Defining hypoxia: a systems view of VO_2, glycolysis, energetics and intracellular PO_2. J. Appl. Physiol. 68:833-842; 1990.

29. Cooke, R.; Franks, K.; Luciani, G.; Pate, E. The inhibition of rabbit skeletal muscle contraction by hydrogen ions and phosphate. J. Physiol. 395:77-97; 1988.

30. Cooke, R.; Pate, E. The inhibition of muscle contraction by the by-products of ATP hydrolysis. In: Taylor, B., ed. Biochemistry of exercise. VII. Champaign, IL: Human Kinetics; 1990: 59-72.

31. Dawson, M.J.; Gadian, D.G.; Wilkie, D.R. Mechanical relaxation rate and metabolism studied in fatiguing muscle by phosphorous nuclear magnetic resonance. J. Physiol. 299:465-484; 1980.

32. De Groot, M.; Massie, B.M.; Boska, M.; Gober, J.; Miller, R.G.; Weiner, M.W. Dissociation of [H⁺] from fatigue in human muscle detected by high resolution ³¹P-NMR. Muscle & Nerve 16:91-98; 1993.

33. Dixon, D.; Corbett, A.; Haynes, D.H. Effect of ATP/ADP/phosphate potential on the maximal steady-state uptake of Ca^{2+} by skeletal muscle sarcoplasmic reticulum. J. Bioenergetics & Biomembranes 14:87-96; 1982.

34. Dixon, I.M.; Hata, T.; Dhalla, N.S. Sarcolemmal Na⁺-K⁺ ATPase activity in congestive heart failure due to myocardial infarction. Am. J. Physiol. 262:C664-C671; 1992.

35. Donaldson, S.K. Mammalian muscle fiber types: comparison of excitation-contraction coupling mechanisms. Acta Physiol. Scand. 128 (Suppl. 556):157-166; 1986.

36. Donaldson, S.K. Fatigue of sarcoplasmic reticulum: failure of excitation-contraction coupling in skeletal muscle. In Taylor, A.W.; Gollnick, P.D.; Green, H.J.; Ianuzzo, C.D.; Noble, E.G.; Métivier, G.; Sutton, J.R., eds. Biochemistry of exercise. VII. Champaign, IL: Human Kinetics; 1990:49-57.

37. Dudley, G.A.; Tullson, P.C.; Terjung, R.L. Influence of mitochondrial content on the sensitivity of respiratory control. J. Biol. Chem. 262:9109-9114; 1987.

38. Dux, L.; Green, H.J.; Pette, D. Chronic low-frequency stimulation of rabbit fast-twitch muscle induces partial inactivation of the sarcoplasmic reticulum Ca^{2+}-ATPase and changes in its tryptic cleavage. Europ. J. Biochem. 195:92-100; 1990.

39. Edman, K.A.P.; Lou, F. Myofibrillar fatigue versus failure of activation during repetitive stimulation of frog muscle fibres. J. Physiol. 457:655-673; 1992.

40. Edwards, R.H.T. Physiological analysis of skeletal muscle weakness and fatigue. Clin. Sci. Mol. Med. 54:463-470; 1978.

41. Enoka, R.M.; Stuart, D.A. Neurobiology of muscle fatigue. J. Appl. Physiol. 72:1631-1648; 1992.

42. Everts, M.E.; Clausen, T. Activation of the Na-K pump by intracellular Na in rat slow- and fast-twitch muscle. Acta Physiol. Scand. 145:353-362; 1992.

43. Fabiato, A.; Fabiato, F. Effects of pH on the myofilaments and the sarcoplasmic reticulum of skinned cells from cardiac and skeletal muscles. J. Physiol. (London) 276:233-255; 1978.

44. Favero, T.G.; Pessah, I.N.; Klug, G.A. Prolonged exercise reduces Ca^{2+}-release in rat skeletal muscle sarcoplasmic reticulum. Pflügers Arch. 422:472-475; 1993.

45. Fitts, R.H.; Courtright, J.B.; Kim, D.H.; Witzmann, F.A. Muscle fatigue with prolonged exercise: contractile and biochemical alterations. Am. J. Physiol. 242:C65-C73; 1982.

46. Fuglevand, A.J.; Zackowski, K.M.; Huey, K.A.; Enoka, R.M. Impairment of neuromuscular propagation during human fatiguing contractions at submaximal forces. J. Physiol. 460:549-572; 1993.

47. Funk, C.I.; Clark, A., Jr.; Connett, R.J. A simple model of aerobic metabolism: applications to work transitions in muscle. Am. J. Physiol. 258:C995-C1005; 1990.

48. Godt, R.E.; Nosek, T.M. Changes of intracellular milieu with fatigue or hypoxia depress contraction of rabbit skeletal and cardiac muscle. J. Physiol. 412:155-180; 1989.

49. Gollnick, P.D.; Bertocci, L.A.; Kelso, T.B.; Witt, E.H.; Hodgson, D.R. The effect of high intensity exercise on the respiratory capacity of skeletal muscle. Pflügers Arch. 415:405-413; 1990.

50. Gollnick, P.D.; Korge, P.; Karpakka, J.; Saltin, B. Elongation of skeletal muscle relaxation during exercise is linked to reduced calcium uptake by the sarcoplasmic reticulum in man. Acta Physiol. Scand. 142:135-136; 1991.

51. Gollnick, P.D.; Saltin, B. Significance of skeletal muscle oxidative enzyme enhancement with endurance training. Clin. Physiol. 2:1-12; 1982.

52. Green, H.; Helyar, R.; Ball-Burnett, M.; Kowalchuk, N.; Symon, S.; Farrance, B. Metabolic adaptations to training precede changes in muscle mitochondrial capacity. J. Appl. Physiol. 72:484-491; 1992.

53. Green, H.J. Manifestations and sites of neuromuscular fatigue. In: Taylor, A.W.; Gollnick, P.D.; Green, H.J.; Ianuzzo, D.; Noble, E.G.; Métivier, G.; Sutton, J., eds. Biochemistry of exercise. VII. Champaign, IL: Human Kinetics; 1990: 13-35.

54. Green, H.J. Neuromuscular aspects of fatigue. In: Shepherd, R.; Jacob, I., eds. Human adaptation to prolonged exercise. Can. J. Sport Sci. 12(Suppl. 1):7-20; 1987.

55. Green, H.J. How important is endogenous muscle glycogen to fatigue in prolonged exercise? Can. J. Physiol. Pharmacol. 69:290-297; 1991.

56. Green, H.J.; Ball-Burnett, M.; Chin, E.R.; Pette, D. Time dependent alterations in sarcolemma Na^+-K^+ ATPase content of low-frequency stimulated rabbit muscle. FEBS Lett. 310:129-131; 1992.

57. Green, H.J.; Chin, E.R.; Ball-Burnett, M.; Ranney, D. Increases in human skeletal muscle Na^+-K^+ ATPase concentration with short term training. Am. J. Physiol. 264:C1538-C1541; 1993.

58. Green, H.J.; Patla, A.E. Maximal aerobic power: neuromuscular and metabolic considerations. Med. Sci. Sports Ex. 24:38-46; 1992.

59. Grover, A.K.; Khan, I. Calcium pump isoforms: diversity, selectivity and plasticity. Cell Calcium 13:9-17; 1992.

60. Hackney, D.D.; Clark, P.K. Steady state kinetics of high enzyme concentration. The myosin Mg ATPase. J. Biol. Chem. 260:5505-5510; 1985.

61. Hägg, G.M. Interpretation of EMG spectral alterations and alteration indices at sustained contraction. J. Appl. Physiol. 73:1211-1217; 1992.

62. Henneman, E. The size principle. A deterministic output emerges from a set of probabilistic connections. J. Exp. Biol. 115:103-112; 1985.

63. Hochachka, P.W. Fuels and pathways as designed systems for support of muscular work. J. Exp. Biol. 115:191-200; 1985.

64. Hochachka, P.W. The lactate paradox. Analysis of underlying mechanisms. Ann. Sports Med. 4:184-188; 1988.

65. Hochachka, P.W. Muscles as molecular and metabolic machines. Boca Raton, FL: CRC Press; 1994: 69-93.

66. Hochachka, P.W.; Matheson, G.O. Regulatory ATP turnover over broad dynamic work ranges in skeletal muscles. J. Appl. Physiol. 73:1697-1703; 1992.

67. Holloszy, J.O.; Coyle, E.F. Adaptations of skeletal muscle to endurance exercise and their metabolic consequences. J. Appl. Physiol. 56:831-838; 1984.

68. Huang, W.-H.; Askari, A. Regulation of (Na^+, K^+) ATPase by inorganic phosphate: pH dependence and physiologic implications. Biochem. Biophys. Res. Commun. 123:438-443; 1984.

69. Hultman, E.; Bergström, M.; Spriet, L.L.; Soderlund, K. Energy metabolism and fatigue. In: Taylor, A.W.; Gollnick, P.D.; Green, H.J.; Ianuzzo, C.D.; Noble, E.G.; Métivier, G.; Sutton, J.R., eds. Biochemistry of exercise. VII. Champaign, IL: Human Kinetics; 1990: 73-92.

70. Hultman, E.; Spriet, L.L.; Söderlund, K. Energy metabolism and fatigue in working muscle. In: MacLeod, D.; Maughan, R.; Nimmo, M.; Reilly, T.; Williams, C., eds. Exercise, benefits, limits and adaptations. Northway, England: E.F.N. Spars; 1987: 63-84.

71. Inesi, G.; Millman, M.; Eletr, S. Temperature induced transitions of function and structure in sarcoplasmic reticulum membranes. J. Mol. Biol. 81:483-504; 1973.

72. Inesi, G.; Sumbilla, C.; Kirtley, M.E. Relationship of molecular structure and function in Ca^{2+}-transport ATPase. Physiol. Rev. 70:749-760; 1990.

73. Ji, L.-L.; Stratman, F.W.; Lardy, H.A. Enzymatic down regulation with exercise in rat skeletal muscle. Arch. Biochem. Biophys. 263:137-149; 1988.

74. Jones, D.A. Muscle fatigue due to changes beyond the neuromuscular junction. In: Porter, R.; Whelan, J., eds. Human muscle fatigue: physiological mechanisms. London: Pitman Medical; 1981: 178-196.

75. Jones, N.L.; Heigenhauser, G.J.F. Effects of hydrogen ions on metabolism during exercise. In: Lamb, D.R.; Gilsolfi, C.V., eds. Energy metabolism in exercise and sport (perspectives in exercise science and sports medicine). Carmel, IN: Brown and Benchmark; 1992: 107-148.

76. Juel, C. The effect of β_2-adrenergic activation on ionic shifts and fatigue in mouse soleus muscle stimulated in vitro. Acta Physiol. Scand. 134:209-216; 1988.

77. Kim, M.; Akera, T. O_2 free radicals: cause of ischemia reperfusion injury to cardiac Na^+-K^+ ATPase. Am. J. Physiol. 252:H252-H257; 1987.

78. Krogh-Lund, C.; Jørgensen, K. Changes in conduction velocity, median frequency, and root mean sware-amplitude of the electromyogram during 25% maximal voluntary contraction of the triceps brachii muscle, to limit of endurance. Europ. J. Appl. Physiol. 63:60-69; 1991.

79. Kugelberg, E.; Lindegren, B. Transmission and contraction fatigue of rat motor units in relation to succinate dehydrogenase activity of motor unit fibres. J. Physiol. 288:285-300; 1979.

80. Kukreja, R.G.; Okabe, E.; Schrier, G.M.; Hess, M. Oxygen radical-mediated lipid peroxidation and inhibition of Ca^{2+}-ATPase activity of cardiac sarcoplasmic reticulum. Arch. Biochem. Biophys. 261:447-457; 1988.

81. Lacapere, J.J.; Bennet, N.; Dupont, Y.; Guillian, F. pH and magnesium dependence of ATP binding to sarcoplasmic reticulum ATPase. J. Biol. Chem. 265:348-353; 1990.

82. Leberer, E.; Härtner, K.T.; Pette, D. Reversible inhibition of sarcoplasmic reticulum Ca-ATPase by altered neuromuscular activity in rabbit fast-twitch muscle. Europ. J. Biochem. 162:555-561; 1987.

83. Lindinger, M.I.; Heigenhauser, G.F. The role of ion fluxes in skeletal muscle fatigue. Can. J. Physiol. Pharmacol. 69:246-253; 1991.

84. Lindinger, M.I.; Sjøgaard, G. Potassium regulation during exercise and recovery. Sports Med. 11(6):382-401; 1991.

85. MacLennan, D.H. Molecular tools to elucidate problems in excitation-contraction coupling. Biophys. J. 58:1355-1365; 1990.

86. Mainwood, G.W.; Renaud, J.M. The effect of acid-base balance on fatigue in skeletal muscle. Can. J. Physiol. Pharmacol. 63:403-416; 1985.

87. Matushita, S.; Dux, L.; Pette, D. Separation of the active and inactive (non-phosphorylating) Ca^{2+}-ATPase in sarcoplasmic reticulum subfractions from low-frequency stimulated rabbit muscles. FEBS Lett. 294:203-206; 1991.

88. Matushita, S.; Pette, D. Inactivation of the sarcoplasmic reticulum ATPase in low frequency stimulated muscle results from a modification of the active site. Biochem. J. 285:303-309; 1992.

89. Mayne, C.N.; Anderson, W.A.; Hammond, R.L.; Eisenberg, B.R.; Stephenson, L.W.; Salmons, S. Correlates of fatigue resistance in canine skeletal muscle stimulated electrically for up to one year. Am. J. Physiol. 261:C259-C270; 1992.

90. McCully, K.K.; Clarke, B.J.; Kent, J.A.; Wilson, J.; Chance, B. Biochemical adaptations to training: implications for resisting muscle fatigue. Can. J. Physiol. Pharmacol. 69:274-278; 1991.

91. McKenna, M.J.; Schmidt, T.A.; Hargreaves, M.; Cameron, L.; Skinner, S.L.; Kjeldsen, K. Sprint training increases human skeletal muscle Na^+-K^+ ATPase concentration and improves K^+ regulation. J. Appl. Physiol. 75:173-180; 1993.

92. Medda, P.; Fassold, E.; Hasselbach, W. The effect of monovalent and divalent cations on the ATP-dependent Ca^{2+}-binding and phosphorylation during the reaction cycle of the sarcoplasmic reticulum Ca^{2+}-transport ATPase. Europ. J. Biochem. 165:251-259; 1987.

93. Meissner, G. Adenine nucleotide stimulation of Ca^{2+}-induced Ca^{2+} release in sarcoplasmic reticulum. J. Biol. Soc. 259:2365-2374; 1984.

94. Meissner, G. Adenine nucleotide stimulation of Ca^{2+} release by sarcoplasmic reticulum. Effects of Ca^{2+}, Mg^{2+} and adenine nucleotides. Biochem. J. 25:236-244; 1986.

95. Meissner, G.; Hendersen, J.S. Rapid calcium release from cardiac sarcoplasmic reticulum vesicles is dependent on Ca^{2+} and is modulated by Mg^{2+}, adenine nucleotide and calmodulin. J. Biol. Chem. 262:3065-3073; 1987.

96. Mellgren, R.L. Calcium-dependent proteases: an enzyme system active at cellular membranes. FASEB J. 1:110-115; 1987.

97. Metzger, J.M. Mechanism of chemical mechanical coupling in skeletal muscle during work. In: Lamb, D.R.; Gisolfi, C.V., eds. Energy metabolism in exercise and sport (perspectives in exercise science and sports medicine) vol. 5. Cornell, IN: Brown and Benchmark; 1992: 1-51.

98. Metzger, J.M.; Moss, R.L. pH modulation of the kinetics of a Ca^{2+}-sensitive cross-bridge state transition in mammalian single skeletal muscle fibres. J. Physiol. (London) 428:751-764; 1990.

99. Meyer, R.A.; Adams, G.R.; Fisher, J.M.; et al. Effect of decreased pH on force and phosphocreatine in mammalian skeletal muscle. Can. J. Physiol. Pharmacol. 69:305-310; 1991.

100. Miller, R.G.; Boska, M.D.; Moussavi, R.S.; Carson, P.J.; Weiner, M.W. ^{31}P nuclear magnetic resonance studies of human energy phosphates and pH in human muscle fatigue: comparison of aerobic and anaerobic exercise. J. Clin. Invest. 81:1190-1196; 1988.

101. Miller, R.G.; Gianinni, D.; Layzer, R.B.; Koretsky, A.P.; Hooper, D.; Weiner, M.W. Effects of fatiguing exercise on high-energy phosphates, force and EMG: evidence for 3 phases of recovery. Muscle & Nerve 10:810-821; 1987.

102. Moss, R.L.; Reiser, P.J.; Greaser, M.L.; Eddinger, T.J. Varied expression of alkali light chains is associated with altered speed of contraction in rabbit fast-twitch skeletal muscles. In: Pette, D., ed. The dynamic site of muscle fibers. New York: Walter de Gruyter; 1990: 355-368.

103. Nassar-Gentina, V.; Passonneau, J.V.; Rapoport, S.I. Fatigue and metabolism of frog muscle fibers during stimulation and in response to caffeine. Am. J. Physiol. 241:C160-C166; 1981.

104. Nimmo, M.A.; Snow, D.H. Time course of ultrastructural changes in skeletal muscle after two types of exercise. J. Appl. Physiol. 52:910-913; 1982.

105. Nosek, T.M.; Fender, K.Y.; Godt, R.E. Is it diprotonated inorganic phosphate that depresses force in skeletal muscle fibers? Science 236:191-193; 1987.

106. Parkhouse, W.S. The effects of ATP, inorganic phosphate, protons and lactate on isolated myofibrillar ATPase activity. Can. J. Physiol. Pharmacol. 70:1175-1181; 1992.

107. Patla, A.E. Some neuromuscular strategies characterizing adaptation process during prolonged activity in humans. Can. J. Sport Sci. 12(3):33S-44S; 1982.

108. Pette, D.; Düsterhöft, S. Altered gene expression in fast-twitch muscle induced by chronic low-frequency stimulation. Am. J. Physiol. 262:R333-R338; 1992.

109. Rüegg, J.C. Excitation-contraction coupling in fast- and slow-twitch muscle fibers. Int. J. Sports Med. 8:360-364; 1987.

110. Rüegg, J.C. Calcium in muscle activation. New York: Springer Verlag; 1988.

111. Sapega, A.A.; Sokolow, D.P.; Graham, T.J.; Chance, B. Phosphorus nuclear magnetic resonance: a non-invasive technique for the study of muscle bioenergetics during exercise. Med. Sci. Sports Ex. 19:410-420; 1987.

112. Scherer, N.M.; Deamer, D.W. Oxidative stress impairs the function of the sarcoplasmic reticulum by oxidation of sulfhydryl groups in the Ca^{2+}-ATPase. Arch. Biochem. Biophys. 246:589-601; 1986.

113. Sejersted, O.M. Electrolyte imbalance in body fluids as a mechanism of fatigue during exercise. In: Lamb, D.R.; Gisolfi, C.V., eds. Energy metabolism in exercise and sport (perspectives in exercise science and sport medicine). Carmel, IN: Brown and Benchmark; 1992: 149-206.

114. Selinsky, B.S.; Yearle, P.L. Effects of potassium on lipid-protein interactions in light sarcoplasmic reticulum. J. Biochem. 29:415-421; 1990.

115. Seow, C.Y.; Stephens, N.L. Fatigue of mouse diaphragm muscle in isometric and isotonic contractions. J. Appl. Physiol. 64:2388-2393; 1988.

116. Simoneau, J.A.; Kaufmann, M.; Pette, D. Asynchronous increases in oxidative capacity and resistance to fatigue of electrostimulated muscles of rat and rabbit. J. Physiol. 460:573-580; 1993.

117. Sjøgaard, G. Role of exercise induced potassium fluxes underlying muscle fatigue: a brief review. Can. J. Physiol. Pharmacol. 69:238-245; 1991.

118. Sorrentino, V.; Volpe, P. Ryanodine receptors: how many, where and why? Trends in Pharmacol. Sci. 14:98-103; 1993.

119. Spriet, L.L. Anaerobic metabolism in human skeletal muscle during short-term intensity activity. Can. J. Physiol. Pharmacol. 70:157-165; 1992.

120. Stevens, E.D. Effect of pH and stimulus phase on work done by isolated frog sartorius muscle during cyclical contraction. J. Muscle Res. Cell Motil. 9:329-333; 1988.

121. Stevens, E.D.; Syme, D.A. The relative changes in isometric force and work during fatigue and recovery in isolated food sartorius muscle. Can. J. Physiol. Pharmacol. 67:1544-1548; 1989.

122. Sweeney, H.L.; Bowman, B.F.; Stull, J.T. Myosin light chain phosphorylation in vertebrate striated muscle: regulation and function. Am. J. Physiol. 264:C1085-C1095; 1993.

123. Thompson, L.V.; Balog, E.M.; Riley, D.A.; Fitts, R.H. Muscle fatigue in frog semitendinosus: alterations in contractile function. Am. J. Physiol. 262:C1500-C1506; 1992.

124. Tibbits, G.F. Role of the sarcolemma in muscle fatigue. In: Taylor, A.W.; Gollnick, P.D.; Green, H.J.; Ianuzzo, C.D.; Noble, E.G.; Métivier, G.; Sutton, J.R., eds. Biochemistry of exercise. VII. Champaign, IL: Human Kinetics; 1990: 37-47.

125. Timmerman, M.; Ashley, C. Excitation-contraction coupling. Bridging the gap. J. Muscle Res. Cell Motil. 9:367-369; 1988.

126. Turcotte, R.A.; Belcastro, A.N. Biochemical adaptation of cardiac and skeletal muscle to physical activity. Int. J. Biochem. 23:221-226; 1991.

127. Turcotte, R.A.; Oueslati, H.; Gardiner, P.F. Ca^{2+} activation properties of myofibrillar ATPase from fatigued rat plantaris. Comp. Biochem. Physiol. 100A:187-192; 1991.

128. Vøllestad, N.K.; Sejersted, O.M. Biochemical correlates of fatigue. A brief review. Europ. J. Appl. Physiol. 57:336-347; 1988.

129. Vøllestad, N.K.; Sejersted, O.M.; Bahr, R.; Woods, J.J.; Bigland-Ritchie, B. Motor drive and metabolic responses during repeated submaximal contractions in humans. J. Appl. Physiol. 64:1421-1427; 1988.

130. Weiner, M.W.; Moussavi, R.S.; Baker, A.J.; Boska, M.D.; Miller, R.G. Constant relationships between force, phosphate concentration and pH in muscles with different fatiguability. Neurol. 40:1888-1893; 1990.

131. Westerblad, H.; Allen, D.G. Changes in myoplasmic calcium concentration during fatigue in single mouse muscle fibers. J. Gen. Physiol. 98:615-635; 1991.

132. Westerblad, H.; Duty, S.; Allen, D.G. Intracellular calcium concentration during low-frequency fatigue in isolated single fibers of mouse skeletal muscle. J. Appl. Physiol. 75:382-388; 1993.

133. Westerblad, H.; Lännergren, J. Slowing of relaxation during fatigue in single mouse muscle fibres. J. Physiol. 434:323-336; 1991.

134. Westerblad, H.; Lee, A.J.; Lamb, A.G.; Bolsover, S.R.; Allen, D.G. Spatial gradients of intracellular calcium in skeletal muscle during fatigue. Pflügers Arch. 4152:734-740; 1990.

135. Westerblad, H.; Lee, J.A.; Lännergren, J.; Allen, D.G. Cellular mechanisms of fatigue in skeletal muscle. Am. J. Physiol. 261:C195-C209; 1991.

Index

A

Acetoacetate, 88, 120
Acetylcarnitine, 163
Acetyl-CoA, 41, 113, 141, 192, 194
Acetyl-CoA carboxylase, 112-113
Acetyl-CoA/CoA-SH ratio, 48
Actin, 134, 153, 222, 236, 238, 239
Acyl-CoA binding protein (ACBP), 111
Acyl-L-carnitine esters, 110-111
Adenine nucleotide degradation, 42, 150, 151, 157, 227, 229
Adenosine, 151, 162, 239
Adenosine deaminase, 155
Adenosine 5'-diphosphate (ADP), 2, 29, 30, 31-32, 44, 45, 46, 140, 164, 165, 191, 193, 196, 239
Adenosine 5'-monophosphate (AMP), 2, 28, 29, 30, 31-32, 44, 45, 46, 48, 101, 165, 193, 239
Adenylate cyclase, 101, 102, 103
Adenylate kinase (AK), 2, 147, 212
Adenylosuccinate, 153, 156
Adenylosuccinate lyase (AL), 146-147, 153, 154, 155, 156, 165
Adenylosuccinate synthetase (AS), 146-147, 153, 154, 156
Adipocytes, 100, 103-104, 105, 107, 109, 115
Adipose tissue lipolysis, 48, 49, 52, 88-89, 99-104, 121, 198
ADP. See Adenosine 5'-diphosphate (ADP)
Adrenal medullary hypertrophy, 200
Adrenocorticotropic hormone, 100, 196
Aerobic metabolism, and anaerobic capacity, 12-13
Alanine, 87, 88, 131, 137, 141, 143, 144, 146, 154, 159, 163-164, 167
Alanine aminotransferase, 166
Alanine transaminase, 163-164
Albumin, 104-105, 106, 107, 111, 121
α-adrenergic blockade, 49, 53, 84, 100-102, 103
Amino acids
  effect of endurance training on, 191
  hepatic metabolism of, 86-88, 91

oxidation of, 141-143
skeletal muscle metabolism of, 131, 176
Amino metabolism, 143-146
Ammonia (NH₃)
  central and peripheral effects of, 160-164
  impact on trained muscle, 165-166
  production of, 88, 131, 132, 137-138, 143-146, 147, 148, 154, 156, 158-159, 160, 165-166, 167, 213
  as a proton buffer, 150, 151
Ammonium ions, 44, 132, 144, 150, 151-153
AMP. See Adenosine 5'-monophosphate (AMP)
AMP deaminase (AMPD), 145, 146-147, 148-153, 156, 157, 159, 164, 165, 213
Anaerobic capacity
  effects of sprint training on, 20-22, 33
  estimates of, 10-13
Anaerobic metabolism
  activation of AMPD fueled by, 151
  activation of anaerobic pathways, 3-5
  amount of total ATP provision, 3, 8
  anaerobic energy from glycogenolysis/ glycolysis, 2, 3, 4-5, 7-8, 18, 19, 25-32
  capacity for anaerobic ATP provision, 5, 8-13
  capacity of skeletal muscle to provide anaerobic ATP, 8-10
  effects of sprint training on, 20-22
  estimating anaerobic capacity, 10-13
  in human skeletal muscle fiber types, 13-17
  during intermittent high-intensity exercise, 17-20
  need for, 1-2
  of phosphocreatine, 2-4, 5, 7-8, 12-13, 22-25
  rates of anaerobic ATP provision, 5-8
  "serial mobilization" theory of, 4
  sources of anaerobic ATP, 2-3
Animal models of metabolism, 178. See also Cats; Dogs; Frogs; Horses; Mice; Rabbits; Rats; Sheep
Arteriovenous (AV) glucose difference, 49
Asparagine, 159
Aspartate, 137, 141, 147, 153, 154, 164, 166
Aspartate transaminase, 164

ATP. *See* 5'-adenosine triphosphate (ATP)
ATP/ADP ratio, maintenance of, 150

B

BCAA. *See* Branched chain amino acids (BCAA)
BCAA aminotransferase (BCAAT), 137, 138-139, 160
BCOA. *See* Branched chain oxo acids (BCOA)
BCOADH. *See* Branched-chain oxo acid dehydrogenase (BCOADH)
BCOADH kinase, 140
BCOADH phosphatase, 140
β-adrenergic blockade, 49, 53, 84, 100-102, 103, 109, 117, 118-119
β-hydroxyacyl-CoA dehydrogenase (HAD), 112
β-hydroxybutyrate, 88, 120, 121
β-oxidative enzymes, 112
Blood pH, 161
Brain, and glucoregulatory hormones, 79
Branched chain amino acids (BCAA), 132, 133, 137-143, 146, 158, 159-160, 162, 164, 167
Branched-chain ketoacid dehydrogenase (BCKADH), 191
Branched-chain oxo acid dehydrogenase (BCOADH), 140, 141, 142, 143, 145, 158, 159, 166
Branched chain oxo acids (BCOA), 137, 138, 140-143, 160, 166

C

Caffeine, 48, 223, 227, 237
Calcium (Ca), 45, 46, 51, 221-230, 234, 236, 237-238, 240, 245
Calmodulin, 29, 32, 45, 225
Carbohydrate metabolism
  and endurance, 41, 182-183
  impact of diet on, 56-57
  impact of endurance training on, 56, 177
  impact of environment on, 57
  influences on, 56-58
  and lactate metabolism, 55
  and muscle glucose uptake during exercise, 41, 49-55
  and muscle glycogen breakdown during exercise, 41, 42-49
  regulated by AMPD, 151
Carbohydrates (CHO)
  dietary supplementation of, 42, 47, 54
  and glycogen levels, 27
  impact on lipid metabolism, 113
  impact on skeletal muscle amino acid metabolism, 158-159
  importance of, 41
  oxidation of, 19
Carbon dioxide (CO_2), 142, 181-182, 241
Cardiac myocytes, 107
Carnitine acyltransferase I (CAT-I), 194-196

Carnitine palmitoyltransferase I (CPT-I), 112-113
Catecholamines, 53, 57, 83, 100, 103, 117, 121, 122, 198
Cats
  fatigue studies in, 241
  hepatic fuel metabolism in, 78
Chylomicrons, 119, 120
Citrate, 30, 44, 45, 48, 54, 55, 113, 163, 193-194
Citrate synthase (CS), 112, 183, 192
Coeliac ganglion blockade, 85, 89
Cori cycle, 188
Cortisol, 85, 196
Coupling proteins, 102
Creatine (Cr), 2, 23-25, 33, 213, 239
Creatine phosphate (PCr), 52, 212, 238
Creatine phosphate kinase (CPK), 2, 4
Creatine phosphokinase (CPK), 212, 243
Cross-sectional studies, 178-179, 185, 198, 200
Cycle ergometer, 17, 20, 28, 188, 189, 191
Cycling
  effect of endurance training on, 184, 188, 189, 191, 193-194
  effect on fatigue mechanisms, 236
  glycogen utilization during, 56
  impact on adipose tissue lipolysis, 100
  lipid metabolism during, 116, 117, 119, 120
  peripheral glucose uptake during, 78
Cyclo-oxygenase products, 162
Cytochalasin B binding, 51
Cytosol, 46

D

Deltoid muscles, 44
Detraining, effects of, 179, 196, 200
Diacylglycerol lipase, 103
Dibutyryl cyclic-AMP, 118
Diet, impact on carbohydrate metabolism, 56-57
Dietary protein, 136-137
Dietary supplements
  of amino acids, 160
  of carbohydrates, 42, 47, 54, 158
  of creatine, 23-25, 33
Dogs
  adipose tissue lipolysis in, 100, 102, 103, 105
  amino acid metabolism in, 87-88
  endurance training of, 188
  hepatic fuel metabolism in, 76, 77, 82, 83, 84, 89
  impact of ammonia on ventilation in, 160-161
  lipid metabolism in, 112, 115
  muscle carbohydrate utilization in, 42
  muscle glycogenolysis in, 49

E

Electrolytes, 213-214

Electromyography (EMG), 215, 222, 231-232, 236
Endogenous ATP, 2
Endogenous tissue protein, 136-137
Endurance
    and carbohydrate metabolism, 41, 113
    and hepatic fuel metabolism, 76, 77, 85
    and lipid metabolism, 99, 102
Endurance training
    experimental models of, 178-180
    impact on fatigue resistance, 245-247
    impact on FFA concentration and FFA uptake, 112
    impact on glycogen utilization, 56
    impact on lipid metabolism, 116, 117, 120
    impact on metabolism, 177-210
    impact on skeletal muscle amino acid metabolism, 165-166
    mechanism of affects of, 191-201
Environment, impact on carbohydrate metabolism, 57
Epidural anesthesia, 79-81
Epinephrine
    effect of endurance training on, 196, 198-200
    impact on anaerobic metabolism, 27-28
    impact on carbohydrate metabolism, 27-28, 43, 45, 46, 48-49, 53, 57
    impact on hepatic fuel metabolism, 83-84, 85, 89, 90
    impact on lipid metabolism, 109, 118
Essential amino acids (EAA), measurement of, 133
Ethanol, 76
Euglycemia, 74, 83
Exercise
    duration of, 56, 76, 99, 105, 111, 115, 116, 120, 121, 122, 135, 142, 144
    impact on adipose tissue lipolysis, 100
    influence on carbohydrate metabolism, 56
    intensity of, 42-43, 56, 76, 90, 99, 102, 111-112, 116, 122, 133, 135, 142, 144, 179-180, 186-187
    intermittent high-intensity, 17-20
    recovery from, 14, 16, 17-20, 23-25
    type of, 135

F
Fasting, 57, 76, 103, 113, 119, 120, 136
Fatigue
    causes of, 19-20, 211-256
    central versus peripheral, 161-164, 221-223
    and defense of ATP concentration, 212, 242-245
    definition of, 211
    effect of ammonia on, 161-164, 167
    effect of endurance training on, 245-247
    and energy metabolism, 241-242
    and glycogen depletion, 41
    mechanical manifestations of, 215-217

metabolically induced, 212-214
    metabolic determinants of, 211-256
    models of, 217-220
    myofibrillar determinants of, 222, 223, 236-241
    and sarcolemma-T tubule system, 214, 221, 230-236
    and sarcoplasmic reticulum, 214, 221, 222-230
    sites of, 221-223
    triggering mechanism for, 227
Fatty acid binding proteins
    cytoplasmic ($FABP_C$), 110-111, 122
    plasma membrane ($FABP_{PM}$), 107-108, 122
Fatty acyl-CoA esters, 110-111
Feedback mechanisms, for regulation of hepatic glucose output, 77-78
Feed-forward mechanisms, for regulation of hepatic glucose output, 78-82
Fibrinogen, 88
Fibronectin, 88
5'-adenosine triphosphate (ATP)
    anaerobic metabolism of, 1-39
    and carbohydrate metabolism, 44
    and fatigue, 212-215, 242-245
    in muscle fiber types, 13-17
    recovery (resynthesis) of, 14, 18, 41-42
5-amino-4-imidazolecarboxamide riboside (AICAr), 155
5-hydroxytryptamine, 162
5'-nucleotidase, 151
Flexor digitorum brevis (FDB) muscle, 113, 116
Free amino acid pools, 136-137, 143, 166-167
Free fatty acids (FFA)
    effect of endurance training on, 188-191
    and hepatic fuel metabolism, 47, 48, 54-55, 88, 89, 91
    and lipid metabolism, 99-115
    and skeletal muscle amino acid metabolism, 159, 192
Frogs (*Xenopus*), fatigue studies in, 237
Fructose 1,6-diphosphate (F-1,6-DP), 29, 30, 31, 32
Fructose 2,6-diphosphate (F-2,6-DP), 30, 31
Fructose 6-phosphate (F-6-P), 29, 30, 31, 32, 44, 45
Fumarate, 45, 141, 153, 156, 163, 164

G
GABA, 161
Gastrocnemius muscle, 192
Gender differences. *See* Men; Women
Glucagon, 57, 82-83, 100, 136, 196, 200-201
Glucocorticoids, 136
Glucose
    and carbohydrate metabolism, 41, 47, 49-55
    effect of endurance training on, 182-187, 193

Glucose *(continued)*
  impact on lipid metabolism, 104, 112-113, 121
Glucose 1,6-biphosphate (G-1,6-P$_2$), 44, 45
Glucose 1,6-diphosphate (G-1,6-DP), 30, 31
Glucose-fatty acid cycle, 54-55
Glucose-6-phosphate (G-6-P), 26, 48, 50, 53, 54, 55, 193-194
Glutamate, 137-138, 141, 144, 154, 161, 163-164, 167
Glutamate dehydrogenase (GDH), 138, 139-140, 145, 164, 166
Glutaminase, 145
Glutamine, 42, 87, 131, 143, 144, 145, 146, 154, 160, 161, 166, 167
Glutamine synthase, 145, 161, 166
Glycerol
  and hepatic fuel metabolism, 88, 89, 91
  and lipid metabolism, 100, 102, 103, 104, 118
Glycerol kinase, 100, 105
Glycine, 159
Glycogen
  anaerobic metabolism of, 2, 3, 4-5, 7-8, 18, 19, 25-32
  and carbohydrate metabolism, 41, 42-49
  effect of endurance training on, 182-187, 246
  in muscle fiber types, 13-17
  recovery of, 19
  and skeletal muscle amino acid metabolism, 158, 159, 160, 164
Glycogen-glucose 1-phosphate (G-1-P), 26
Glycogen loading, 41
Glycogen phosphorylase (PHOS), 26-29, 33, 42, 44, 45-46, 48-49, 53
Glycogen synthase, 45
Growth hormone, 85, 100, 136, 196

H
Hadacidin, 155, 156, 157
Heat stress, 57
Hepatic amino acid metabolism, 86-88
Hepatic fuel metabolism
  from glycogenolysis and gluconeogenesis, 75-85, 131, 198
  and hepatic uptake from gluconeogenic precursors, 86-89
Hepatocytes, 107
Heptic glycogenolysis, 49
Hexokinase, 44, 50, 54, 193
Hexose biphosphates, 44, 45
Hexose monophosphates, 44
Hormones
  effect of endurance training on, 189, 197-201
  regulation of carbohydrate metabolism by, 198
  regulation of hepatic glucose output by, 82-83, 85, 90
  regulation of lipid metabolism by, 100-104, 109-110, 118-119, 121, 198
  regulation of muscle glucose uptake by, 52-53
  regulation of muscle glycogenolysis with, 48-49
Hormone-sensitive triacylglycerol lipase (HSL) system, 103-104, 118, 121
Horses, fatigue studies in, 244
Hydrogen ions (H$^+$), 28, 29, 31-32, 33, 44, 45, 140, 145, 149, 151, 213, 214, 229, 238, 239, 241, 244, 246
Hydroxyproline, 159
Hypercapnia, 199
Hyperglycemia, 104
Hyperinsulinemia, 48, 52, 103
Hyperoxic gas, 152
Hypoglycemia, 41, 73, 199, 200
Hypoinsulinemia, 103
Hypothalmus, 79
Hypoxanthine, 151
Hypoxia, 51-52, 55, 57, 83

I
Immunohistochemistry, 51
Indirect calorimetry, 177, 181, 185
Inosine, 151, 239
Inosine monophosphate (IMP)
  accumulation of, 41, 42, 45, 46
  effect on fatigue, 239
  production of, 2, 151, 156, 164, 165-166, 213
  reamination of, 154-155
  regulation of phosphorylase *b* by, 29, 152-153
Insulin
  effect of endurance training on, 196, 198, 200-201
  impact on carbohydrate metabolism, 49, 52-53, 57
  impact on hepatic fuel metabolism, 82-83, 88, 90
  impact on lipid metabolism, 101, 102-103, 104, 109, 113, 118-119, 121, 122
  impact on tryptophan uptake, 162
  regulation of protein synthesis by, 136
Integrated electromyography (IEMG), 222, 231, 232-233
Intestinal hormones, 100
Intracellular metabolism, 111-115, 122
Intralipid, 119, 159
Intramuscular triacylglycerol (TG) metabolism, 115-119
In vitro studies, modeling from, 218, 220
In vivo studies, modeling from, 219-220
Isoforms GLUT1 and GLUT4, 51, 52
Isokinetic cycle sprinting, 17-18, 19-20
Isoleucine, 132, 133, 141. *See also* Branched chain amino acids (BCAA)
Isometric activity, modeling of, 215
Isoproterenol, 53, 118-119
Isozymes, 148

K

Ketogenesis, 75, 88-89, 91
Ketones
    ketone bodies metabolism, 120-121, 122, 192
    and skeletal muscle amino acid metabolism, 159
Krebs cycle, 181
Krebs cycle enzymes, 112
Krebs cycle intermediates (KCI), 113

L

Lactate
    accumulation of, 19-20
    anaerobic metabolism of, 3, 4-5
    effect of endurance training on, 187-188
    effect on fatigue, 239, 244, 246
    escaped into the blood, 5, 7, 8, 10, 44
    and hepatic fuel metabolism, 89
    impact on lipid metabolism, 105
    metabolism of, 42, 55, 187-188
    and skeletal muscle amino acid metabolism, 152, 162
Lactate shuttle hypothesis, 55
Lactic acid, 162, 246
Leucine, 132, 133, 136, 137, 140, 141, 142, 158-160, 166, 191. *See also* Branched chain amino acids (BCAA)
Lipid metabolism
    effect of endurance training on, 56, 177, 189-190, 193-194
    intramuscular triacylglycerol metabolism, 115-119
    ketone bodies metabolism, 120-121
    and maximal oxygen uptake (VO$_2$ max), 42
    plasma free fatty acid (FFA) metabolism, 99-115
    plasma triacylglycerol metabolism, 119-120
Lipoprotein lipase (LPL), 118, 120, 122
Liver
    and amino acid metabolism, 160
    glycogenesis and gluconeogenesis in, 42, 73-85
    protein synthesis in, 133, 140
Liver nerves, 83, 84-85, 90
Longitudinal studies, 178-179, 180, 185, 198, 200
Longitudinal tubules (LT), 225, 226, 228, 230
Lysine, 159

M

Malate, 45, 113, 163
Malonyl-CoA, 112-113, 122, 194-196
Mannoheptulose, 82
Marathon runners, 162
Maximal accumulated O$_2$ deficit, 11-12, 32-33
Maximal oxygen uptake (VO$_2$ max), 5, 17-18, 22, 42, 43, 179-180
Maximal voluntary contraction (MVC), 7, 8, 222, 241, 244

McArdle's disease, 42, 78, 158, 160, 163
Men
    carbohydrate metabolism of, 57-58
    creatine supplementation in, 24
Mercaptopicolinic acid, 76
Methionine, 159
Methylxanthines, 223
Mice, fatigue studies in, 237
Michaelis-Menten saturation kinetics, 51
Microdialysis probe, 100
Monoacylglycerol lipase, 103
Motor unit action potentials (MUAP), 231
Motor units, 216, 220
Muscle fatigue. *See* Fatigue
Muscle pain, 162
Muscles
    capacity to provide anaerobic ATP, 8-10, 13-17
    contractile and noncontractile proteins in, 134
    fast-twitch glycolytic (FG) fibers, 111, 116, 119, 120, 246
    fast-twitch oxidative glycolytic (FOG) fibers, 111, 116, 119, 120, 246
    fast-twitch red gastrocnemius (RG) fibers, 149
    fast-twitch versus slow-twitch, 111, 116, 119, 120, 145, 148, 226, 241, 245, 246
    fast-twitch white gastrocnemius (WG) fibers, 149
    mechanics of, 215-217
    pH of, 46, 118, 214, 227, 229, 230, 239, 241-242, 246
    respiratory capacity of, 192-196, 201
    slow-twitch oxidative (SO) fibers, 111, 116, 119, 120, 246
    slow-twitch red soleus (SOL) fibers, 149
    type I versus type II fibers, 13-17, 22, 33, 43, 46, 115, 152, 183, 194
Muscle wisdom, 232
Myofibrillar determinants of fatigue, 222, 223, 236-241
Myophosphorylase deficiency, 78, 158
Myosin, 134, 148, 149-150, 153, 222, 236, 238, 239, 245

N

Neuromuscular fatigue. *See* Fatigue
Nitrogen metabolism, 88, 145-146
Nociceptors, 162
Norepinephrine, 83, 197, 198-200
Normoxia, 83
Nuclear magnetic resonance (NMR), 22, 220, 241-242

O

Oleate, 54, 55, 112, 114, 188
Oleic acid, 88, 113
Ornithine, 159
Orthophosphate, 150
Oxaloacetate, 137, 163

Oxygen (O₂)
and anaerobic metabolism, 1
and lactate production, 55
maximal accumulated O₂ deficit, 11-12, 32-33
maximal oxygen uptake (VO₂ max), 5, 17-18, 22, 42, 43, 179-180

P

Palmitate, 55, 107-108, 113, 188
Palmitoyl CoA, 112
Pancreatic hormones, 85
Parathyroid hormone, 100
PCr. *See* Phosphocreatine (PCr)
Peptide mapping studies, 103
Percutaneous needle biopsy technique, 41
pH
of blood, 161
of muscles, 46, 118, 214, 227, 229, 230, 239, 241-242, 246
Phentolamine, 101-102
Phenylalanine, 134
Phlorizin, 78
Phosphatase, 46
Phosphate, inorganic (Pᵢ), 2, 26, 27, 29, 30, 31-32, 46, 153, 162, 193, 213, 229, 238, 241, 243, 246
Phosphocreatine (PCr)
anaerobic metabolism of, 2-4, 5, 7-8, 12-13, 22-25
and muscle fatigue, 243
in muscle fiber types, 13-17
recovery of, 14, 18, 23-25
in resting muscle, 22-23
in skeletal muscle amino acid metabolism, 164
Phosphodiesterase, 102, 104, 109
Phosphoenolpyruvate, 30, 141, 164
Phosphofructokinase (PFK), 26, 29-32, 33, 44-45, 48, 54, 150, 151-153, 193-194, 244
Phosphorylase (PHOS). *See* Glycogen phosphorylase (PHOS)
Phosphorylase *b* (PHOS *b*), 29, 152-153
Phosphorylase kinase, 45, 46, 48
Pituitary hormones, 100
Plantaris muscle, 145, 240
Plasma triacylglycerol (TG) metabolism, 119-120
Potassium (K⁺), 230, 233-236, 242
Proline, 159
Propranolol, 101-102, 119
Prostaglandins, 162
Protein kinase, 102, 103, 104
Protein kinase C, 51
Protein synthesis and degradation, 132-136
Purine nucleotide cycle (PNC), 132, 146-157, 159, 166, 213
Pyruvate, 41, 42, 45, 141, 144, 163-164, 187-188, 192

Q

Quadriceps femoris muscle, 116
Quadriceps muscles, 10

R

Rabbits
fatigue studies in, 229, 235
skeletal muscle amino acid metabolism in, 140, 148
Radioactivity, 115
Rats
adipose tissue lipolysis in, 100, 101, 103-104
blood glucose levels in, 47
carbohydrate metabolism in, 43
effect of epinephrine on, 53
endurance training of, 165, 166, 178, 183, 188, 191, 192, 193, 200
fasting of, 57
fatigue studies in, 240
free fatty acid levels in, 48
hepatic fuel metabolism in, 73, 75, 76, 77, 78, 79, 82
hormone regulation in, 48-49, 83-84, 100
insulin in, 52
lipid metabolism in, 107-108, 111, 113, 116, 118, 119, 120
liver nerves in, 85
muscle glucose uptake in, 53, 54, 55
muscle glycogenolysis in, 28
purine nucleotide cycle in, 147-148, 155
skeletal muscle amino acid metabolism in, 145, 149, 157, 165, 166
Vₘₐₓ of glucose transport in, 51
Respiration. *See* Ventilation
Respiratory exchange ratio (RER), 111, 115, 180-182, 187
Respiratory quotient (RQ), 180-182, 187
Running
and creatine supplementation, 25
and fatigue, 240
glycogen utilization during, 56
lipid metabolism during, 112, 116, 120
peripheral glucose uptake during, 78
protein synthesis and degradation during, 133, 134
skeletal muscle amino acid metabolism during, 162
Ryanodine, 226

S

Sarcolemma and T tubule system, 214, 221, 230-236
Sarcoplasmic reticulum (SR) complex, 20, 29, 46, 51, 214, 221, 222-230, 237, 245
Serine, 159
Serotonin, 162
Sheep, hepatic fuel metabolism in, 82
Skeletal muscle metabolism of amino acids
amino acid metabolism in muscle, 136-143
amino metabolism in muscle, 143-146

central and peripheral effects of ammonia, 160-164
impact of endurance training on, 165-166
influence of other substrates on, 157-160
protein synthesis and degradation, 132-136
purine nucleotide cycle, 132, 146-157
Skiing, lipid metabolism during, 120
Sleep, hepatic fuel metabolism during, 81-82
Somatostatin, 82, 85
Splanchnic glucose, 73-74, 76, 78
Sprinting, sustaining of, 152
Sprint training
effect on ammonia production, 165
effect on anaerobic capacity, 20-22, 33
effect on fatigue mechanisms, 236
Succinate dehydrogenase (SDH), 112, 196
Succinyl-CoA, 141
Sweating, 146
Swimming
effect of endurance training on, 200
lipid metabolism during, 116, 119
Sympathoadrenergic activity, 83-85

T
Terminal cisternae (TC), 225, 226, 231
Tetraplegic subjects, hepatic fuel metabolism in, 79
3-methylhistidine (3-MH), 134, 135
3-O-methyl glucose, 55
3-phosphoglycerate, 30
Thromboxanes, 162
Thyroid-stimulating hormone, 100
Tibialis anterior muscle, 25, 140, 237
Transverse tubular system (T tubules), 214, 221, 225, 230-236
Triacylglycerol (TG) metabolism
intramuscular, 115-119, 122
plasma, 119-120, 122
Triacylglycerols (TG), plasma and intramuscular, 99, 103-104, 111, 113-114, 115-120, 122

Tricarboxylic acid (TCA) cycle intermediates, 41, 45, 141, 154, 156-157, 163, 164, 167, 194
Triceps brachii muscle, 20
Triglyceride-fatty acid cycling, 105
Triglycerides, 48, 136, 188-191
Tropomyosin, 236
Troponin, 236
Troponin C, 45, 223, 224
Tryptophan, 162
Turbocurarine, 79
2-oxoglutarate, 137, 164
2-phosphoglycerate, 30
Tyrosine, 133, 134
Tyrosine kinase, 52

U
Urea formation, 88, 91, 145-146

V
Vagotomy, 85
Valine, 132, 133, 141. See also Branched chain amino acids (BCAA)
Vastus lateralis (VL) muscle, 5, 25, 44, 116, 183
Ventilation, effect of ammonia on, 160-161
Very low density lipoproteins (VLDL), 119, 120, 190
VO₂ max. See Maximal oxygen uptake (VO₂ max)

W
Western blot analysis, 51
Whole-body anaerobic capacity, measurement of, 11, 33
Whole-body glucose turnover, 73
Whole-body protein synthesis rates, 133
Wingate cycling test, 13
Women
carbohydrate metabolism of, 57-58
total creatine (TCr) in, 24
Wrestlers, endurance training of, 188

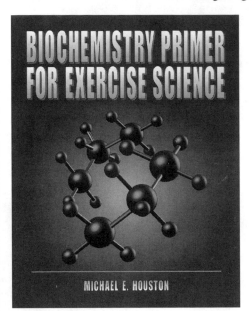